VIRAL MOTHERS

D0877858

LI

Viral Mothers

Breastfeeding in the Age of HIV/AIDS

Bernice L. Hausman

The University of Michigan Press • *Ann Arbor*

Copyright © 2011 by Bernice L. Hausman
All rights reserved
Published in the United States of America by
The University of Michigan Press
Manufactured in the United States of America
⊗ Printed on acid-free paper

2014   2013   2012   2011   4   3   2   1

A CIP catalog record for this book is available from the British Library.

Library of Congress Cataloging-in-Publication Data

Hausman, Bernice L.
    Viral mothers : breastfeeding in the age of HIV/AIDS / Bernice L.
Hausman.
        p.   cm.
    Includes bibliographical references and index.
    ISBN 978-0-472-07131-9 (cloth : alk. paper) — ISBN 978-0-472-
05131-1 (pbk. : alk. paper)
    1. Breastfeeding—Social aspects.   2. Breastfeeding—Health
aspects.   3. Breast milk—Contamination.   4. Mother and child.
I. Title.

RJ216.H284   2010
649'.33—dc22   2010021767

For my family

Acknowledgments

IN THESE BRIEF PAGES, I hope to remember everyone who has contributed to this project, either by supporting me directly or by helping me to understand more fully what I am trying to say.

Jerry Niles, former dean of Virginia Tech's College of Liberal Arts and Human Sciences, funded my trip to the International AIDS Conference in 2006. Two department chairs, Lucinda Roy and Carolyn Rude, graciously understood when I needed to sequester time for research and writing. I conducted primary research at the University of Wisconsin College of Medicine, in Madison, and the University of Kansas School of Medicine, in Kansas City. My research in Kansas City included work on tuberculosis at the Clendening History of Medicine Library and Museum, where the staff was very helpful in finding sources for me. In fall 2003 Virginia Tech's International Supplemental Travel Grant provided funding for me to conduct research at the Welcome Library in London, as part of a conference trip to Manchester University. I also did research at Penn State University Medical College in Hershey in summer 2002 while I attended a National Endowment for the Humanities Summer Institute on Medicine, Literature, and Culture directed by Susan Squier and Anne Hunsaker Hawkins. That experience gave me some initial insight into the project, and I thank the participants and the directors for their help in getting me started. A semester's leave from teaching during spring 2009, approved by Virginia Tech provost Mark MacNamee, allowed me to complete revisions to the manuscript.

Audiences around the continent have been instrumental in helping me develop my arguments. I presented papers from the *Viral Mothers* project at conferences of the Society for Literature and Science, the American Society for Bioethics and the Humanities, the Association for Research on Mothering, the Modern Language Association, the International Society for the Study of Narrative Literature, the Southeastern Women's Studies Association, the Berkshire Conference on the History of Women, the Rhetoric Society of America, and the Cultural Studies Association. I also presented material from the book at the Breastfeeding and Feminism Symposium at the University of North Carolina, Chapel Hill; the Gender, HIV, and Child Survival conference at York University, Toronto; and the Feminism(s) and Rhetoric(s) conference in Little Rock, Arkansas. In addition, I spoke about *Viral Mothers* at the annual convention of the International Lactation Consultant Association; at a benefit conference for the Bay Area Lactation Consultants in Oakland, California; at an annual Perinatal Conference in Roanoke, Virginia; before an audience of women's studies students and faculty at Appalachian State University in Boone, North Carolina; and to various faculty and graduate students at Virginia Tech. I made a poster of the project for the Deans' Forum on Infectious Diseases at Virginia Tech, where the idea of "cultural studies" was a bit confusing for scientists more familiar with "culture media" used to grow cells. Emily Satterwhite, Becky Taylor, and Phil Olson took the time to read and comment on an early version of the denialism chapters, at an ASPECT working papers session. All of these opportunities have prompted fascinating discussions, and the questions generated by audience members have challenged me to greater clarity and depth in my writing.

There are many individuals who made comments that led to improvements in the book. Penny Van Esterik, Paige Hall Smith, Jackie Wolf, the late Mary Rose Tully, and Miriam Labbok constitute the most knowledgeable group of breastfeeding experts I could hope for. Each has responded to specific questions when I needed direct answers fast, and together they support my interdisciplinary efforts with their own disciplinary expertise. Penny especially has been a model for me of how to do feminist research on breastfeeding that is also a form of breastfeeding advocacy. Liew Mun Tip, formerly from the World Alliance for Breastfeeding Advocacy, shared a room with me at the AIDS conference in Toronto and offered her thoughts on my project when we both weren't exhausted and sleeping. Gretchen Michlitsch, Lissa Knudsen, and Amy Koerber presented with me at the Feminism(s) and Rhetoric(s) conference, and Gretchen, Edith Frampton, and Lynn Makau made up a panel I chaired at the 2006 Breastfeeding and Feminism symposium at Greensboro. They are the next generation of biocultural breastfeeding scholars.

Gary Downey suggested that I needed to develop connections across and between the figures that I analyze. He also patiently listened to me discuss my ideas about risk and culture and helped me think more clearly about this approach. Pam Morrison alerted me to the article on Zambia discussed in chapter 13, and her enthusiasm about my brief article on choice that was published in the *International Breastfeeding Journal* motivated me to write the final chapter of the book. Craig Brookins and Sylvain Boko chose me as the Virginia Tech representative on the ACC trip to Africa in June 2007, an opportunity of a lifetime. Steven Epstein responded graciously to an emergency request for information. The anonymous readers for the University of Michigan Press gave me invaluable advice for revision.

I share almost all of my good ideas, and a number of my bad ones, with Nancy Cervetti, who never fails to support my every endeavor and takes me shopping when I go to visit her. Gena Chandler makes life on the second floor of Shanks Hall livable, as does Mary Denson. Both are forced to listen to me when I need a sounding board and my usual victims are not available; neither has ever made me feel annoying or intrusive, although I know that I can be both. Brad Lewis has influenced me more than he realizes, as his clear and humble prose offers me models to think with that are exactly what I need all the time. Jonathan Metzl snuck me into the program for the Against Health conference at the University of Michigan, where I learned some important things and met Susan Kippax of the National Centre in HIV Social Research of Australia. Fiona Giles sends me information and insight across the Pacific, keeping me in touch with the wilder side of breastfeeding research. Marian Mollin became a Hokie with me through the nightmare of April 16 and is my touchstone for radical attitudes.

Judy Grady arranges all of my conference and research travel, making that part of my life much easier than it would be otherwise. The rest of the staff in the English department—Dee Hezel, Denise Royal, Tammy Shepherd, and Stephanie Snyder—have all supported some aspect of this project, either by making copies, sending faxes, or just listening to me complain. Staff members at the interlibrary loan office of the Carol Newman Library were gracious and helpful with all of my numerous requests. Connie Stovall purchased a number of books necessary for my research.

I had the pleasure of working with four fantastic graduate assistants for different parts of this project. Heather Switzer is the first graduate student I have formally advised as dissertation chair, and she has contributed enormously to the success of *Viral Mothers*. She read the entire first draft of the manuscript, gave me indispensable comments, and continues to offer important advice about all aspects of the project. She is my Africa expert, teaching me almost everything I know about African women's lives and the ways in which we white Americans might do research concerning Africa with integrity. The Center for the Study of Rhetoric in Society in the English Department at Virginia Tech provided funds for Heather to conduct library and field research for me. Jongmin Lee chased down articles over one summer and kept tabs on developing news headlines. Jin You also did a lot of library legwork, but her main contribution was helping me refine my arguments and clarify their theoretical coherence. She read almost every chapter of the revised manuscript before it was sent to the second set of readers. As I went through her notes one last time, I was amazed at the insight and appropriateness of her spare, pointed comments. Brian Gogan designed the poster for the Deans' Forum on Infectious Diseases. He also read and commented on the methodology discussion that appears in the introduction. His recommendation of Wayne Booth's book *The Rhetoric of Rhetoric* could not have come at a better time, and my discussion of rhetoric and ideology is greatly improved as a result of his input.

My most consistent supporters for this project were the women in my writing group: Mitzi Vernon, Kathy Jones, Kelly Belanger, and Ann LaBerge. What an amazing experience this has been. We were so busy that we read less of each other's work than we would like, but being accountable to each other kept us on track in the midst of our otherwise hectic schedules. When I needed criticism, I knew I could count on these women for straight responses. In the last few weeks of preparing the second draft, their brief comments on just a few sections helped me to see how reorganizing the introductory chapters of the book would solve a number of conceptual and structural problems that I had not been able to figure out on my own. Our motto was "It is our world and we decide."

My parents send me original clippings of every article on breastfeeding or infant formula published in the *New York Times* and the *Wall Street Journal,* and my father, especially, does not complain when I criticize medicine. They are my original, and most loyal, supporters. My children, Rachel and Samuel, will be teenagers when this book is published; they were eight and six when I began. While they usually forbid me to talk about the subject of my research when I present to their classes on "career day," they think it's cool to have a mom who writes books. I think it's cool to have kids who understand when I need to be left alone, who cheerfully put up with frozen waffles for dinner, and with whom I can intelligently converse about my writing. Clair makes my writing life possible, primarily by loving me, but also by answering my editing questions and letting me talk through the impossible conceptual tangles that I get myself into. This book is dedicated to my family, whose members sustain me, love me, and believe in me in ways that will always take my breath away.

Portions of the chapters "MTCT" and "Viral Mothers" were published previously in "Contamination and Contagion: Environmental Toxins, HIV/AIDS, and the Problem of the Maternal Body," *Hypatia* 21, no. 1 (Winter 2006): 137–56.

Portions of "Informed Choice" were published previously in "Women's Liberation and the Rhetoric of 'Choice' in Infant Feeding Debates," *International Breastfeeding Journal* (2008), http://www.internationalbreastfeedingjournal.com/content/ 3/1/10.

Portions of "West Nile Virus" were published previously in Bernice L. Hausman, "Risky Business: Framing Childbirth in Hospital Settings," *Journal of Medical Humanities* 26, no. 1 (Spring 2005): 23–38, and are published here with the kind permission of Springer Science and Business Media.

A different version of "West Nile Virus" is being published as "Risk and Culture Revisited: Breastfeeding and the 2002 West Nile Virus Scare in the United States," in *Giving Breast Milk: Body Ethics and Contemporary Breastfeeding Practice,* edited by Rhonda Shaw and Alison Bartlett (York, ON: Demeter Press, 2010), and is published here with permission.

The three figures in the book have been reproduced from other sources.

Figure 1: Breastfeeding and alcohol consumption chart printed with permission from *The Complete Guide to Everyday Risks in Pregnancy and Breastfeeding,* by Gideon Koren, MD, FRCP (C), 206. Copyright Gideon Koren, 2004. Published by Robert Rose Inc.

Figure 2: Photo accompanying "Bottled Up: As Unicef Battles Baby-Formula Makers, African Infants Sicken," by Alix M. Freedman and Steve Stecklow, *Wall Street Journal,* December 5, 2000, A18. Reprinted courtesy of UNAIDS.

Figure 3: Cover photo of Partners In Health, *2004 Annual Report,* Boston: Partners In Health, 2005. Reprinted with permission.

Contents

CHAPTER 1

Introduction

I HAVE WRITTEN *Viral Mothers* as an exploration of anxieties about breastfeeding and contamination. I began this research thinking to focus solely on HIV/AIDS[1] and maternal transmission of the virus through breastfeeding, but I found other, somewhat similar, preoccupations salient in local and global conversations about mothers. These anxieties, as I came to think of them, are manifested in dominant ideological formations, revealed in public health approaches to maternal behavior, and realized in mothers' own practices. They seem most pervasive in wealthy countries, where biomedical research and health-conscious advice guide maternal behaviors, but are also evident in public health debates about women who live in the poverty environments of the global south. In modern life, breastfeeding is a practice that seems to sharpen cultural ambivalence about mothers and their bodies.

In *Viral Mothers,* I examine why the maternal body is a focus of intense concern in modernity, or how modernity causes us to focus on the maternal body as a problem in particular ways. I am not claiming that the focus on mothers' bodies is a new problem. Rather, I am arguing that modernity poses particular problems for mothers' bodies *and* that mothers' bodies pose problems within and for modernity. Maternal bodies seem to constitute a special case that demonstrates and exemplifies contemporary obsessions with contagion and contamination as particularly modern risks.

Breastfeeding has always been a focus of concern in modern social formations. In Enlightenment France, Jean-Jacques Rousseau discussed the shaping of citizens that occurred initially at the maternal breast. According to philosopher Rebecca Kukla, "Even Rousseau's critics, such as Mary Wollstonecraft, did not dare to call into question the Rousseauian tenet that nursing is a civic duty crucial to the production of sympathetic and well-ordered citizens."[2] Yet advancing industrialization allowed for the development of proprietary infant foods in the nineteenth century, calling into question women's unique contribution to the nutrition and development of human offspring. The impact of globalization with respect to foods to replace breast milk was first publicly noted by physician Cicely Williams in 1939 in her famous "Milk and Murder" speech but was realized most fully in the Nestlé boycott of the 1970s and 1980s.[3] Most recently, the crisis of mother-to-child transmission of human immunodeficiency virus (HIV) through breastfeeding has initiated a new round of debates about infant feeding in the resource-poor contexts of the global south. It is clear that the anticipated achievements of 1980s breastfeeding activism—the preservation of breastfeeding as the dominant mode of infant feeding around the world, aided by the passage of international codes, policy guidelines, and other agreements—have been severely challenged by HIV/AIDS.

The medical community has known since the late 1980s that HIV is passed through breast milk from infected mothers to their babies. In highly industrialized countries, HIV-positive mothers are advised not to breastfeed their babies. Because replacement feeding is considered ordinary in these contexts, this public health protocol receives little attention. But breastfeeding has continued to be a predominant and culturally normative practice in poor countries. In addition, until the 1990s breastfeeding was thought to be a partial solution to problems of infant health and welfare in resource-poor contexts. Now, in areas of high rates of HIV infection and high infant mortality, decisions concerning infant feeding are terribly conflicted. As a result, breastfeeding receives significant attention in the medical literature concerning AIDS in poor countries, and there has been an enormous shift in international public health conversations concerning infant formula manufacturers and replacement feeding.

As a result, mother-to-child transmission of HIV (MTCT) garners tremendous attention from breastfeeding advocates. The global community of breastfeeding supporters is worried about what it perceives to be a renewed zeal to introduce breast milk substitutes in areas beset by high HIV-prevalence rates. In the minds of advocates, such prevention efforts to end MTCT reveal a lack of understanding of the fundamental health contributions of breastfeeding in these contexts. They worry that AIDS researchers and policymakers will make changes to infant feeding policies to stop transmission of the virus while not attending to overall infant morbidity and mortality, which breastfeeding advocates think will increase if breastfeeding rates decrease in the global south.[4]

AIDS itself is a quintessential illness of modernity. An incurable, fatal, slow-acting virus, it has challenged advanced biomedical research and public health systems with its biological, epidemiological, and social complexity, demonstrating that modern medical institutions have not conquered or tamed microbes and their devastating potential. It emerged in equatorial west Africa in the late 1950s, with decolonization and the momentous transformations in the politics, cultural life, and economic and social organization of African countries. Following labor migration routes in Africa, HIV/AIDS is an illness dependent on an imperialist history and the structured inequities of the colonial labor systems established in the late nineteenth century and the first half of the twentieth. Yet the establishment and spread of HIV/AIDS have also traced the dislocations and political unevenness of the postcolonial period.[5] The epidemiology of HIV/AIDS differs around the world, testifying to the divisions that characterize modern global society.

The transmission of HIV through breastfeeding is a medical and public health issue that touches on and augments contemporary concerns about bodies, germs, and the environment. These concerns affect all people around the globe as we struggle with the meanings of health, risk, and embodiment in modernity. *Viral Mothers* addresses and explores current constructions of mothers in order to understand the dense cultural meanings evoked by postnatal transmission of HIV. In so doing, the book pays special attention to fears of contamination and contagion that emerge as consequences of a medicalizing modernity.

Ideology and Rhetoric

Viral Mothers is a book about representations—the discourses, rhetoric, and images that contribute to and emerge from public debates about mother-to-child transmission of HIV through breastfeeding. It therefore addresses the representational staging of an argument about maternity. Because of this, the book itself is not an argument about real women, but a set of critical commentaries concerning conflicting ideas about motherhood, particularly the embodied practice of breastfeeding. These ideas struggle to resolve the problem of the maternal body within modernity. *Viral Mothers*

traces and analyzes this struggle over ideas in the context of power relations, cultural forces and meanings, and everyday practices. As such, it is a
book primarily addressing ideologies and the controversies they engender.

Any wide-ranging critical study of ideology and its effects, especially
one that attempts a broadly sweeping analysis across continents and disciplinary domains, risks oversimplification. While the book is set up as a series of case study commentaries focusing on ideological configurations, my
interpretive gestures are synthetic, to demonstrate regularities across representations. It is my hope that whatever fine complexity is lost in this endeavor is made up for in the revelation of those representational similarities
that guide contemporary global thinking about mothers' bodies and their
potentially dangerous relation to fetuses and infants.

My own work is not ethnographic, although I have attended professional conferences in order to listen to the discourses about infant feeding
and HIV that are current and to engage, in a limited manner, the kind of
"visceral learning" cited by Emily Martin as a basis for anthropological research.[6] I am not trained in ethnography, so my efforts at participant observation are self-taught and less systematic than those of a professional anthropologist. I use my experiences of observation as ways into particular
nodal points of meaning that would otherwise be difficult to identify or analyze, but these experiences themselves never make up the main subject the
research itself focuses on.

My methodology involves identifying and analyzing pervasive and
dominant themes in contemporary discourses about infant feeding, maternity, and HIV. The problems that I am addressing in this book are generally
taken up by people and organizations devoted to *practical plans,* either direct research, the implementation of research findings, clinical practice, or
the development of public health guidelines. My project is to demonstrate
how language use matters in each of these contexts, how seemingly technocratic approaches depend on images, beliefs, and unseen cultural patterns
in order to make sense or be effective. The larger field within which this research finds a home is cultural studies, with a particular focus on rhetoric.

Rhetoric is an interdisciplinary field of study focused on persuasive discourse, in the form of language, visual imagery, or nonverbal behavior.
Rhetorical inquiry usually focuses on language use but also pays attention
to these other elements of meaning-making that contextualize language.
While lay understanding of the term *rhetoric* often suggests that it means

the purposefully manipulative use of language to gain devious ends, rhetoricians are usually more open and positive about the study of rhetoric. Wayne Booth, quoting Lloyd Bitzer, provides this as one among many definitions: "Rhetoric is a mode of altering reality, not by the direct application of energy to objects, but by the creation of discourse which changes reality through the mediation of thought and action."[7] Postmodern perspectives would alter that statement to emphasize the rhetorical construction, not rendering, of reality.

In cultural studies, the kind of persuasive discourse that I analyze goes by the name of *ideology. Ideology* is a name for forms of knowledge and meaning that shape people's direct experience and determine its significance. Ideological analysis exposes how particular kinds of meaning are naturalized and made normative in given cultural contexts. Such analysis asserts that the work of ideology overall is to obscure contradictory and problematic elements of material life from ordinary people in order to forestall their inquiry into, and resistance to, the status quo. Ideological analysis is not a democratic approach to knowledge. Ideological analysis presumes that most individuals do not have access to critical modes of thinking that will break through layers of mystification that circumscribe and define experience. Rather, this method assumes that dominant ideologies operate in the service of dominant groups, although individuals who serve these ideologies are largely unaware of their roles.

For Marxists, or quasi-Marxists like myself, ideology inheres in material practices. Ideas themselves are important as elements of culture, but it is through practices of daily life that ideologies are made real for people and become natural ways of being a person. Actions and habits that go without question thus are instances of the naturalization that ideology accomplishes. But studying ideology is largely conducted through the analysis of discourses available as text or speech. Because of this, the field of rhetoric is a significant arena for the study of ideology since rhetorical scholars examine persuasive language in concrete contexts of use, using various forms of documentary evidence. Rhetorical analysis is one method of critical thinking that can break through or uncover the mystification produced by ideologies, largely by focusing on the signifying activity that supports supposedly natural modes of being and thinking. Rhetorical study can demonstrate how cultural consensus is created, common sense comes into being, and norms of behavior are established and sustained. Semiotics, the study of sign systems, is a mode of rhetorical analysis that examines the representational apparatus of cultural meanings, especially advertising, mass media, and other discursive forms that dominate the public sphere.

There are advantages and constraints to the semiotic analysis of ideology. Let me first enumerate the constraints. Ideological analysis can be crude and stereotyping, even as it attempts to explode the stereotypes that can characterize ideological figurations. It is not fine-grained enough to address lived experience or the idiosyncrasies of individual lives. It can encourage a simplistic analysis that poses ideology against material reality, as if everyone's experiences are not forged through complex accommodations and resistances to dominant formations. It is not democratic, and suspects all belief systems of conformity to the status quo. It is skeptical rather than empathetic. The semiotic analysis of ideology can make it seem like individual people do not matter at all because they are understood to be pawns in the larger game of power being played out in the discursive contexts of culture. In addition, its evidence base can seem thin, because ideological analysis targets symptomatic, rather than representative, examples.

But analyzing dominant ideologies through the discursive systems of culture is a way of identifying and critiquing norms of behavior and belief that do not serve the interests of most people. In being a form of skeptical reading, the semiotic analysis of ideology helps us to see modes of being in the world as connected to interests that we did not even realize were operating in our lives. Ideology obscures from people the difficulty or unsustainability of the actual conditions of their existence or sometimes just the fact that those conditions are not given but constructed by and naturalized through particular discursive mechanisms. Its critique can reveal to us ways of moving forward and altering those conditions. Ideological analysis is founded on the belief that ideas, representations, and meanings matter to the material conditions of people's lives, and that direct critique of ideology's hold on perception and practice can effect individual and social transformation. Ideological analysis has, as its goal, not just understanding, but change.

Ideological analysis informs us of existing constraints on our own modes of thinking, discovery, and practical action, suggesting that such constraint always acts in the service of politics and power. In *Viral Mothers*, I want to show, in very specific terms, how mothers are disadvantaged by dominant ideologies about maternal embodiment and practice. I am less interested in how mothers imagine themselves than in those forces shaping their beliefs and experiences. My emphasis, then, is tilted toward the forces and away from the women themselves, toward understanding the myths and not women's responses to the myths. This is not because I do not care about women and their lives. My method results from my belief that individual experience is forged within ideological contexts that are determining and limit the kinds of freedoms available to individuals. Constraint—living within boundaries not of one's own making—is the common experience of most people's lives. Thus analysis of the constraining forces—the systems of ideas, practices, and meanings that constitute dominant ideologies—is one way of understanding human experience, albeit not by direct participation in people's lives or ethnographic encounters.

The focus on ideology has another significant effect on the analysis produced. *Viral Mothers* is not a book that will show us how to separate real concerns from imagined ones. Unveiling ideologies does not allow us access to a real or true level of experience beneath or beyond cultural constructions.[8] In this book I argue that valid concerns about mothers' bodies are always imagined and experienced through ideologies of maternity. Identifying the work of ideology does not do away with these concerns, nor reduce them to insignificance, but it does demonstrate the cultural importance of meaning systems disseminated by powerful institutions and evident in everyday practices and beliefs. Exposing ideological constructions allows us to imagine ways of resisting dominant modes of understanding and experience. Resistance is the first step in transforming cultural constraints toward more liberating alternatives.

Globalization

Most of the dominant ideologies I examine in this book emerge from the global north, in particular the United States, and often they are simply targeted back to inhabitants of the highly industrialized contexts that characterize the developed world. My own expertise is in cultural studies of the United States and its medical institutions and practices, with a focus on gender, sexuality, and maternity. But one purpose of this project, for me, has been to expand my understanding of how particular beliefs about mothers and their bodies influence physicians and policymakers all over the world. Because biomedicine has its roots in the cultures of the global north, figurations of maternity that guide medical thinking about mothers' bodies, illnesses, and risks emerge from those same contexts. Moreover, medical ideas about mothers from the global south are highly inflected by norms of maternal behavior forged in the global north. Just as American culture seeks global outlets as a way of marketing American goods and services, biomedicine transports cultural imperatives as it crosses borders and seeks to improve health outcomes around the world.[9]

The terminology to describe the divergence of human circumstance globally is fraught with political contestation. In the first sentence of the previous paragraph, I purposely used three sets of terms that often are used interchangeably to identify the world's wealthy nations: *developed, highly industrialized, global north*. Other terms include the *West* and *First World*. Terminology in use to identify the world's poorer nations includes *global south, Third World, non-West, underdeveloped*, or *developing*. In the body of this book, I have settled on *global north* and *global south* as names that designate levels of industrialization, wealth, and global economic power. Noting that "like all binaries . . . it is problematic if taken too seriously," philosopher Alison Jaggar describes her use of *global north* and *global south* as follows.

> The collapse of the Soviet bloc has made the older terminology of First, Second and Third Worlds inapplicable, and it is now often replaced by talk about the global North and the global South. Roughly, the "global North" refers to the world's highly industrialized and wealthy states, most of which are located in the northern hemisphere—though Australia and New Zealand are exceptions. The "global South" refers to poorer states that depend mostly on agriculture and extractive industries and whose manufacturing industry, if it exists, is likely to be foreign owned. . . . Northern states often have a history as colonizing nations, and Southern states often have been colonized.[10]

There are other reasons to jettison *Third World* and *developing*. The first/third distinction suggests a hierarchy of value, just as developed/developing does. That the global north sets the paradigm for development is not at issue, but the meaning of its power is. Indeed, one of the advantages of the global north/south terminology is the fact that as a distinction it does not map actual north/south geographies exactly but is meant to signify a distinction in power and wealth. The north/south distinction is one within the context of neoliberal globalization, not merely in relation to geographic positioning, as

Jaggar's description makes clear. Those who use the global north/south terminology are calling attention to critiques of development paradigms and the hierarchization of modernization implicit in official development institutions like the World Bank and the International Monetary Fund.

The West/non-West distinction is interesting to consider in this regard. Like global north/south, it suggests a geographical difference that is actually a political and economic difference. But its usefulness seems to have diminished, and its specificity is unclear: does West/non-West refer to Euro-America against the Eastern Bloc, or Euro-America against Asia? And all of the terms, I should point out, ignore differences *within* the totalities described: not all communities in the global north share in its overall wealth and have access to its power. Unevenness characterizes modernities around the world.

In *Viral Mothers,* the analysis of modern constructions of maternity in the global north is derived primarily from explorations of the U.S. context. In the discussion, I make this focus on the United States explicit. The United States represents a limit-point of the modern trends investigated here and, arguably, emblematizes the expectations of modern paradigms. One goal of this book is to show how preoccupations developed in the ideological contexts of highly industrialized countries can be seen to inflect policy considerations about and representations of women in the global south, particularly in sub-Saharan Africa, the epicenter of the AIDS epidemic. A fuller consideration of these issues would use a more truly global lens. But even in the more narrow comparative analysis provided here, we can see that debates (in the media and in policy contexts) about what mothers in the global south should do when they are HIV positive are articulated in relation to an "economy of statements" that constrain and produce expectations of modern maternity in the global north.[11]

Countries of the global north, and perhaps especially the United States, export ideology in the service of neoliberal goals. Jaggar offers another useful definition.

Neoliberalism is the name given to the version of liberal political theory that currently dominates the discourse of globalization. Neoliberalism assumes that material acquisition is the normal aim of human life, and it holds that the primary function of government is to make the world safe and predictable for the participants in a market economy. Although its name suggests that it is a new variety of liberalism, neoliberalism in fact marks a retreat from the liberal social democracy of the years following World War II back toward the non-redistributive laissez-faire liberalism of the seventeenth and eighteenth centuries.[12]

As Bradley Lewis points out, and as I develop more fully in the next chapter, globalizing biomedicine is a new development in this old internationalist strategy. Instead of a military-industrial complex, the global north is expanding its "medical-biotech-pharmaceutical sector."[13] That neoliberal developments would spread to (and through) global health-care initiatives is no surprise, given the increasing proportion of GDP that health-care expenditures take up in the economies of the global north. Lewis argues that the exportation of northern biomedical practices and products to the cultures of the global south is also the exportation of "cultural solutions," suggesting that medicalization is a specific and normative response to social circumstances and concerns. That is, the globalization of health care is much more than just an attempt to improve the well-being of impoverished individuals around the world. It entails the domination of local modes of thinking and acting by the energy- and capital-intensive regimes of medicalized bureaucracies.[14]

Viral Mothers is not a book of political economy. Yet ideological analysis focuses our attention on those discourses and practices that sustain political economy. It is impossible to analyze culture without paying attention to the structures and agents that are shored up and perpetuated by ideology. Global biomedical endeavors are not ideology free, and are intimately linked to other globalization efforts that are more commonly thought of as political economy. Within biomedical systems of thought "health" is a natural state of the human body, and medicine is a scientific response to illness or impairment. Medical treatment from a professional is thus what one commonly seeks in response to an accident, falling ill, or becoming disabled. But such a response can only occur when a medical infrastructure exists to make such action normal. And the medical infrastructure depends on the attitudes and actions of individuals to utilize, respect, and pay for the treatments and procedures administered by medical professionals. Advanced medical practices, technologies, and pharmaceuticals are an ordinary aspect of life in the global north for many people, but it is precisely what is accepted as ordinary that ideological analysis targets for interpretation and critique.

Medicine as a Value System

Biomedicine is an arena of knowledge and practice bounded by specific constraints: its dependence on medicalization as a basic paradigm that improves lives, its focus on statistically identifiable risks and rational choices with respect to known risks, its obscured relation to the conditions of advanced industrialized development (and thus to an intensely energy-dependent infrastructure not available in many parts of the world). Most inhabitants of highly industrialized countries are subjected to biomedical paradigms that define good living—at a cost to other cultural systems of meaning and value. When we analyze biomedicine as a cultural system, we can see that it has won overall (or official) consensus in the global north but that it conflicts consistently with other cultural systems both within the global north and in other contexts around the world.

This is not to say that biomedicine makes no valuable contribution to health or the public good. The point here is not to vilify medicine or healthcare personnel, nor to subject the vast global project of public health to criticism for its importation of values from the global north to the global south. Rather, what I aim to do is to demonstrate and work from the understanding that many discussions purporting to be focused on medical risk or health are really about cultural meanings and values. Insofar as biomedicine can be figured as a value system, it is a value system that pretends to not be one because it defines itself as science. Science is often thought to be interested in truths that are outside of or untouched by culture. To demonstrate that medicine is a cultural system with a value system, we must reveal its repudiated, disavowed discourse about values. In this project, the discourse of values underlies attitudes and perceptions that apply to mothers and their bodies. Such revelation is one result of attention to the discursive construction of both medical knowledge and the dissemination of medical ideas and practices globally.

Focusing on the rhetorical presentation of biomedical arguments and evidence is one way of addressing the value-laden nature of scientific discourses. Biomedicine presents its information about the body in the form of scientific studies, public health policies, and clinical practice. Biomedical resources clearly operate as important sources of information about the body. But medical information is also an element of the "circuits of culture," an idea originally articulated by Stuart Hall and developed by Bradley Lewis with respect to medicine. Biomedical knowledge is produced by people and rendered in certain forms.[15] And ideas are not only produced and represented, they are *consumed,* they provide opportunities for *identification,* and they are *regulated* (or mediated) in a variety of ways (both officially and unofficially). As Lewis writes, "What is considered 'true' and 'good' in medicine is not determined simply by science, but also by complex currents of culture."[16]

In *Viral Mothers* I focus on the cultural consensus necessary for medical facts to be accepted as such, emphasizing the circuit of consumption in the production of scientific truth. Scientific studies are persuasive to individuals and groups for many reasons, some of which have little to do with data itself. Because of this, cultural consensus is crucial to the verification of scientific knowledge in the public sphere. We can discover the normative ideals driving scientific and medical research and the dissemination of its findings, exploring the complex nature of public consensus that responds to, validates, and supports biomedical conclusions culturally.

Reading *Viral Mothers*

Viral Mothers is divided into three parts, each with internal chapters. "Frames," the first part, provides a set of conceptual and theoretical frameworks for the subsequent analysis. The second part, "Risk and Purity," focuses on the elaboration of these themes in public discourses about maternity in the United States. The third part, "Breastfeeding and Global Public Health," demonstrates how configurations of risk and purity—developed in the highly medicalized global north—contribute to accusations of denial and the construction of false paradigms of choice for mothers in the global south. These themes—*risk, purity, denial,* and *choice*—define the terms through which the viral mother is constituted in discourse and enacted publicly as a set of identifiable, culturally legible, concerns.

In "Frames," the chapter "Viral Mothers" introduces the concept of the viral mother as an imago dominating perceptions of breastfeeding in the age of HIV/AIDS. "Modernity" presents the basic theoretical foundation for *Viral Mothers,* offering a wide-ranging discussion of medicalization and globalization in the uneven, contested, multiple, yet relentless conditions of modernity. "Modernity" addresses issues within a theoretical framework informed by cultural studies and critical theory, in a language that may be challenging to some readers. While I have tried to make the discussion accessible, "Modernity" may seem less inviting than other chapters. Readers are welcome to skip the chapter, or skim through it selectively, looking for definitions of modernity, medicalization, discipline, and biopower as they see fit.

In "Risk and Purity in the Contemporary United States," I explore the public articulation of risks to breastfeeding and risks of not breastfeeding in the United States, as well as fears of environmental contaminants in mothers' bodies. This part includes six chapters, including a theoretical introduction, "Theorizing Risk, Imagining Purity," which overviews theories of risk selection and notions of a risk society. "West Nile Virus" examines concerns about West Nile viral infection through breast milk during fall 2002 in the United States. "The 2004 U.S. National Breastfeeding Awareness Campaign" explores the controversies over risk messages in an Ad Council public health campaign, and "Guilt" demonstrates how the threat of maternal guilt functions culturally to forestall public acknowledgment of the health risks of not breastfeeding. These chapters focus on the United States as a cultural whole influencing perceptions of risk and infant feeding practices. I argue that the strong susceptibility to certain kinds of medicalized risk discourses, and seeming indifference to others, depends on cultural consensus rather than the absolute value of scientific facts. As a result, cultural norms emphasize microbial threats—and their passage through breast milk—but downplay medically established risks of not breastfeeding.

Current concerns with environmental contaminants in breast milk are the subject of the last two chapters of this part. Here I connect issues of viral contagion and toxic contamination by showing how the transfer of dangerous substances from mother to infant is set against an idealization: a pure maternal body. The notion of a pure maternity that relies upon clear distinctions between what is inside the body and what is outside cannot accommodate breastfeeding as a material practice. It is an idealization that relies on medicalization and engenders distrust for mothers who do not practice their maternity under the supervision of physicians or medical ideas. This part, also largely focused on the United States, is divided into two chapters: "Pollution Taboos and Pregnancy Advice," which analyzes pregnancy advice books concerning their presentation of chemical contaminants, emphasizing how expectant mothers are introduced to maternity through highly disciplined and medically regulated practices; and "Contamination and the Sacred Maternal Body," which examines ambivalent representations of breast milk in environmentalist discourses. These two chapters demonstrate the importance of the concept of risk in imagining an idealized, pure maternal body, which is contrasted to real mothers' bodies that are fully permeable, with no plausible barriers that can be set up to protect a baby from its mother's contaminating influence.

In "Breastfeeding and Global Public Health: Denial, Choice, and HIV/AIDS," I shift focus from the United States as a context generating ideologies of risk and purity to specific representations of and within global public health that are affected by those ideologies. The first chapter of this part is an overview of the issues at stake in mother-to-child transmission (MTCT) of HIV. "MTCT" offers the reader a basic understanding of global public health guidelines concerning infant feeding, especially concerning the Nestlé boycott and the advent of HIV/AIDS, and introduces various ways in which denial figures into perceptions of viral mothers. "Denialist Rhetorics" examines AIDS denialism and demonstrates how it operates from the margins of science as a challenge to hegemonic biomedical beliefs. Without supporting its claims, I examine how denialism functions rhetorically and can be identified as a particular style of argumentation. The final chapter on denialism, "Situating Denialism," explores the official AIDS denialism of the South African government in order to understand, through analogy, breastfeeding advocates' usage of denialist discourses.

Scholars have understood South African denialism as reflecting the ongoing struggles of the new black majority government confronting the legacies of racist science and struggling to handle the burgeoning epidemic, in the midst of other forms of denial in the world system. Breastfeeding advocates assert that too many AIDS researchers are blind to—in denial of—the crucial contributions that breastfeeding makes to health, everywhere, but particularly in the global south. These chapters focus on denial's function as a judgment on mothers, at the same time that it operates rhetorically as a challenge to certain kinds of authority. As accusations of denialism are made with respect to the global AIDS pandemic and breastfeeding advocacy, an analysis of the discourses involved demonstrates why it is so important to understand the discursive mechanisms that make these charges so difficult to refute, and also so damaging to global efforts to fight HIV/AIDS.

The final two chapters of the book continue the global focus of this part by looking at how maternal choice is represented in mass media and public health discourses. "Representing African Women" looks at news reports in the U.S. media that portray replacement feeding as preferred choices for HIV-positive African women. This is a significant shift from the days of the

Nestlé boycott, when bottle feeding in the "Third World" was equated with dead babies. The final chapter examines global public health guidelines for infant feeding that emphasize "Informed Choice" for HIV-positive mothers, setting these against the way choice in infant feeding is presented to American women by infant formula manufacturers. Discussing controversies over infant feeding practices in the medical and public health literature, I show how two groups are split over how to address poverty as an agent of infection in the global south. This chapter ends the book with a meditation on the real fear of breastfeeding advocates in the time of AIDS—that breastfeeding will disappear as an ordinary relation of mothers and babies. The conclusion to chapter 14 is a conclusion to *Viral Mothers* as a whole.

While each chapter can stand on its own as an independent analysis, the book's discussion overall builds from beginning to end. In dividing the book into parts and composing the argument through shorter chapters, I lay out the complex ideological web constraining women's lives, as well as the connections between and among these ongoing contestations about maternal experience. As should be clear in the book's organization, I am particularly concerned about the globalization of specific biomedical values, especially as they trade on mothers' vulnerability and widespread lack of power. HIV/AIDS is an illness that defies easy answers, especially with respect to MTCT in the global south. Analyzing discourses about it is no simple task, and does not lead to obvious or unambiguous conclusions.

Yet I have written this book because I believe that cultural studies scholarship can address the seemingly intractable, and tragic, problems posed by HIV in the modern world. Medicine is fully embedded in, and not outside of, the cultural spheres in which it operates. Cultural studies scholarship can help to solve the world's problems by framing its analysis as contribution, not just critique. It is in this spirit, and in the context of this framework for engaged research, that I present *Viral Mothers*.

PART 1

Frames

CHAPTER 2

Viral Mothers

THE IMAGE of the viral mother focuses attention on the maternal body as a conduit for disease, drug addiction, or contamination that ends up in the body of an innocent—and pure—infant. The cultural construction of the viral mother is based on the specific development paradigm that frames maternal experience in the United States and much of the global north. Not all mothers in industrialized contexts have the same experience, of course, as there are national and cultural distinctions that obtain, as well as diversities within national boundaries, but overall an ideological frame work defines and constrains their experience with a certain set of expectations and requirements.

The viral mother is perceived to be a risky conduit for disease because the other vectors of disease are thought to be adequately controlled through immunization, clean water, medical care, and other preventive measures. The viral mother is so because she conceivably could have avoided the infection or contamination of her infant but, having engaged in risky, immoral, or illegal behaviors, she endangers the infant anyway. Choice is thus an aspect contributing to her deviance. Viral mothers in the global south, made abject through their lack of choice, have tended to be rendered as victims. In the public health context, choice offers women a version of neoliberal agency, but, one might argue, does not alter the difficult calculus of morbidity and mortality that constrains outcomes.

This chapter introduces the figure of the viral mother. My attempt here is synthetic and expansive, to offer to the reader some of the preliminary ideas that led me to ask questions about breastfeeding, infection, and contamination in the modern world. The viral mother functions as a cultural imago, an idealized mental image that organizes perception and both constrains and contributes to maternal experience. The negative of an ideal of pure motherhood, the viral mother simultaneously represents modern fears of contaminating mothers and modern desires for mothers to be lifted out of the dirty circumstances of material life. This chapter examines the ideological context of that ideal, as well as the actual challenges HIV poses to its realization, in order to begin to imagine alternative ways of construing mothers and their bodies.

Breast Milk as Medicine

Breastfeeding advocates and global public health workers understand that mothers in the poverty environments of the global south do not inhabit the same kinds of spaces as most mothers in the global north. Certain mothers are more vulnerable to the predations of multinational corporations, although all mothers are, at some level, susceptible to the promotion of products claiming both ease and health. It is on this basis that the first and current boycotts against the Nestlé corporation, the world's largest producer of infant formula, were initiated.[1] Global breastfeeding advocates put forth the argument that breast milk operates to protect babies in poverty environments, where breast milk substitutes endanger the health of babies.[2] Usually, this argument is made on the basis of the immunological protectiveness of breastfeeding and breast milk, which medicalizes maternal nursing and frames the experience with medical views of health.

The portrayal of breast milk as medicine represents, in part, the response of breastfeeding advocates to the fact that infant formulas bear the imprimatur of science as an industrial food imagined to improve on nature. As a result of the International Code of Marketing of Breastmilk Substitutes, formula companies are not supposed to advertise infant formulas as better than breast milk.[3] An article in the U.S. Food and Drug Administration's Web-based consumer magazine is entitled "Infant Formula: Second Best but Good Enough," suggesting the rhetorical complexity of evaluating and representing breast milk substitutes in ways that comply with international law and medical knowledge as well as corporate interests.[4] And for many women, infant formulas do seem "good enough." Most U.S. women, for example, know that breast milk is healthier for infants than infant formulas, but most U.S. women also don't nurse longer than a few months.[5] Thus there are ways in which infant formulas do seem to enhance women's lives so that women themselves are motivated to use them: they make it possible for mothers to be separated from their infants but know that they are fed, they allow mothers to remove their own bodies from the feeding picture, and they allow mothers to efficiently outsource child care and other traditionally female burdens onto partners, husbands, or other caregivers.

Meanings of breastfeeding and infant formulas are not consistent across cultures or even within a given culture. In the United States, breastfeeding is often configured as a gift; it is highly romanticized and associated with leisure and material resources. This association does not always translate to other contexts. In some societies formula is presented as a gift that defines paternity.[6] Infant formulas inevitably seem to represent "science" or at least modernity, however, since they necessitate paraphernalia, measurement, refrigeration, warming, and, often, switching of brands in order to find what "agrees with the baby." In low-income countries, feeding with formula may be available only to the urban elite, with access to piped water, sanitation, and the resources necessary to sustain infant feeding through consumption of a commodity. In the United States, breastfeeding is associated with high income and education, but using infant formulas helps mothers lessen or do away with the amount of time they spend on a culturally anomalous practice. In societies where breastfeeding is a more widespread and culturally dominant practice, formula feeding is unusual and, since the 1990s, is often associated with the stigma of AIDS.

Breastfeeding advocates fight against the widespread abandonment of breastfeeding with numerous medical studies demonstrating the biological superiority of maternal nursing and breast milk. Breastfeeding itself is represented in infant care manuals in the United States as an activity for which mothers need medical guidance and supervision. Medicalizing breastfeeding—in this context, bringing it into the field of medicine's authority—is one way advocates have worked toward a positive relationship with the mainstream of the medical profession. Medicalization was also an early response to the abandonment of breastfeeding in the late nineteenth century by U.S. women as physicians perceived connections between bottle feeding and infant morbidity.[7] Yet the medicalization of infant feeding has had an ambivalent effect on breastfeeding as a practice and on breastfeeding advocacy. Breastfeeding advocates often are caught in the odd position of touting the biological advantages of breastfeeding while at the same time pointing out most medical professionals' lack of knowledge concerning lactation. Advocates criticize medical practitioners for not knowing more about lactation and for providing false information to women, but usually stay within the general medical paradigm of infant feeding. After all, much of breastfeeding advocacy itself is indebted to a medical model of demonstrating the contribution that breastfeeding makes to health.

Breast Milk as Virus

If breastfeeding advocacy touts the medical benefits of breastfeeding to such an extent that breast milk seems to be a medicine itself, the focus on viral transmission through breastfeeding confounds this representation. Recent attention to HIV and West Nile virus and analogies to the mother's body as a conduit for disease in general have made breastfeeding seem risky even in the United States. The suggestion that breast milk conveys virus, and thus is itself viral, casts doubt on the perception that breast milk is a medicine or acts like a medicine to enhance health outcomes for babies and children. Good mothers don't put their babies at risk. News reports of the passage of virus from mother to baby serve to foment anxiety and the further medicalization of nursing practices, as mothers are encouraged, if they have any questions, to ask their doctors for advice about whether to continue nursing. Nursing constructed under these circumstances is always on the verge of ending, with messages about risk putting a consistent and negative pressure on a practice defined almost entirely through discourses of health enhancement.

The assault on the paradigm of breast milk as medicine has proved difficult for breastfeeding advocates to address in the context of HIV transmission. One current response has been to demonstrate that, at least in the poverty environments of the global south, breast milk is still more medicinal than viral, in that it continues to be protective against gastrointestinal illnesses (rotovirus, for example) and pneumonia (top killer of children under five around the globe), both of which are more likely to kill babies than is HIV infection. Supporters also advocate for exclusive breastfeeding, although it is not a customary practice of nursing anywhere and must be taught to mothers and supported like any other culturally anomalous health-care practice.[8]

The conundrum of breast milk as medicine or virus reiterates the enigma of HIV itself, a virus that attacks the immune system and lives within it, destroying the body's ability to fight off disease, because breastfeeding has been thought of as helping infants gain immunity at a time when their bodies (and immune systems) are underdeveloped. In order to address the challenges of maternal HIV infection and pediatric AIDS, we need to supersede this problematic opposition that currently informs public health perspectives on breastfeeding. The medicine-virus opposition, perhaps because it fits so well with other dichotomous renderings of maternal adequacy, deflects attention from other ways of understanding breastfeeding and its relation to disease.

The viral mother is cast against the image of a pure mother whose idealized maternal behavior contrasts strongly with the material circumstances of most women's lives, as well as with the physiology of breastfeeding itself. Maternal nursing is a physiological exchange between two human beings who live in a dirty world; it is necessarily of that world and thus implicated in its filth. Not acknowledging the concrete materiality of most mothers' circumstances impedes reasonable public health efforts. Conceptual oppositions that encourage a view of breast milk as risky as a result of maternal impurity are part of the problem. Indeed, understanding the mother's body to be fully contextualized and materially responsive to its cultural and physical habitat should result in acknowledging maternal corruption rather than defending against it. Such a perspective also suggests breastfeeding is a practice that offers its own signifying power: for most viral illnesses, it is precisely through infection that nursing confers its immunizing advantage.

That this is not true in the case of HIV, a virus that attacks the immune system itself, is another tragic dilemma of breastfeeding in the age of HIV/AIDS. And yet the image of the pure mother is an important ideal that still (negatively) affects approaches to breastfeeding in cases of maternal HIV infection. Idealizations of maternal purity make it difficult to understand or even address mothers' real circumstances, especially when those circumstances offer no good resolution to infection, disease, or contamination.

From Hygiene to Permeability: The Case of Tuberculosis

The viral mother has a history. In the early twentieth century, in the United States and Europe, her precursor was the hygiene mother, whose main enemy was tuberculosis infection. She may have breastfed her baby swathed in a medical mask, or prepared infant milk according to a complex formula given to her by the doctor. If she were suffering from an active TB infection, she may have been separated from her infant, especially if she was poor. Barriers, separation, and cleanliness were the hallmarks of her maternal practices as a potential source of infection for her own baby.

The mother constructed under the regime of "hygiene" embodied and practiced her maternity differently than the contemporary mother, whose embodiment is influenced by the hegemony of pharmaceutical medicine, with its dependence on a belief in the continual permeability of the body.[9] The hygienic mother can be blocked off from her infant, separated from it and sanitized, while the contemporary mother's boundaries are more flexible. Mothers today are subjected to greater scrutiny with regard to their own practices of cleanliness and purity, which extend inside to their bodies and wombs. In the early twentieth century, the hygiene mother was set against the traditional, ignorant, often immigrant mother, whose practices were perceived to be unhealthful in the degree to which they adhered to unthinking traditions and dangerous cultural patterns. The traditional mother could, however, be educated and transformed into a hygienic mother, one goal of Progressive Era antituberculosis campaigns.

In 1882, physician and researcher Robert Koch determined that consumption was a bacterial illness, caused by a tubercle bacillus, and that the disease was communicable and spread through sputum droplets in the air.[10] Sheila Rothman points out that there were two main medical responses to the discovery of the tubercle bacillus, with respect to public health strategies: eradication of contagion and the sanatorium cure.[11] Both aspects of the antituberculosis campaigns relied on hygiene and rest as their main strategies for combating the spread of the illness and treating the illness in individuals. There were not many medicines for any diseases, so the fact that there were none to treat tuberculosis at this time (not until the mid-twentieth century) was not anomalous in the context of medicine in general. The hygiene movement and its requirements for sanitary living were significant to both the experience of tuberculosis and the development of the public health bureaucracy.

Rest and the corollary practice of eating a rich diet were the basis of sanatorium treatments and an important part of the general antituberculosis movement. Milk diets were popular, as was the addition of eggs to an ordinary diet.[12] The focus on rest, which continued into the era of antibiotic treatment, encouraged alternatives to breastfeeding as a strategy to shore up the mother's energy and ensure that she was able to husband her energies to fight her own infection. Hygiene was the other arm of public health efforts to limit the spread of tuberculosis. In *Fevered Lives*, Katherine Ott argues that sputum and dust were the focus of this aspect of the campaign: "Sputum and dust came to symbolize tuberculosis and in turn became the focus of most legislation. Of all the aspects of consumption (from cough to sweating to diarrhea and weight loss), sputum and dust represented the most fearful and insidious manifestations of bacteria, germs, and chaotic modern life."[13]

Given that almost all adults in the hygiene period were tuberculin positive, having had and recovered from infection that may not have registered as an illness, purity for mothers is not legible in relation to the TB epidemic. Rather, there is the mother who cleans, who sanitizes, and who regulates the sanitary activities of her family. She consciously protects her infant from her own possible contagiousness. If she herself has active tuberculosis, she rests and drinks a lot of milk, and she may be segregated from the family or removed entirely to a sanatorium. Since the tubercular mother's infectious capacity is not through her breast milk itself but simply through routine contact, the effect of the antituberculosis campaigns on breastfeeding was accomplished by the establishment of a public health bureaucracy, the normalization of infant removal (primarily of the poor), and the regularization of public health and visiting nurse education. This last point is important, since it seems that over time public health nurses were more successful at supporting replacement feeding even though breastfeeding was always presented as best for most mothers and babies.[14]

The public health efforts in the antituberculosis campaigns contributed to the hygiene movement and accelerated expectations of mothers' abilities to keep homes germ free. Eventually, scientific motherhood as an ideal of maternal behavior and submission to medical authority transformed into the version of highly functioning middle-class motherhood we see in the United States and much of the global north today: the mother who purifies her body in the context of pregnancy and worries over the possibility of breast milk contaminated by environmental toxins leaching from plastics or pesticides.

The tubercular mother, like the mother with HIV, was perceived to be poor, and thus the antithesis of the mother whose purity is the result of careful and deliberative ingestion. Middle-class mothers now represent with their own bodies the ecosystems it is necessary to sanitize, harkening back to the hygiene era of swiping nipples with alcohol or boric acid, but instead of antiseptics we have disciplinary practices that cleanse the body through eating organic foods, using chemical-free body products, and otherwise consuming naturally. It is not enough to avoid feeding the baby coffee, as in the hygiene era of public health; now mothers must also abstain from caffeinated beverages themselves.

We are no longer in the hygiene era, but we are affected by it and live with its legacies—the widespread usage of antibacterial soaps, hand sanitizers, and antibacterial household sprays testifies to this fact. We live in the era of pharmaceutical medicine, when not only are diseases matched with drugs to treat them, but drugs are developed and then shopped around to find the right disease to treat. Yet viral illnesses are particularly difficult to address in the era of pharmaceutical medicine, since viruses have proved resistant to cure except through vaccination (and some are difficult to develop vaccines for). For retroviruses like HIV, treatment is expensive, not curative, and always at risk of increasing mutant strains of the virus. A significant number of HIV-positive individuals either cannot tolerate the prescribed antiretroviral treatments or else go through a number of highly toxic therapies before determining which one they can tolerate. Enhanced antibiotic medicines—and widespread abuse of antibiotics—eventuate in a situation in which more and more bacteria develop resistance. Tuberculosis is a case in point, its normal tendency toward antibiotic resistance exacerbated by HIV.

Today, as historically, active tuberculosis infection contraindicates maternal-infant contact because of the threat of droplet infection. Separation makes sense only if the infant has not already been exposed, and it is not breast milk that threatens the infant's health, but the mother's sputum.[15] Yet current perceptions of permeable maternal bodies inform ideas about how tuberculosis poses a risk to breastfeeding babies. In much contemporary advice about tuberculosis contraindicating breastfeeding, the tubercular mother is figured as a viral mother because, however erroneously, her breast milk itself is implied to be harmful for her baby.[16]

Imagining Mothers with HIV

Cindy Patton argues, in *Globalizing AIDS,* that tropical medicine and epidemiology make use of the theme of mobility to describe the spread of HIV. For tropical medicine, which is a historical framework of colonialism focused on place, mobility is what brings colonized, tropical spaces closer to "here," threatening "here" with what should stay "there." For epidemiology, which addresses vectors of transmission, mobility is what allows one to trace the disease vectors and make predictions about the future of disease spread. In Patton's analysis, both tropical medicine (a historical mind-set) and epidemiology (a contemporary method of public health) frame approaches to the global HIV/AIDS pandemic, highlighting the theme of mobility—where the disease is, where it came from, how it got from A to B. Given the importance of migration, migrant work, and truck routes in the spread of HIV in Africa and elsewhere, mobility is key to understanding the disease and its progress.[17] Mobility is what allows the virus to develop in central Africa but have its most devastating effects in southern African countries. It is also what allowed a virus incubated in central Africa to come to public attention by sickening gay men in the United States.

Because mother-to-child transmission of HIV typically does not start a chain of infection—an HIV-positive infant does not tend to pass the disease on to others—mobility is not the central issue or theme of MTCT. The mother can be conceptualized as potentially spreading HIV through sex to other adults, but her child is an end point. Tropical and epidemiological approaches to mother-to-child transmission through breastfeeding do affect perceptions of maternal embodiment, as the mother's body can be rendered as a place (environment) or as a vector of transmission. The latter rendering reiterates some trends that discuss "father-to-child" transfer through the mother, which portray the mother as passive victim and cipher. When mothers become vectors through which the virus passes, they are no longer subjects. Feminist HIV activists have been complaining for years about women's relative invisibility—except as mothers and possible vectors of infections to their infants, or as prostitutes and the immoral spreaders of venereal disease—as AIDS victims.[18]

Investigating mother-to-child transmission through breastfeeding shows us the difficulty of conceptualizing the mother's body in the age of medicalization. Mothers' bodies have always confounded and fascinated doctors and others. But medicalization demands purity, safety, sterility, and reliability; it dislikes permeability, corruption, and contamination. The function of the maternal body as environment explodes the expectations generated in the context of modern notions of risk. Maternal bodies are always already contaminated, and with respect to breastfeeding this phenomenology is crucial, providing immunity through breastfeeding and colonizing infants with neighborly bacteria. HIV/AIDS can be understood to offer us this vision of the mother's body as contagious and yet necessary, but the epidemic also suggests the very material difficulties associated with bloodborne viruses and maternity. The problem of transmitting HIV to infants is an existential problem of the mother's body, its status as a necessary environment for fetuses as well as for most of the world's infants and toddlers and its uncertain condition as positive or negative, infected or infection free.

Discourses on environmental contamination and breastfeeding alert us to the problem of purity as a way of referencing maternal bodies. Yet solutions to environmental toxins seem remote, less likely to accomplish, and, in some ways, less pressing. The illnesses and deficits purported to result from environmental contaminants are those that raise awareness most forcefully in the highly industrialized contexts of the global north—cancer, lowered intelligence, and growth deficiencies, for example. This is not to diminish the biological accounting of the effect of environmental contaminants on human bodies, but to locate the rhetorical effect of the discourses drawing our attention to them and outlining their risks. Solutions to HIV transmission seem more insistent and necessary, given the global numbers of people with the disease (33 million people living with HIV by the end of 2007, with 2.1 million people having died of AIDS-related illnesses in 2007 and over 25 million dead since 1981),[19] as well as the fact that the successful development of a vaccine for HIV is still unrealized.[20] HIV/AIDS also brings back the specter of contagion as a major mechanism of disease, confounding the dream of twentieth-century medicine to eradicate the major viral illnesses, like smallpox and polio, and to control others, like measles, through global vaccination programs.

What does it mean to consider how public health debates seek to protect infants from potential dangers that track their way through mothers' bodies? We might begin by characterizing this problem as the way modernity, through medicalization, impinges on the embodied practices of maternity. Like Barbara Duden we may be struck by how little power mothers themselves have to define their own bodily processes and to develop their own responses to the inevitable unknowns of pregnancy and motherhood.[21] In our current context of increasing medicalization of maternity globally, how a mother uses her body in relation to her infant or her fetus is necessarily tracked, debated, and, in many parts of the world, decried. In both the global north and south, maternal behaviors are perceived to risk debilitation or fatal illness in their infants. This trend places mothers under constant medical surveillance and suspicion.

As an alternative, we can accept that ordinary mothers are impure, and, more generally, we can refuse purity as a way to conceptualize good maternal embodiment and practice. As an impure body, the lactating mother poses certain problems to her nursing infant. This is true for mothers with tuberculosis as well as mothers with the common cold, let alone HIV-positive mothers. We can see HIV as a unique condition, because it is incurable and because it attacks the immune system itself. Or we can address HIV as one among many disease states that signify in relation to other meanings circulating within and across cultures. Or we can do both, recognizing "AIDS exceptionalism" at the same time that we acknowledge the linkages that make HIV-positive mothers like other viral mothers.

Conclusion

The global political economy of contamination and disease influences the way we understand maternity and its particular embodiments. If mothers are both locations of and vectors for viral and bacterial disease, as well as environmental toxins, then their complex embodied functions as habitats for fetuses, infants, and toddlers must be read against overtly politicized figurations of mothers' own environments.[22] Breastfeeding suggests mothers are liminal bodies invested in particular ecological contexts, exchanging compounds and contributing toward growth and, at times, the spread of disease. For HIV-positive mothers—indeed, for all mothers whose milk contains residues of DDT and PCBs and other environmental toxins (that is, virtually all mothers)—breastfeeding is a conundrum that represents the contemporary maternal condition. It is *pharmakon,* both medicine and poison.[23] In this sense, all mothers are viral mothers. Our sometimes desperate gestures to purify ourselves, however promoted by medicine and public health, are enacted against the material conditions of modern embodiment. As such, they represent the impossible dreams of a sacred motherhood separated from the world, its dirt, and its communicable diseases.

CHAPTER 3

Modernity

FEARS ABOUT maternal bodies have crystallized in the figure of the viral mother, as we saw in the previous chapter. Her perceived permeability to infection and contaminants, a vulnerability that is difficult to manage except through increasingly stringent protocols of purification, is both origin and effect of modern medicalization. In affluent societies, we see these protocols enforced by institutions and social norms, and embraced by (some) women as disciplined subjects. Their impact on women in poverty environments is ambivalent and uneven, but they affect public health attitudes toward maternal behaviors and practices.

This chapter explores modernity as a basis for medicalizing maternity. As modernity has developed over the course of centuries, concerns about mothers' bodies have intensified and changed. Historical concerns about maternal fitness have become sutured to biomedical paradigms. Yet medicine's fraught relation with breastfeeding—heralding its value while contributing to its abandonment—demonstrates the quintessentially ironic doubleness of modernity. Bringing more human experience within the domain of medicine—the general definition of medicalization—produces important achievements in public health, but it also enforces a regulatory biopolitics of the body that engenders significant side effects.

A noncritical usage of the term *modernity* leads to problems, largely because it has been conceptualized as a break from so-called traditional patterns.[1] The resulting dichotomy of modern/premodern can exacerbate perceptions of certain behaviors, practices, and phenomena—even those enacted in the present—as antiquated, traditional, and thus nonrelevant to modern life.[2] Current attempts to theorize multiple modernities try to overcome the modern/premodern dichotomy as a limiting framework, yet throughout *Viral Mothers* it nevertheless generates conceptual tensions.

Poor mothers in the global south often are figured as existing in a pre-modern state with respect to infant feeding.[3] Those aspects of modern societies that support replacement feeding—piped clean water, adequate energy supplies to households, routine medical care—are also ones that have transformed the lives of most people in the global north and the elite in the global south. Breastfeeding, marked by international agencies as crucial to health outcomes for poor children in the global south, is perceived as an activity of mothers who must feed their babies from their own bodies to make up for the lack of modern infrastructures in their environments. Modern mothers in the global north have choices and can breastfeed as a health enhancement for their children, rather than a health necessity.

That there is some truth to this configuration does not make its dichotomies less troubling. In this chapter, I elaborate the meanings of modernity in relation to global north/south dichotomies in order to set up the book's exploration of breastfeeding as a locus of modern anxieties. After defining modernity and exploring the issue of multiple modernities, I focus on medicalization. The medicalization of maternity gives us the figure of the viral mother, a modern, ironic image that embodies both risk and redemption.

Defining *Modernity*

Modernity refers to the historical break with traditional social, economic, religious, and political structures thought to emerge in the seventeenth and eighteenth centuries in Europe in tandem with Enlightenment philosophies.[4] The development of capitalism and market economies, the advent of industrialization, the establishment of democratic politics and secular governments, the rise of the nation-state, and the flowering of reflexive sensibilities are all identified as part of the emergence of the modern cultural and political situation. The break with tradition is one way of heralding modernity's focus on the new and the transformative. The idea of progress through the development of science and technology and the application of scientific principles to daily life are characteristic of modern modes of being. The Enlightenment emphasis on rationality and contractual social relations inaugurated modernity's belief in the individual and the human capacity to live through reason, defined in relation to science and general laws. Understanding and control of nature through consciously scientific processes and practices is distinctly modern. This is the basis of much of public health practice, as well as the disciplining body projects related to medicalization.

One central task of scholars addressing modernity as a concept has been to identify the relationship of political and economic transformations to modes of lived experience, expression in the arts, and sensibilities around bodies, behaviors, and interpersonal relations. If modernity is a condition brought about by the advent of liberal capitalism, democracy (or its presumptions as an ideal), and the industrial revolution, it is accompanied by cultural changes. These cultural aspects are crucial to what modernity is. Without them, modernity is only a description of changing circumstances, but not the experience or understanding of them. Charles Taylor suggests "social imaginary" as a way of conceptualizing these cultural impacts or experiential requisites. Raymond Williams came up with "structure of feeling."

Williams defines a structure of feeling as the "felt sense of the quality of life at a particular place and time: a sense of the ways in which the particular activities combined into a way of thinking and living." The structure of feeling is not learned and is material, evidenced in the arts and in what Williams terms "documentary culture," the archive of discursive and textual remnants available for analysis.[5] Structure of feeling is somewhat similar to Charles Taylor's notion of a "social imaginary," "that largely unstructured and inarticulate understanding of our whole situation, within which particular features of our world show up for us in the sense they have." The modern social imaginary is the basis for the transformed social forms of modernity, which Taylor identifies as "the market economy, the public sphere, and the self-governing people, among others."[6]

Modernity, thought through the concepts of social imaginary and structures of feeling, involves the abstraction of the individual as the most important component of the social formation, and the egalitarian interaction of individuals in a social relation structured by the idea of the mutual benefit of all adherents. Taylor suggests that individuality and egalitarian interaction involve "disembedding," or the separation of subjects from the contexts and traditions previously thought to define their purpose and sensibility. Modern society thrives when its members act in harmony, but that harmony is understood to be achieved when each strives for her or his own good. Such good is understood to "accrue to individuals and society as a whole" through the spread of self-discipline and training.[7]

Sociologist Anthony Giddens, like Taylor, identifies disembedding as a central characteristic of modernity. The two other aspects he identifies are the separation of time and space and the reflexive appropriation of knowledge. As a result of disembedding, trust in abstract systems becomes necessary to daily life: when social relations are "lifted out" of the "local contexts of interaction" and are "restructur[ed] across indefinite spans of time-space," trust "is vested . . . in abstract capacities" like money.[8] That is, when local contexts and face-to-face interactions (i.e., traditional or premodern conditions) no longer provide security grounding decisions or actions, individuals must develop trust in the abstract systems governed and sustained by others whom they do not know personally. Expert systems are one kind of abstract system demanding the trust of modern subjects. Individuals must believe in the knowledge base of those others who increasingly determine the possibilities and constraints of their lives.[9]

Both Giddens and Ulrich Beck focus on reflexivity as a constituent aspect of modernity, although each has a slightly different rendering of it. Reflexivity, for Giddens, challenges the Enlightenment faith in rationality and scientific progress, even as it emerges from the emphasis on reason characteristic of Enlightenment thinking.[10] Beck's notions of reflexivity are less focused on intellectual "reflection"—the idea that the knowledge domains of modernity are self-reflexive and thus always in flux—than on the dialectical push-pull of modernization: "in the modernization phase since the Second World War, the *advancement* and the *dissolution* of industrial society *coincide*. This is exactly the process of reflexive modernization."[11] For Beck, the consequences of disembedding and individualization involve the requirement that people create their own biographies and are thus personally responsible for life choices, remaking them continuously. Reflexive modernity for Giddens, on the other hand, involves the effects of individualization but is focused more on knowledge and the fate of the rational in post-Enlightenment culture.[12]

For Ulrich Beck, modernity inaugurates a risk society, one in which risks are distributed as effects of the overall social formation. In this view, the conditions of modernity continually create risks larger than the individual and as a result of which individuals are more fully dependent on the abstract, expert systems beyond their control. Focusing on toxins, pollutants, and radioactivity as invisible risks that "exist in terms of the (scientific or anti-scientific) knowledge about them," Beck also addresses intensifying individualization as a core aspect of modernity. Individualization is related to disembedding, as it is an effect of the dissolution of traditional community ties and modes of belonging beyond the family, including class affiliations.

Significantly, individualization makes life the result of deliberative choices.[13]

Overall, the idea of reflexive modernity offers a perspective on the ironic situation of individual subjects within modern systems. Individuals are both created by and subjected to the constraints of the social formation. This doubleness is characteristic of modernity, and it will emerge as a theme in almost all of the scholars whose work I examine in the rest of this chapter. Michel Foucault's concepts of discipline, biopolitics, and medicalization—all forms of biopower—are no exception.

Modernity and Biopower

Michel Foucault sought to define and elucidate the unique nexus of power/knowledge defining modernity. While he did not consider the interior experiences of the self as productive foci for analytic inquiry, Foucault did aim to understand modern subjectivity. For those scholars following the Foucauldian paradigm, discipline and biopolitics, along with governmentality, are the dominant forces that shape modern experience, characterizing the bureaucratic social formations of modernity and their characteristic modes of subjectivity.

The prototype of discipline is the Panopticon, or the prison designed by Jeremy Bentham to instill self-regulation within prisoners by making them feel that they are always watched by an unseen guard. Discipline instills in individual subjects the necessary behaviors and self-consciousness to conform to social norms. For Foucault, its main institutional sites in the nineteenth century were the army, schools, and prisons. Biopolitics describes the power invested in bodies that works not through repression but through the production of certain kinds of bodies and bodily experience. The sexualized body, or body infused throughout with a sexuality particular to it and at the core of subjective identity, is an example of biopolitics in operation. Disciplinary power, or anatomopolitics, works through the self-regulatory mechanism of internalization. Biopolitics, on the other hand, is bound up with bureaucratic management and works through the regulation of populations. In this definition, both discipline and biopolitics are forms of biopower, a mechanism of modern social formations having to do with the internal regulation of the subject and the management of bodies within new modes of normalization. Governmentality incorporates both discipline and biopolitics as elements of modern political strategies aimed at subjects.[14]

Medicalization is a form of biopower with both disciplinary and biopolitical implications. As a general sociological term, *medicalization* describes how "general social problems" are turned into "technical medical concerns." In addition, it suggests that medicine as an institution becomes "a basis of social control."[15] In this common understanding of the term, individuals are thought to be complicit with institutions and companies in expanding the purview of medicine.[16] Foucault, on the other hand, sees medicalization as a more foundational vector of power within modernity. Medicalization, in his view, opens up a new way of making modern people—it does not just act on individuals already constituted, but makes them who they are.

Thus, for Foucault medicalization is the simultaneous establishment of a domain of subjectivity and a regulatory mechanism within that domain. Medicalization results from modern conditions of biopower, but it is also a powerful instance of biopower's continuing constitution of subjects through the management of health (a concept that is itself partly an effect of this new domain).

Medicalization, like discipline and biopolitics more generally, is more powerful for the ways in which it works invisibly, through normalization, than for its more visible, authoritarian efforts. While medicalization certainly works through the institutionalization of physicians' power, Foucault argues that emerging concepts of health—concretized in medical ideas, practices, and perceptions about life—began to dominate the bureaucratic management of populations and environments in the eighteenth century.[17] Within circumstances of widespread medicalization, attitudes and behaviors oriented toward health are simply normal and good. It becomes difficult to see them as established and enforced through institutions, operating below or beyond our daily attention through intimate, routine practices.

Discipline, biopolitics, and medicalization are inseparable from modernity, for Foucault and his followers, among whom I count myself. Although from this presentation all of these concepts must seem irreparably negative, they signify a doubled sensibility similar to Giddens's and Beck's ideas about reflexive modernity, if only because the production of subjectivity is the same mechanism as subjection. For Foucault, the modern situation does not admit of alternatives, although it is perhaps not the straitjacket that some ascribe to his representation of it. Discipline, biopolitics, and medicalization represent the characteristic modes through which power circulates and produces subjects within modernity. While it is not possible to step fully outside the practices, discourses, and institutions through which biopower operates, Foucault did, in his later writings, suggest that change is possible when we are able to identify "the shortcomings in our own self-understanding and practices."[18] Nevertheless, it is true that in the development of these concepts and his demonstration of their operation as modern regulatory mechanisms, Foucault offers a stunning critique of Enlightenment modernity, suggesting irrationality behind a facade of reason, regulation instead of freedom, external control in place of self-authorization and independence from norms.

These various vocabularies for defining and understanding modernity agree that momentous historical changes occurred in Europe and America in the period following the Enlightenment and that these changes involved transformations of perception as well as of politics and economics. Most also agree that modernity is not a completed project.[19] Not all theorists of modernity are as pessimistic as Foucault, but many seem to corroborate his view that the pretensions of modernity—to reason, to progress, and to the triumph of scientific knowledge—constrain as much as they produce.

But is modernity a phenomenon bounded by the quasi-geographical "West"? The question of modernity's reach is a vexed one, laden with controversy concerning the trajectory of development required by international monetary institutions and the value of local cultures. Modernity denotes progress in cultural as well as political and economic terms. To be labeled nonmodern signifies a seeming inability to get in step with the project of Enlightenment. For champions of modernization along the model laid out by Europe and North America, modernity is not bounded to specific cultural norms or customs. Those cultures not "developing" along the lines already laid down are perceived to be resistant to modernity's promises and demands.[20] That modernity has only one path and one goal, however, is implied by its designation as what has emerged from a distinct break with past eras and with tradition, writ large. This perspective is made possible by a refusal to see modernity as linked to the customs and cultures of Europe and North America. Certainly, it is difficult to accommodate such a view in the context of globalization and the transformations it has engendered. And yet it is also problematic to ignore the uneven impact of modernity and modernization globally—the domination of the global north in the world system. The next section of this chapter concerns scholarship addressing multiple modernities by exploring perspectives on modernity and the global south.

Modernity and/in the Global South

When modernity is linked with decolonization and the promise of Euro-American-style development in the global south, it cannot be separated, conceptually, from modernization. Modernity seems to be what happens when nations in the global south develop their way out of poverty and into capitalist accumulation. Modernity, thought through modernization theory as a particular process of development that offers cosmopolitanism, choices, individuality, and presentness, is the end goal of a winning historical trajectory.[21]

This view, of course, values the perspective of the so-called modern nations toward their own development, and confuses historical contingencies for optimizing formulas.[22] It also confuses cultural values with a set of absolute values. This is, in part, because Euro-American-style modernity is linked to technological progress and scientific and biomedical advances that are represented as value-neutral. Thus modernity as a mode of experience and living is understood to have to emulate patterns established in Europe, the United States, and other industrialized nations, rather than being the uneven mode of living for everyone in an interconnected global system. Modernity has always, it seems, depended on a view of the "primitive" as its vital other.[23]

Current conversations challenging this view of modernity question the strict historical teleology of the modernization thesis, exploring ways to theorize multiple concurrent modernities in a global context. Debates about multiple modernities and modernity and (or in) the global south are characterized by contestation and frustration with a conceptual system that neglects the contributions of intellectuals from poor countries to ideas about, as well as the experience of, modernity. Alfred Zack-Williams suggests that it is precisely the "modernization paradigm" itself that creates the African as a premodern other unable to incorporate the advantages of modernity. Such a view, he argues, suggests that "cultural pathology," rather than political economy, is the basis for Africa's resistance to modernization. As a response, Zack-Williams offers an analysis emphasizing the "hybridity" of Africa's response to modernity and modernization, within the context of political economy.[24]

This response to the Euro-American-centered view of modernity is typical of those struggling with the issue of modernity in the global south, in that it accepts the origins of modernity in Europe but refuses to separate continents like Africa from a world system that at that time allowed modernity to emerge as it did. My account of this discussion is not going to overview all positions, nor evaluate the findings of existing scholarship on this issue. Instead, I chart a response to the question "What does modernity mean globally?" that moves along the lines suggested by Zack-Williams. This response presumes that it is inappropriate to evaluate cultures according to how modern they have become or how much modernity they have failed to achieve. In discussing modernity and its global reach, it is far too easy to imagine that when a group or nation differs from the cultural systems of the global north it is the fault of people who are not ready to take up modernity as a cause and a mode of living rather than the effect of unequal distribution of resources and power. The discussion here focuses on ways to understand what Zack-Williams calls the hybridity of modernity in the global south, presuming, as he argues, that "structural explanations based on the reality of . . . political economy" are preferable to those based on "cultural pathology."[25] Within these hybrid conditions, however, how might we talk about modernity and its cultural effects?

We are all modern because the conditions of global capitalism and the widespread dissemination of media demand adherence to certain common understandings about the self and experience that are no longer localized. The conditions of modernity are global but uneven because they are structured by unequal social relations and the domination of some peoples and their systems over others. Modernity is not simply a condition that occurs as a spontaneous combustion when people are "ready" for it; it demands capital investment and resources, as well as particular kinds of political structures and legal traditions. As Charles Taylor demonstrates, it is accompanied by a social imaginary "making possible the practices [it] make[s] sense of and thus enable[s]," such as market economies, a rational public sphere, and democratic practices.[26]

It is interesting that many theorists of modernity seem to forget that modernity is uneven even in the global north.[27] In some ways, modernity acts as a horizon that defines experience and sets both possibilities and constraints on behavior and social expectation. It acts, in other words, like a dominant ideology and, like ideology, has uncertain, variable, overdetermined, but widespread effects. Along these lines, Björn Wittrock characterizes modernity as both a global condition and a "set of promissory notes." As a global condition, it "has been characterized by a high degree of variability in institutional forms and conceptual constructions," even in Europe where it began. This variability within Europe is often neglected, making it easier to imagine a singular modernity and the convergence of all societies toward this one model. Wittrock suggests that the idea of multiple modernities involves a singular notion about what modernity as a concept stands for ("notions of self-reflexivity, agency, and historical consciousness"), but he argues that specific cultures individually adapt aspects of these promissory notes ("a set of hopes and expectations that entail some minimal conditions of adequacy that may be demanded of macrosocietal institutions").[28]

It is important, however, to understand how the varied contexts of the global south are specifically affected by a modernity emerging from the particular social, cultural, political, and economic conditions of Europe and North America in the seventeenth and eighteenth centuries. Constraints on modernity in the global south include centuries of cultural and economic domination by nations of the global north and continuing conditions of poverty for large portions of the population, especially following the institution of structural adjustment policies (SAPs) in the 1970s.[29] Cultural differences are thus arrayed within a system of structured domination and continued subordination. Indeed, modernity in the global north, some might argue, has depended on the subjugation of the global south to a world economic system not favorable to its terms of growth and cultural transformation. In this sense, the purported nonmodernity of the global south is just as modern as the modernity it strives for. Modernity historically has relied on the nonmodern other both conceptually and practically to bolster itself as what is desired globally as well as what is particular to certain privileged cultures. The global south serves as the primitive other of modern, Euro-American cultures, the underside and ironic double of prosperity, cosmopolitanism, and the rational democratic state. It is what modern societies need to rescue and change, but also what they need to remain the same, in order to sustain and enhance their own modernity.

Modernity is both an imposition on the global south (the demand to expand markets, for example) and desired by its inhabitants (development of infrastructure and markets, improved education systems, health-care availability, political reform). Modernity can never be only negative or positive. It is a mix of achievement (egalitarian social relations) and devastation (the violent wars of the twentieth century, ethnic cleansing). The "underdevelopment" of the global south can be seen as a side effect of the modernization of the global north, which has certainly not delivered on many of its promissory notes. Continued underdevelopment has been the case for many countries subjected to modernization programs.[30]

Concepts of hybrid modernity suggest divergent social imaginaries. Another way of saying this is to suggest that what is deemed "rational" will differ in differing contexts. After all, it is the social imaginary that creates the grounds for rationality. This is one reason why modernity "feels different" in different contexts, or why people from divergent cultures cannot always make sense of the other's actions and behaviors. The familiar structure of feeling is simply not the same. This is not to say that all instantiations of modernity are relative and thus good. Rather, it is to suggest that specific cultures and societies struggle with and within modernity as a broad global system of meanings, practices, and social structures, each producing its own version of modern life. That some modernities seem more traditionally oriented than others reflects the hybrid nature of modernity everywhere—its unevenness and variability, and the structures of domination that characterize its global phenomenology.

The next and final section of the chapter explores medicalization, specifically analyzing its disciplinary and biopolitical functions within modern cultures. I also consider medicalization in the context of hybrid modernities characteristic of the global south, analyzing how medicalization works in the relations between countries of the global north and south to distinguish identities, risks, and susceptibility to disease.

Modernity and Medicalization

Biomedicine provides an excellent example of how modernity functions in the global south, producing and naturalizing inequalities and regulating bodies into particular behaviors, roles, and identities, and recreating the iatrogenesis common in the north. Charles Briggs holds that "medical epistemologies and technologies have long been seen as produced in Euro-America for export to less-industrialized countries as bases for regulating bodies and diseases," in part because these nonmodern sites are understood as repositories of illnesses that could eventually infect modern citizens of the global north. This is close to what Bradley Lewis sees as a crucial problem of "the new global health movement," which does not understand biomedicine as an element of international domination but simply assumes that health is a right and health care is an unalterable good. Ivan Illich is even more suspicious: "The struggle against death, which dominates the lifestyle of the rich, is translated by development agencies into a set of rules by which the poor of the earth shall be forced to conduct themselves."[31] These perspectives identify medicine as an active element in the institutional enforcement of particular norms and judgments on peoples subjugated around the world.

It is often difficult to see medicine in this role, because its positive value is perceived to be self-evident. Bradley Lewis counters the common view that "Rx for the world" is wholly good by focusing on the side effects of medical treatment and practice. Borrowing from Emily Martin (who borrows from Jacques Derrida) the notion of the *pharmakon* as both remedy and poison, Lewis interrogates current attempts to spread biomedicine's benefits to the global south more fully.[32] Pharmaceutical medicine always comes with side effects, effects on the body that are consequential to treatment but held apart from the "main action" of the drug. These side effects are the negative pole of the pharmakon duality. Lewis, in "The New Global Health Movement," emphasizes the side effects in order to "rebalance our appreciation of the downsides of global health."

He offers five "macrolevel complications" that should give us pause: "(1) downplaying social and political causes of disease; (2) increasing healthcare costs and profits; (3) worsening environmental damage; (4) reintroducing old prejudices through the back door; and (5) globalizing medical biopower in the service of a deeply problematic New World Order." At the basis of his critique is the idea that medicine is not simply a technical practice but an institution with values and interests. These interests work to obscure the fact that negative side effects are ever-present elements of modern medical treatment. The medical creation of health problems (iatrogenesis) is a significant factor limiting health attainment in the global north, yet it is not readily acknowledged or publicly known in contexts where technological advancements and aggressive approaches to disease prevention are championed and accepted as normal.[33] The configurations of biopower obscure the iatrogenesis of the system as a whole, normalizing it.

Medicalization, as a constituent element of modernity, transforms human experience by defining more and more aspects of that experience as diagnosable illnesses or conditions meriting the attention of medical professionals. Lewis's critique of the new global health movement demonstrates how medicalization enlarges the number of people around the globe who see and understand themselves as individuals in need of complex, expensive, pharmaceutically enhanced medical treatments. Medicalization increases the number and severity of the interventions practiced on individuals in the name of health, and normalizes such interventions as ordinary experience.[34]

Charles Briggs, along with Lewis and Illich, suggests that the issue is not the provision of health care globally, but the emphasis on and appropriation of certain forms of technologically intensive biomedicine and the values that are embedded in them (as well as the capital and resources required for their use). Lewis is not interested in ending efforts in global public health but wants to recognize and account for the "complications and large-scale trade-offs" in "future policy and funding decisions."[35] My point is not to set modern medicine against traditional healing and to consider which has more to offer those suffering ill health. Nor is the point to identify the supplanting of traditional knowledges by modern technocratic methods as a cultural tragedy. Rather, my aim here is to reiterate that modernity, in all its manifestations, is double-edged. In affluent contexts saturated with biomedical values, we tend not to see what Lewis identifies as the side effects of biomedicine as a whole, because we are already invested in and normalized by its institutional reach. The crisis over health care and private insurance in the United States (addressed by legislation in 2010) has caused some recognition of the linkages between health care and capitalism and the sociocultural impact of a technology-dependent health-care infrastructure, but probably not enough to really motivate a recognition of the iatrogenesis endemic to the system. This is because the problem is understood as one of access to the system, rather than within the constraints of the system and its implicit values.

Foucault pointed out that medicalization emerges as a strategy for the management of life in the new biopolitics of modernity. The personal regulation of bodies through discipline has become a hallmark of modern embodiment in many contexts of the global north, where individuals go to great lengths to form and maintain their bodies according to medicalized models of comportment and fitness. This modern disciplinary embodiment differs from nonmodern forms in part through its dependence on medicalization. Lewis identifies several developments in "medical biopower . . . as a global force" that have become evident since Foucault's death in 1984, one of which is "the exponential increase in biotechnology."[36] If we, like Lewis, understand pharmaceuticals to fall under the rubric of biotechnology, as do diagnostic imaging and other testing techniques, we can see that medicalization itself has intensified significantly in the later twentieth century and into the twenty-first. The ubiquitous medicalization currently characteristic of U.S. medicine is evident in the typical, widespread use of preventive medicines and extensive, routine screening for disease.

These practices are justified through the language of risk. I discuss theories of risk at length in chapter 4. Here I want to briefly introduce how medicalization is related to risk and also how this relationship plays out in global north/south relations. Charles Briggs explores how risk figures in relation to modernity in the context of epidemic disease in the global south. Writing about the Venezuelan cholera epidemic in the 1990s, he states, "The practices that place populations 'at risk' from cholera seem to emerge from tradition and culture, thereby extracting the epidemic from its historical and political-economic context." The same could be said for HIV/AIDS. Much of John Iliffe's book *The African AIDS Epidemic* is argued against the idea that the epidemic in Africa is worse than elsewhere in the world as a result of indigenous or traditional cultural practices ("dry sex," for example). He shows, instead, as does Helen Epstein in *The Invisible Cure,* how the epidemic was linked to the effects of modernization efforts in Africa in the twentieth century, specifically to migratory routes for laboring men and armies and to vaccination campaigns.[37]

In addition, Iliffe argues that among the factors placing Africans at risk of HIV/AIDS were the structural adjustment policies of the 1970s, which forced impoverished governments to economize on health services by forcing user fees, among other practices. These policies "did less to raise money than to deter the poor from using" health services and, by extension, to keep HIV/AIDS obscured as an emerging disease during the decade that it grew to epidemic proportions. Briggs suggests a similar linkage between illness and modernity in Venezuela: "If we equate modernity with the penetration of the nation-state into the delta and the lives of its residents and resource exploitation by national and transnational corporations, then cholera emerged in the historical memory of people in the delta precisely as a part of the experience of modernity."[38]

Figurations of risk within medicalization imagine that individual and population vulnerability can be managed through monitoring, preventive techniques, and scientifically informed approaches to bodily regulation. While it is true that these basic elements of public health policy and practice do contribute to improved health outcomes in many instances, they often ignore health risks emerging from political economy, unequal social relations, and other aspects of the social formation not directly under the control of individuals. Charles Briggs points out that the field of health promotion began adopting social marketing techniques in the 1970s and 1980s. He labels these as "neoliberal schemes of privatization" that figure health care "as a commodity sold by private institutions to 'consumers' who make rational, knowledgeable, self-interested choices."[39] The emphasis on "personal responsibility" in health care also implies that those who become ill are victims of their own negligence: they did not take care of themselves through adequate preventive practices, self-surveillance, or bodily discipline. In the United States, the emerging recognition that income affects individuals' ability to exercise their health-care rights does little to dispel the dichotomy structuring the field of signification: health is a normal state of the body to be maintained through technology-intensive regimes of management and surveillance, while illness is the effect of resistance to modernity, ignorance, and lack of discipline. Modern peoples manage their individual health for the good of their communities; nonmodern folk put everyone at risk.

In these ways, citizens of the global south can be figured as the repositories of health risks that threaten those in the global north. There is widespread resistance to the theory that HIV initially developed in equatorial Africa from those who are suspicious that such a version fits too readily into ideological constructions identifying Africa as the "dark continent" (or "heart of darkness") harboring diseases that will kill Europeans and North Americans. Many contemporary disease outbreaks or anticipated outbreaks are imagined to threaten the U.S. population from afar: sudden acute respiratory syndrome (SARS, from China), bird flu (H5N1, from Asia), Ebola and Marburg viruses (from equatorial Africa), West Nile virus (WNV, from Uganda), and, most recently, swine flu (H1N1, from Mexico). That these diseases may have been incubated elsewhere does not diminish this critique, as the "outbreak narratives" that articulate the risk fantasies of the global north neglect its contribution to the ill health of citizens of the global south through the structured inequalities of globalization. Indeed, Bradley Lewis anticipates an increase in the biomedical side effects experienced by people in the global south as a result of the new global health movement. Iatrogenesis may be a significant factor in modern health-care systems as they scale up in impoverished countries around the world. Lewis identifies capital- and technology-intensive biomedicine as itself a potential risk to the health of the people it is meant to improve, suggesting that conditions of modernity make the assessment of true health risks difficult because the mechanisms involved in identifying risks also create them.[40]

Conclusion

Medicalization is thus fully consonant with the reflexivity Anthony Giddens and Ulrich Beck characterize as distinctively modern. Other aspects of modernity discussed earlier clearly contribute to the shape of medicalization in the current period. The normalization of medicalization in the global north depends upon the disembedding of individuals described by Charles Taylor, Anthony Giddens, and Ulrich Beck, primarily because medicalization is individualizing and requires people to develop rationalistic, purposeful relationships with their bodies. Medicalization as a norm of behavior also depends on trust in abstract, expert systems, as described by Giddens. Subjecting the self to biomedical perspectives and care has become central to contemporary structures of feeling and contributes to modern social imaginaries, although medicalization is not discussed by either Raymond Williams or Charles Taylor in this regard. Medicalization demands new ways of thinking about the body in relation to the emerging concept of health and new ways of living in the body that are unthought but nevertheless learned and passed on. Medicalization demands that embodied behaviors always be related to ideals about health and the professional expectations of health-care practitioners.

Through medicalization, risk becomes a primary conceptual frame for modern subjectivity. But risks are perceived through distinctly cultural lenses, which focus attention on certain dangers while ignoring others. Biomedicine replicates the value and belief systems of industrialized countries and tends to downplay the risks of its own systemic effects, especially iatrogenesis. This theme—medicine as pharmakon—pervades the discussion provided in *Viral Mothers,* suggesting time and again that the products of modern bioscientific efforts offer poisons along with treatments. These poisons can often be accounted for and counteracted in the affluent medical systems of the global north but prove to be more of a challenge in the global south.

If biomedicine is blind to the iatrogenesis it engenders, it also ignores the disciplinary regimes it demands. These two effects of modernity—discipline and iatrogenesis—contribute to the fundamental situation of the viral mother. Their ironic effects influence both her negative image and the strategies created to save her.

PART 2

Risk and Purity
in the Contemporary
United States

CHAPTER 4

Theorizing Risk, Imagining Purity

RISK BECAME a focus of social and cultural analysis in the 1980s, as scholars identified it as an emerging concern of late modernity. The robust academic literature on risk includes a subcategory devoted to risk discourses in medicine. Some of the contributions discuss how to better communicate risk as a method of improved management of natural and constructed dangers to human life.[1] Others address the rise of a "risk epidemic" in medical publications and try to ascertain both the causes and effects of such a phenomenon.[2] My concerns in understanding perceptions of risk in relation to breastfeeding are related to these issues. I focus on the primary theoretical literature on risk as a way of addressing how breastfeeding is perceived as risky maternal behavior in the United States. Questions about effective risk communication concern a secondary level of application and assume that specific, quantifiable risks exist as epistemologically stable facts. What is of interest to me is the first-order identification of particular risks associated with infant feeding, the obvious public neglect of other risks identified by biomedical research, and the overall influence of risk as a paradigm regulating modern maternal behaviors.

In this part of *Viral Mothers,* I examine why certain dangers are identified and experienced as risks, while other well-researched dangers are not perceived similarly. In addition, risk organizes ideas about maternal embodiment that are significant to perceptions of maternal purity. Risk selection is important to understanding cultural expectations of maternal purity, but exploring how risk perceptions influence constructions of modern motherhood also necessitates other approaches to risk. As I will discuss below, the focus on risk selection embraces the culturalist approach to risk associated with the work of anthropologist Mary Douglas, while the focus on risk and modernity relies on the "risk society" ideas developed by sociologists Anthony Giddens and Ulrich Beck. Both approaches inform my understanding of "Risk and Purity in the Contemporary United States."

Introducing Risk

Research on the cultural uses of risk, in particular how it functions in concrete contexts and how it is related to the fundamental beliefs and institutions of specific cultures, was developed initially by Mary Douglas and Aaron Wildavsky in their 1982 book *Risk and Culture*. In that text, Douglas and Wildavsky were interested in the perceived risks attached to technological development and environmental degradation, asking specifically "why, at this time, pollution has been singled out for special concern" as a social risk?[3] Developing this question, they ask, "How can we explain this sudden widespread, across-the-board concern about environmental pollution and personal contamination that has arisen in the Western world in general and with particular force in the United States?"[4] Their answer at the time was that the historical particularities of American culture, as well as specific changes in the economy and the workforce in the third quarter of the twentieth century, created an ideal context for the perception of pollution risks: "Since perceptions of environmental impurities form part of a critique of the existing social system, we would expect people who stand outside industrial society [such as the increasing number of educated workers in the service sectors of the economy] to be more concerned about risk from pollution."[5]

Slightly more than a quarter of a century later, it would seem that concerns about the environment have intensified, evidenced, for example, in exploding interest in organic foods and other products deemed to be natural or unadulterated, as well as the burgeoning attention paid to individual body burden of environmental contaminants. In keeping with this attention to environmental pollutions, health has become a focal point for risk discourses.[6] This observation fits with the claims made by Edward J. Burger Jr. in "Health as a Surrogate for the Environment," in which he demonstrates that many of the significant political fights made and won concerning the environment in the 1960s and 1970s were articulated with respect to the health effects of environmental degradation or contamination. Human health is often used rhetorically to press environmentalist claims, as opposed to more direct arguments concerning the earth itself.[7]

Health also takes center stage in the contemporary experience of risk for other reasons: the increasing scientization of medical practice through the elevation of what is called evidence-based medicine, the development of an increasingly successful number of chemical approaches to disease, and an extended life span that makes chronic illnesses like heart disease, cancer, and stroke "the most important health risks we [U.S. citizens] face."[8] Indeed, the end of the twentieth and start of the twenty-first centuries witnessed an increasing number of so-called lifestyle diseases coming to the foreground of medical attention in the United States and much of the global north—obesity, mood disorders, sleep disorders, to name a few—all of which constitute conditions that previously stood outside of medical practice or were not considered major health risks. Risks to health become more pressing in contexts of increasing medicalization, in which prevention becomes a more insistent focus of clinical practice and public health education. That is, risks to health become more salient—or, in more radical terms, are more likely to be created—within highly medicalized cultures. Modern, medicalized bodies attend to the risks identified by expert systems and professionals. Modern individuals heed medical advice about health as a matter of course.

Critics within medicine point to specific changes in medical practice that encourage an emphasis on risk. Epidemiologist Philip Alcabes argues, "Risk reduction is the new religion," a public health moralism ushered in by (1) the abandonment of social-reform epidemiology, which emphasized social determinants of health over individual behavior, and (2) the publicizing of too many studies that make people think they can control for health risks in their personal habits, even though the actual improvements to health are evident only across populations. These changes to the practice of epidemiology have led to a belief that one can lead a "risk-free life," a belief that seems to increase perceptions of risks to health, in addition to constituting a fully individualized approach to public health problems.[9] John-Arne Skolbekken suggests that the increasing number of medical publications using the language of risk has multiple causes, one of which is the "present statistical paradigm of scientific medicine" and the methodology of biostatistics, recently improved through developments in computer technology. Pointing out that these are only tools, he argues that health promotion, the strategy of public health agencies to improve health and wellness, is a likely cause of the current emphasis on risk: "Our belief in past successes has left us with a substantial optimism as we take on new challenges in the pursuit of eliminating risks and promoting health. The elimination of various infectious diseases as the major cause of death in the western world in the first half of this century, has undoubtedly generated such optimism, and may be seen as one of the reasons for the raise [*sic*] of health promotion as an important ideology of health."[10]

Understanding how risk itself contributes to or is intensified within medicalization provides only a partial interpretation of the significance of risk in discourses about breastfeeding. As a maternal behavior brought (rather insistently) into the domain of medicine through modernity, breastfeeding is a likely focus of medical management through the analysis of risk. Yet medical research has, in the last twenty-five years or so, consistently demonstrated the contributions that breastfeeding makes to maternal and infant health. An understanding of risk in relation to breastfeeding has to account for why breastfeeding, in the context of such research, continues to draw attention to its potential risks, while the risks of not breastfeeding seem publicly denied or neglected, at least in the United States. This is especially interesting given current attention to organic, natural, and local foods and increasing skepticism about the industrial food system. An overview of current approaches to risk demonstrates the value of a culturalist analysis in addressing this particular issue.

Approaching Risk

Sociologist Deborah Lupton provides a useful categorization of various theories of risk, as she efficiently and cogently distinguishes different approaches by identifying their points of convergence and divergence.[11] She identifies four primary paradigms for addressing risk in contemporary theory: (1) technical-objective, which is a primarily scientific and managerial approach; (2) risk society, whose main theorists are Ulrich Beck and Anthony Giddens and which is prominent in sociological and political analyses; (3) cultural, identified primarily with Mary Douglas's work and anthropology; and (4) governmentality, associated with the later theories of Michel Foucault. Each paradigm has a different premise concerning the reality of risks and the cultural contribution that makes some dangers stand out as risks to particular constituencies. For example, in the technical-objective paradigm, risks are assessed by scientific means and managed by bureaucracies. The technical-objective approach is based on the idea that real risks exist and their effect on populations can be managed with statistical and other scientific methodologies. For Beck and Giddens, late modern (or late industrial) societies are associated with greater risks, either because of the global reach of technological advancement or because individuals in late modern societies perceive greater risks around them as a result of the enlargement of the technological sector and its social impacts. Thus for these theorists a central paradox of modernity is that the same technological developments that make possible longer lives and better quality of life for many people also involve the understanding or perception of heightened risk and vulnerability.

The cultural and governmentality approaches move even further in the direction of social constructionism, in that they understand specific risks as less connected to objective dangers than to the social formations through which they are identified. In Douglas and Wildavsky's work, particular cultures select specific risks among the panoply of possible risks because those selected represent, symbolically and materially, risks to the institutions on which the culture depends. Real dangers do exist, but out of them people create risks that are socially recognized and attended to because of the cultural beliefs and pressures of community life and its demands on individuals to conform to shared beliefs. Indeed, Douglas and Wildavsky argue that there is no objective perception of risk. In this sense, their work is diametrically opposed to the technical-objective approach.[12] In their view, risks are constructed against a backdrop of ideals, not a natural world of real risks that can be chosen over other, more illusory, dangers: "When we say, therefore, that a certain kind of society is biased toward stressing [a particular risk], we are not saying that other kinds of social organization are objective and unbiased but rather that they are biased toward finding different kinds of dangers."[13] Risks are always both real and socially constructed in this view, as their identification as risks has less to do with actual scientific verifiability than with the social contexts that identify them as risks and elaborate their meanings.

The governmentality approach treats risk as entirely socially constructed. *Governmentality* refers to the process through which modern societies enforce elaborate systems of social regulations that are integrated into the subjective experience of people such that they regulate themselves. Governmentality is an overarching mechanism of biopolitics and discipline, and is associated with modern systems of state government and modern expectations for citizenship and personhood. Because governmentality is what one could call the management style of neoliberalism, which in Lupton's words "champions individual freedom and rights against excessive intervention of the state," the regulation of individuals is obscured as regulation or social control because they initiate it and manage it themselves. Expert knowledges are key vectors for governmentality, since they "provid[e] guidelines and advice by which populations are surveyed, compared against norms and rendered productive." Significantly, individual management of risk becomes, in this theoretical paradigm, a moral barometer: "Risk-avoiding behavior, therefore, becomes viewed as a moral enterprise relating to issues of self-control, self-knowledge and self-improvement. It is a form of self-government, involving the acceptance and internalization of the objectives of institutional government."[14]

The experience of the technological-objective approach to risk is ubiquitous in the United States; it is there every time one sits down to read a newspaper or watch a television news program. Identifying new risks and the possibilities for their mitigation are staples of health and environment reporting. Indeed, the technological-objective approach undergirds public health initiatives like the 2004 U.S. National Breastfeeding Awareness Campaign (NBAC). The NBAC, in promoting breastfeeding, sought to characterize formula feeding in terms of risk rather than breastfeeding as a health enhancement. As I will show in chapter 6, controversy erupted over the use of risk discourses in breastfeeding promotion. The technological-objective approach fails to adequately interpret the controversy, primarily because it depends on a scientific approach to evidence as its mode of managing risk. Because the controversy involved disagreement over the scientific evidence cited in the campaign, identifying the controversy as one of risk selection allows us to see how adjudicating the conflict through a scientific assessment of the purported reality of risk does not address the core issues involved in perceiving risks in the first place.

The technical-objective approach to risk depends on a universalizing rational-choice model of decision making that Douglas and Wildavsky reject as a plausible explanation of how individuals determine their behavior with respect to risk.[15] They find that "the exercise of rational choice must include selection of focus, weighting of values, and editing of problems."[16] These are all elements of the perception and identification of risks, and demonstrate the cultural specificity of risk selection.

Culturalist, governmentality, and risk society theories all offer important critical approaches to understanding the social meanings of risk and the relation of risk to the social formation and its interests. For example, instead of seeing public health efforts like the NBAC as a legitimate attempt to educate citizens of the health implications of infant feeding practices, governmentality theorists are more likely to characterize public health strategies as mechanisms of social control. The governmentality approach suggests that the purpose of the campaign was to enforce new normative expectations of maternal behavior concerning infant feeding practices.

Risk society theorists might address the ways in which the development of infant formulas helped to free women from the traditional demands of maternity and enter market work on a more equal basis with men, but also introduced new risks for infant health and welfare, most of which are difficult to assess or accurately determine. Thus, in this perspective, equivocations concerning the scientific evidence for breastfeeding's contributions to health are an effect of the modernization of infant feeding. Anxiety about infant feeding risks is displaced onto the social context, where there are heated debates about whether common practices of modern life, like feeding babies manufactured infant formulas, are really risky behaviors worthy of full-fledged public health campaigns.[17] Rather than simply accept new risks associated with infant feeding as acceptable trade-offs for women's participation in the labor force, for enhanced equality in labor markets and civil society, and for men's greater participation in child care and parenthood, the risks of formula feeding remain a problem for society and are thus the focus of significant, yet ambivalent, attention.[18]

Selecting Risk

While both the governmentality and risk society approaches offer compelling interpretations of the risk scenarios discussed in the chapters on West Nile virus and the NBAC, neither approach helps us to understand how groups identify particular risks and not others within the context of comparable scientific evidence or expert knowledge.[19] As I will show in chapter 6, Rebecca Kukla's analysis of the NBAC, influenced by governmentality theory, depends upon an initial rejection of scientific claims concerning the risks of formula feeding. But governmentality's interpretive power is not oriented toward the assessment of the plausibility of medical knowledge in order to make a case for certain risks over others as real dangers. If all knowledge is implicitly about power, then how does anyone ever use scientific data to inform personal practices (as all of us moderns, rightly or wrongly, do)? To determine that we are all just dupes of neoliberalism does not really get us very far in understanding how West Nile virus is perceived to be a threat to breastfeeding infants. Both the governmentality and risk society approaches can show us how public health debates over infant feeding are invested in larger social anxieties (and regulatory mechanisms) concerning maternal behavior and women's changing roles, as well as how the risks of infant feeding are implicated in the transformation of infant care in the modern period. But neither theory offers a satisfying explanation of why the widespread publication of scientific evidence about the health contributions of breastfeeding and the risks of formula use continues to be met with the concern that such evidence will make mothers feel guilty about their maternal practices rather than with calls to break down the social barriers that make guilt a common response to the inability to follow medical advice. Neither theory explains the cultural consensus that shuns biomedical information about risks to not breastfeeding. This issue is clearly at stake in investigating why West Nile infection through breastfeeding, an obscure *potential* mechanism of infection that never actually caused an infection, became the focus of media attention in the fall of 2002. Relating this intense interest in a possible breastfeeding risk to the controversy concerning the represented risks of formula feeding in the NBAC is one main focus of this part of *Viral Mothers.*

Understanding these issues and their connections requires a theory that addresses why some risks and not others are identified by specific cultures and groups as worthy of widespread attention. In the process of the analysis, I examine how guilt operates in risk discourses about breastfeeding—as well as in the very public contestation of their meaning—to manipulate the representation of scientific evidence about infant feeding. The articulation of guilt in defense of replacement feeding justifies the repudiation of biomedical evidence. Consequently, understanding risk discourses about infant feeding must address a generalized cultural denial about plausible, scientific findings. The theoretical perspective addressing these complex issues cannot itself be invested in the notion that science is the definitive arbiter of risks, given that it is precisely the question of scientific evidence that is at issue. Instead, the problem is fundamentally rhetorical: what kind of consensus makes it possible to question scientific findings, when science as a value system is otherwise prized culturally? Analyzing risk selection helps to understand how scientific information itself functions rhetorically in identifying and responding to risks.

Anthropological perspectives on risk, exemplified in the cultural approach, do not single out modernity as an intensifier of risk. Pollution risks, for Douglas, exist in every culture, although they are different in each, specific to the particular context and its institutions. While modernization is clearly an issue with respect to the changing social meanings of breast-feeding, culturalist approaches to pollution avoid treating the contemporary period—or specific nations of the global north—as special with respect to how pollution risks function in cultural systems. In this analysis, modernization does change some of the conversations and dilemmas around risk because it introduces scientific evidence as new data in the cultural selection of risks. The culturalist approach understands that "private individuals . . . choose not to be aware of every danger" and "the social environment, the selection principles, and the perceiving subject [are] all one system."[20] Thus within the culturalist approach, scientific evidence concerning risk is simply one element of a cultural system concerning the perception and experience of pollution risks.[21] Such evidence operates in some contexts much like the magical systems of the so-called primitive cultures, in that it provides the reason for otherwise unaccountable phenomena. The culturalist approach helps explain individuals' decisions within communities of common practice and belief.

In addition, the culturalist theory of risk selection is helpful in analyzing the heightened focus on embodied purity for expectant and new mothers. Douglas's approach directs attention to how particular kinds of risks become salient in specific social formations, why cultural anxieties condense in idiosyncratic ways. But the analysis of purity discourses leads in other directions as well, especially since environmental contamination is a key focus of risk society theorists and their understanding of modernity's side effects. Purity discourses emerge in the context of what Ulrich Beck has termed the "risk society," the development of industrial society to the point where it produces risks that put its own existence into doubt.

Risk Society

Risk society theorists accept the baseline reality of the invisible risks to health and well-being caused by environmental contaminants, radiation, and other forms of pollution. Their innovation, in the context of risk theories overall, is to point out how modernization itself produces risks that threaten human survival. These industrially produced risks are the heart of reflexive modernity in Beck's terms. Bradley Lewis similarly identifies the side effects of technology-intensive biomedicine as a downside to modern regimes of health. Pregnant and lactating women become the focus of attention within risk societies because fetuses and infants are seen as the innocent victims of modernity's side effects. They become exemplars of humanity in its most pristine form, and women's bodies are the vehicles for their contamination.

As I discuss in detail chapters 8 and 9, the image of infants contaminated by nursing mothers alarms breastfeeding advocates, who worry that mothers will abandon breastfeeding as a result of the use of such representations to shock audiences into political action. These images are staples of risk society discourses, used as simple examples to demonstrate existing risk or, early in Beck's *Risk Society,* to show the cynicism of current political attempts to explain away body burdens of toxic substances.[22] The images are meant to be alarming: the idea of mothers contaminating infants is thought to go against nature and is used to demonstrate the terrible risk hazarded by human babies. Yet the images, even those in contexts meant to be supportive of maternal nursing, function in relation to expectations of maternal purity that are impossible precisely because of global industrial pollutants. The ideal that mothers should be pure has a long history, its meanings enhanced and intensified by modernity's increasing perception of risk.

Beck makes the point that risk is an idea conveyed through knowledge. Indeed, he writes, "It is not clear whether it is the risks that have intensified, or our *view* of them. Both sides converge, condition each other, strengthen each other, and because risks are risks in *knowledge,* perceptions of risks and risks are not different things, but one and the same."[23] Because risks are anticipated but often not experienced directly (we do not feel the polybrominated diphenyl ethers [PBDEs, which are flame retardants] in our bodies but learn about their potential effects from informational sources), they are constructed objects of knowledge that are all the more powerful because the actual effects they point toward are unknown and, in some senses, unknowable.[24] Imaging techniques and other technologically advanced screening techniques put maternal and fetal bodies under medical scrutiny during gestation, and tight surveillance of mothers' prenatal behaviors has become a norm in cultures of the global north, in an attempt to forestall the uncertainties of pregnancy. In true risk-society fashion, mothers increasingly draw attention as both victims and contaminators.

Beck makes the point that scientists are ill-equipped to deal socially with risk discourses, in part because they perceive laypeople as "hopelessly irrational." He writes that the "technical elite" treat the public as if it were made up of "engineering students in their first semester": "They only need to be stuffed full of technical details, and then they will share the experts' viewpoint and assessment of the technical manageability of risks, and thus their lack of risk." Indeed, he accuses science and scientists of being the progenitors and "legitimating patrons" of the risks that they try to manage through technological means. Specifically, scientists do not have the right kind of knowledge to recognize as valuable the risk perceptions of ordinary people, in part because they do not recognize the value-laden nature of their own speech: "statements on risks contain statements of the type *that is how we want to live*—statements, that is, to which the natural and engineering sciences *alone* can provide answers only by overstepping the bounds of their disciplines."[25]

Conclusion

That women might seek a perception of their embodiment opposed to—or merely not the same as—the one made available through the intensive regime of prenatal care in the global north is often understood as sheer lack of reason or good sense. It seems impossible to refuse risk as a way of experiencing the body within modern medicalization; there is always another test to diagnose or screen, another way to anticipate and thus ward off negative outcomes. In Beck's presentation of risk society, there does not seem a way out of the risk scenarios built into late modernity. His perspective seems to accept a high level of medicalization as normal and necessary to combat the side effects of industrialization. In my view, such a conclusion does not attend enough to the side effects of medicalization itself, the iatrogenesis built into technically sophisticated and pharmaceutically driven medical practice. It does seem to me that fully opting out of the current social formation and its requirements is impossible, but strategic responses that refuse the body's codification as a data set are appealing.

In the chapters that follow, I discuss how risk itself, and then purity, are figured in relation to controversies over breastfeeding in the United States. The cumulative effect of this part of *Viral Mothers* is a significant critique of the dominant paradigms for portraying breastfeeding as a risky behavior and for idealizing the impossible purity imagined as achievable for mothers and mothers-to-be. Throughout these chapters, and the concluding ones in the part on denial and choice, there is a looming question about what to do with knowledge of existing risk that nevertheless seems to do little good for the women and children whom the knowledge is meant to help. My analysis does not fully answer this question, but moves toward it by rethinking risk as a product of knowledge and asking how cultural consensus affirms or denies the meaning of risk in the public domain. By examining risk as a cultural construction that needs consensus to be established as real, we may find ways to reorient expectations of maternal embodiment and behavior that currently frame mothers' struggles globally.

CHAPTER 5

West Nile Virus

ON OCTOBER 4, 2002, a short article about West Nile virus and breastfeeding appeared in my local newspaper, the *Roanoke Times*. The headline was "Infant Likely Got West Nile in Breast Milk." It read in its entirety:

ATLANTA—Federal health officials said Thursday that a Michigan infant has the West Nile virus and probably got it from the breast milk of his infected mother.

The child is healthy and his mother is recovering, the Centers for Disease Control and Prevention said. The CDC said it was virtually certain the virus came from breast milk, though there is no way to be completely sure.

Doctors stressed that breast milk is the healthiest food for babies and that mothers shouldn't quit nursing because of West Nile fears.

Last week, when the case was being investigated, the CDC urged new mothers with the virus to talk with their doctor about whether to continue breast-feeding.[1]

The article was also published on CNN.com, from which I printed it the same day. The CNN article, indicating an Associated Press byline, is a bit longer than the one appearing in the *Roanoke Times*.[2] According to the full article, this particular mother received a blood transfusion on the day she gave birth as well as the following day. Subsequently, the donor blood showed "signs of contamination" with West Nile virus, a fact that was confirmed on the CDC Web page discussing the case.[3]

What would it be like to be a new mother in fall 2002 in America, having just given birth in a highly technical institution (the hospital) and embarking on an entirely new embodied experience, breastfeeding, reading this article after a night of little sleep?[4] Would I ask to be tested for West Nile virus? Would I worry if I'd been blueberry picking a few days or weeks before (as I did before I gave birth to my second child)? How would I feel about breastfeeding? What would I know? How, in other words, would I assess the risk, to myself and to my baby, of West Nile virus, or anything, for that matter, having to do with breastfeeding?

This chapter concerns representations of the risk of West Nile virus infection through breastfeeding, although, of course, its aim is broader than the specific case analyzed here. I address risk discourse as a primary way in which people encounter representations of breastfeeding in the United States. Why, given current scientific attention to and evidence of the contributions that breastfeeding makes to infant and maternal health, is breastfeeding so often identified as a potentially risky behavior? In the United States and elsewhere, a general cultural resistance to the scientific evidence of the risks of not breastfeeding fuels public debates about infant feeding. The risks of not breastfeeding, detailed by medical research, are challenged culturally by representations that imply breastfeeding itself is risky.

Ultimately, through the course of this and the two following chapters in this part, I will argue that the general public's disinterest in admitting the risks of not breastfeeding presents a crucial answer to the limitations of breastfeeding promotion as a public health endeavor. Analyzing the American refusal to acknowledge the publicized health risks of not breastfeeding reveals how the acceptance of those risks would threaten basic institutions and the overall worldview of the culture, just as the analysis of perceived breastfeeding risks points out the cultural enforcement of women's subordination to medical authority. Medicalization as a process (and medicine as an institution) triumphs each time women are encouraged to ask their doctors if it is safe for them to breastfeed. The pretense is that medical authorities make their decisions within the context of an objective base of evidence, rather than a cultural and institutional situation. In this chapter I begin this discussion by demonstrating the cultural factors feeding fears of West Nile virus infection through breastfeeding.

Background

West Nile virus was originally identified in 1937 in Uganda. In 1999, residents of New York City became ill with the first West Nile infections known in the United States. A blood-borne virus, the vector for West Nile is the mosquito, with a host range of 180 species, including birds, dogs, cats, horses, squirrels, and alligators.[5] The virus is a member of a group of viruses called the Japanese Encephalitis Serocomplex of the family Flaviridae, which exists around the globe in temperate and tropical climates. A related virus in the United States is the St. Louis encephalitis virus, "a similar flavivirus [that] caused periodic epidemics in the United States . . . [which] has subsequently [after 1975] caused no large US epidemics, possibly due to herd immunity. The fact that there are only sporadic cases of WNV in the United States suggests a similar pattern."[6] Of those infected with West Nile virus, 80 percent have no symptoms at all; almost 20 percent develop a fever and some neurological symptoms. Fewer than 1 percent of those infected develop severe West Nile fever, and fewer than that die from it. Physician John G. Bartlett, in a *Medscape* summary article, states, "The commonly quoted mortality rate for neurologic cases is 10%, but for the current epidemic in the United States it is 1.6%."[7]

Nevertheless, some localities in the United States have returned to aerial spraying and community fogging to reduce mosquito populations.[8] The Centers for Disease Control produced a series of prevention posters, including one with the caption "West Nile Virus Can Make You So Sick You Can Miss Work or Even Die." While technically true, the message sent with such a poster is that death is a likely or at least common result of West Nile fever. Bartlett's *Medscape* article notwithstanding, most public comments on WNV do not include a discussion about the possibility of herd immunity on the part of humans as a response to the West Nile "epidemic." Citizens are urged to spray themselves with DEET insect repellents and to monitor their own property and their communities for likely areas of mosquito breeding (such as standing water). Clearly, some prevention efforts are logical responses to the introduction of West Nile virus to the United States, but it is not at all clear that drastic measures to eradicate mosquito populations are warranted, given the nature of West Nile fever to infect most people mildly and thus to confer substantial immune advantage through natural means. But the article on breastfeeding and West Nile virus continues the overwhelming trend of most West Nile journalism at that time, which was to overstate the danger to individuals and misconstrue the nature of the disease and its origins.[9]

Breastfeeding and West Nile Virus, 2002

There are two vectors of contagion represented in the short article in my local newspaper: the one that constitutes the article's purported focus, breastfeeding, and the actual mechanism of infection of the mother, blood transfusion. I look first at how breastfeeding and its risks are represented. This short notice of a possible new health risk offers a lot of information about common perceptions of breastfeeding. First, breast milk initially figures more prominently than the activity of nursing itself. The term *breast milk* appears in the story three times, in the first three paragraphs, while *nursing* is used once (third paragraph) and *breastfeeding* once (fourth paragraph). Breast milk, we learn, can be a mechanism for viral transfer but is nevertheless a healthy food for babies. In other words, breast milk, generally thought of as good for babies, can also be bad for babies. Breast milk is separated from breastfeeding, conceptually, in the beginning of the article, although by the end there is the suggestion that one gets breast milk through breastfeeding. Mothers should not quit nursing "because of West Nile fears" but should consult a doctor if they actually have the West Nile virus.

The baby in this instance is identified as being healthy; it is the mother who is recovering. Nothing new is really going on here, as we know that breastfeeding is one way that mothers confer important protections from illness on their infants. Further investigation of the CDC Web site demonstrates that the infant was never ill but did have evidence of viral antibodies in its blood. This infant may have developed the mildest form of West Nile infection, where there are no symptoms and the individual is actually not ill, perhaps because the mother passed antibodies through her breast milk.[10]

Generally, infants are vulnerable to the same germs that their mothers come into contact with.[11] Access to maternal antibodies through breastfeeding is one way that infants ward off illnesses that both they and their mothers are exposed to. Significantly, almost all the articles about West Nile infection in the breastfeeding baby on October 4, 2002, do not mention this common medical understanding of one mechanism through which breastfeeding helps infant immunity. Indeed, breast milk contains antibodies to viruses that are not present themselves in breast milk and thus not transmitted through breastfeeding (like cold or flu viruses).[12] Yet instead of stressing the immune-strengthening properties of breastfeeding and breast milk, the articles generally focus on the potential for breastfeeding as a vector for infection.

While the CDC was "virtually certain the virus came from breast milk," it was actually "not clear how the mother became infected." Since there was contamination of the donor blood with West Nile virus, this was clearly a viable conclusion at the time; it has since been confirmed. Interestingly, the October 4, 2002, articles about breastfeeding came after a month of media reporting about the possibility of West Nile infection spread through organ donation. The October 4 articles are actually related to this thread in health reporting during fall 2002, as a group of articles on September 28, 2002, announce that the virus was found in the mother's breast milk.[13] The concern overall is with a newer virus in the United States and its emerging modes of transmission. First, with organ transplant recipients falling ill, there is concern about the organ donation system and with blood recipients. Then, with a breastfeeding mother ill with West Nile, there is concern about what is termed "vertical transmission," from mother to baby.[14] Isolating the articles on breastfeeding makes it more difficult to see that there is a generalized fear of new vectors of West Nile infection, of which breastfeeding is only one potential mechanism.

Subsequent attention to West Nile transmission through organ donation and blood transfusion has demonstrated that infection through this route is not only possible but often lethal.[15] When we look at breastfeeding as a possible route for transmission, we see that the potential risk to the baby emerges from the situation of modern, hospitalized childbirth and the routinization of donor blood transfusion for mothers who experience anemia postpartum or significant blood loss during delivery. The same advances in medical practice that may have saved this mother's life have made her body into a conduit for viral infection in ways unimaginable in previous historical periods when transfusion was not possible. Yet in the reporting on October 4, 2002, donor blood transfusion is represented as the routine, normal behavior, while breastfeeding is not. In addition, breastfeeding is presented as what is best for babies, but not always. There is an implicit alternative for mothers who wish or need to cease breastfeeding, but blood transfusions are part of an unexceptional backdrop of medical care for childbearing women. Thus, the common understanding of breastfeeding as a health-promoting practice is challenged by the focus on dangers associated with the transfer of bodily fluids. Oddly, we see no attempt to find out if breastfeeding has been identified as a route of WNV transmission in the areas of Africa where it is endemic and where breastfeeding is a widespread practice and often of long duration.[16] Instead, breastfeeding is likened to organ donation and blood transfusion, the exchange of bodily fluids and/or tissue between two separate individuals that is mediated by medicine as a technical practice.

The analogy should give us pause. Such an analogy takes breastfeeding out of its context as a human relationship between mother and child and makes it a medical transaction presided over by a physician. Of course, this is in many ways what breastfeeding has become in modern industrialized societies, but here we see a representation that enforces this meaning at a cultural level. And not only is breastfeeding estranged from its other meanings by the analogy, but organ donation and blood transfusion are naturalized by their association with breastfeeding. This is because breastfeeding is idealized as a natural form of infant feeding, which moderates the technical strangeness of organ donation and blood transfusion through the association. If organ donation and blood transfusion are really like breastfeeding, then they too are natural practices. That all three are medicalized fits a paradigm in which nature is subordinated to the technical expertise of physicians.

In addition, advances in medical research have guided us to think of breast milk as a substance replete with important nutrients and immune factors and the necessary ratio of fats to sugars to proteins for growing human babies. As neonatologist Nancy Wight writes, "The benefits of breastfeeding in terms of species specificity, balanced, changing nutrients and enzymes, host resistance factors, immunologic protection, allergy protection and psychosocial development, make breastmilk the most important and cost effective substance we have in medicine today."[17] In other words, advances in medical research have led us to think of breast milk as both a medicine and a food. Linked to a cultural history of lactation iconography that represents the breastfeeding mother as Madonna (the mother of Jesus, not the pop music diva), as well as to a recent history of medical breastfeeding advocacy that stresses the natural purity of breast milk in contrast to the easy bacterial contamination of infant formulas, the medicinal and nutritional approaches to breastfeeding contribute to perceptions of it as a perfect and unadulterated food and medicine. Historical changes in the technical practice of medicine thus have encouraged us to imagine that West Nile virus would not be found in breast milk or transmitted through breastfeeding because breastfeeding is about the transfer of a pure substance from mother to baby.

The original newspaper article suggests that mothers should not "quit nursing because of West Nile fears," but if they have the virus and are nursing, they should contact their doctors. This information is mentioned in each subsequent article on the topic. Mothers' actions are always under the supervision of physicians and are subject to the expert knowledge of relative risk that the physician controls. What do we think this imaginary physician would say to a mother who now understands her breast milk may contain and transmit an infectious virus? Some version of "Most people bitten by an infected mosquito never get sick," which is the way that the CNN.com version of this article ends? Most infants who breastfeed from mothers ill with West Nile virus will never get sick? The *Morbidity and Mortality Weekly Report* (*MMWR*) in 2002 about breastfeeding and West Nile virus infection states, "Because the health benefits of breastfeeding are well established and the risk for WNV transmission through breastfeeding is still unknown, these findings do not suggest a change in breast-feeding recommendations."[18] This message was transmitted to the public as well as to clinicians, through the CDC's 2002 article on West Nile virus and breastfeeding, but to the public the understanding of "unknown" risk, when compared to the standard of infant formula, may be very different. After all, what are the benefits of breastfeeding when compared to an unknown risk of infection? Ask your doctor. Mothers who are ill with West Nile virus should do what all mothers in all instances should do: what their doctors tell them to do.

Doctors, of course, differ in their understanding of breastfeeding; their perceptions of its benefits and their knowledge of its management are notoriously unreliable, at least according to breastfeeding advocates. Neonatalogist Nancy Wight writes, "In all cases, the risks of breastfeeding with maternal hepatitis should be weighed against the known risks of NOT breastfeeding in each individual case and environment."[19] Similar advice concerning West Nile infection would have been appropriate and is suggested in each article about the case. Typical language is presented in the *Roanoke Times* article: "Doctors stressed that breast milk is the healthiest food for babies and that mothers shouldn't quit nursing because of West Nile fears." Yet the Michigan woman whose baby and breast milk were the focus of all this attention in fall 2002 stopped breastfeeding "on the advice of her physician when she was hospitalized."[20]

The Centers for Disease Control now states unequivocally that "scientists have found no evidence that a mother's West Nile Virus infection harms her breastfeeding infant."[21] I've never seen a newspaper article herald this information, and other Web sites provide more circumspect views of the potential for WNV to infect, and harm, breastfeeding infants. This lack of consistency may be one result of the longevity of some Web-based information, but it also demonstrates the kind of evidentiary controversies that plague breastfeeding research and promotion strategies. Even if there is little evidence of harm through breastfeeding in the context of maternal West Nile infection, there is a theoretical risk that, for virus-phobic American citizens and their physicians, can lead to the selection of West Nile infection through breastfeeding as a real danger. This is because West Nile virus is a risk that Americans, at least, see and appreciate. According to Lynn Payer, Americans are prone to seeing microbes, especially viruses, as primary threats to health.[22] Yet Americans do not see the risks of not breastfeeding, and demonstrate this blindness by questioning the scientific data behind breastfeeding promotion, while questionable West Nile virus risk scenarios flood the news.

Breastfeeding and Risk

So why was breastfeeding selected as a particular risk of the U.S. West Nile virus "epidemic" in 2002 (especially since no American infants at the time, or since, were harmed by breastfeeding from a mother infected with the virus)? The linkage between breastfeeding, organ transplantation, and blood transfusions—the three foci of the U.S. news media attention to WNV during the fall of 2002—shows us that breastfeeding is construed as a potentially dangerous, although generally beneficial, medical practice that involves the transfer of bodily fluids from one individual to another. It can go awry, however, when a foreign substance interferes with the (imagined) aseptic conditions necessary to ensure the safety of the receiving body. Indeed, with respect to organ transplantation, one could argue that the breastfeeding infant is remarkably like the individual whose immune system has been suppressed in order to receive the organ, yet an infant's incomplete immune system needs breast milk in order to survive as its immune system develops over time. The difference is that, according to medical studies that support breastfeeding's unique contribution to health, it is breast milk and the practice of nursing that confer immune advantage to the baby, not at all like the continual necessity of immune suppression for the recipients of donor organs.

How does the selection for West Nile virus and, more specifically, for specific risks attendant to breastfeeding, support a particular worldview? In the terms of Douglas and Wildavsky's original 1982 analysis, viruses constitute pollutions that are singled out by American sensibilities because they have a "fear of pollution, of cancerous contamination from external intercourse."[23] A current concern in the United States has to do with the effects of globalization on the workforce and economy. West Nile virus demonstrates concretely the difficulty of a truly global world in which germs, like capital, jobs, and workers, travel freely. Many of our recent epidemic scares—avian flu, sudden acute respiratory syndrome (SARS), West Nile virus, HIV, and, at this writing, swine flu—are perceived to threaten the United States from without. The fact that potential infection from some of these diseases involves intimate relations between people—breastfeeding, sexual relations—demonstrates the obscured intimacy and strangeness of other, technologically mediated methods of infection such as transfusion and transplantation. The threats from the outside become threats from the inside, which is another real fear—that we will not know when something gets inside us that might kill us. In the context of a society invested in a risk-free life, unexpected threats to health are experienced as threats to the core expectation of the culture that illness can be managed successfully and that health can be guaranteed.

Organ donation and blood products can be regulated. Mothers' bodies are a different story. Some of the most common problems women have with breastfeeding involve difficulty knowing that their babies get enough milk, understanding the supply-demand system that regulates milk production, and trusting themselves to feed their babies adequately. Breastfeeding as an ordinary activity of motherhood involves very basic unknowns about whether any given mother can succeed. These uncertainties about the maternal body—felt by individual mothers and exacerbated in a cultural context in which breastfeeding is not a common public practice—constitute much of the current experience of breastfeeding in the United States. Although the fall 2002 newspaper articles consistently reiterated the "known benefits of breastfeeding" even in the context of WNV, one effect of their information was to implicitly emphasize the unknown risks. While ordinary unknowns of breastfeeding are different from the unknowns of WNV, the fact that ordinary nursing is perceived to be an experience of uncertainty (especially concerning success or failure) contributes to the sense that breastfeeding is, essentially, a risky endeavor.

Moreover, decisions about risks are not made in a vacuum. They emerge from cultural circumstances and do not assess competing risks in an objective, scientific mode. Douglas and Wildavsky remind us, "In risk perception, humans act less as individuals and more as social beings who have internalized social pressures and delegated their decision-making processes to institutions. They manage as well as they do, without knowing the risks they face, by following social rules on what to ignore: institutions are their problem-solving devices." They continue, stating that "most habits, good and bad, are rooted in community life."[24]

In the United States, as in much of the global north, the institution regulating mothers' decisions about infant feeding is medicine, and more specifically pediatrics, yet mothers' experiences of risk and their initial relation to medically mediated risk decisions with respect to their babies come largely from their experience as obstetric patients. Currently most U.S. women do not fear death when they become pregnant, although numbers for maternal and infant mortality and morbidity are stratified according to race.[25] The represented risks of fetal injury or harm, however, continue to drive the medical management of pregnancy and childbirth, as well as to ensure women's complicity with its norms. The risk of doing damage to their babies (as well as fears of giving birth to babies already damaged) propels many women to demand highly technological and interventionist management of pregnancy and childbirth. Thus, the notion that childbirth is risky overrides the commonsense idea that it is nevertheless normal and thus not, in most circumstances, deserving of intense medical scrutiny. The idea that women can take advantage of medical advances yet resist the medicalization of childbirth seems culturally anomalous. Indeed, as Robbie Davis-Floyd argues, many women "participat[ing] most fully in a society's hegemonic core value system . . . are most likely to feel empowered by and to succeed within that system."[26] That is, many, if not most, U.S. women are likely to feel that births complying with the technological model of childbirth are appropriate and warranted, and that such births reflect well on their decision making as mothers. Any sense that there are unknown risks attendant to breastfeeding—in a cultural circumstance in which the known benefits are equivocated publicly—can lead to a rational choice to formula-feed, just as the possible (but unlikely) risks of childbirth encourage women to engage in interventionist practices of unknown benefit to themselves and their infants.

Conclusion

The representation of breastfeeding as a possible conduit for West Nile infection supports the existing social apparatus of medical regulation of pregnancy, childbirth, and infant feeding, in part by raising health risk fears about a practice that is culturally anomalous, but also by emphasizing mothers' subordination to the institutions that already guide maternal practice and experience. Even though the issue of West Nile infection through nursing turned out to be a red herring, it is clear that breastfeeding—and the permeable nature of maternal bodies—play an important role in demarcating widespread fears about globalization and microbes. In the United States, the anxieties elicited by fears of maternal contagion are contained and softened through the mediation of medicine, whose approval is necessary to make mothers' bodies acceptable as the environments of fetuses and infants.

CHAPTER 6

The 2004 U.S. National Breastfeeding Awareness Campaign

CONTROVERSIES OVER biomedical research supporting breast-feeding erupted publicly in the United States when the Department of Health and Human Services (DHHS) sought to launch a breastfeeding awareness campaign in 2003. Accounts and analysis of the National Breast-feeding Awareness Campaign (NBAC), especially the debate over its representation of the risks of not breastfeeding, made their way into feminist scholarship, feminist mass media, and the general mass media, even though many Americans remain unaware of both the campaign and the controversies it engendered. Much of the controversy concerned the proposed use of risk messages in the campaign. Politics, in this case, did encourage the proverbial strange bedfellows, as feminist scholars ended up criticizing the campaign in a manner echoing the forceful (and successful) complaints of infant formula companies.

This chapter concerns the relation of scientific evidence to rhetorics of risk in public health promotion efforts, especially in the context of feminist challenges to breastfeeding promotion. Analyzing the National Breastfeeding Awareness Campaign and the public controversies over its risk messages demonstrates that, at least in the United States, there continues to be ambivalence about breastfeeding's contribution to health. Equivocation over the research support for public health efforts allows various groups to argue that women are made to feel guilty over recommended practices that are not grounded in a solid evidence base. In chapter 7, I discuss how guilt operates in the context of this rhetorical puzzle. Here, I focus on equivocations concerning scientific evidence and how these function rhetorically in a public controversy concerning mothers' bodies.

I look at the initial controversy over the NBAC risk messages that led to changes in the campaign's content, and then analyze three feminist approaches to the final campaign as launched. These particular feminist commentaries on the NBAC (one that laments the weakened risk message and two that criticize the campaign as an assault on women's freedom and moral integrity), along with the original controversy concerning the campaign, illuminate a more general ambivalence in the United States over the value of scientific evidence concerning breastfeeding and formula risks. The feminist critiques of the NBAC are helpful in identifying particularly damaging rhetorical gestures of health promotion, especially the use of images of "bad mothers" to encourage women to nurse their babies. Yet they seem to suggest that if the scientific evidence for breastfeeding's benefits were stronger, risk-based social marketing might be justified.

That the value of maternal bodies and their relation to their offspring is measured through the lens of biomedicine at all demonstrates the problem of medicalization in the modern age. Of course, public health campaigns routinely use biomedical evidence as the standard by which to establish policy and promote particular behaviors in the public at large. But the controversies around the NBAC reveal more than just contemporary enmeshment in medicalized paradigms. These controversies, especially within feminist scholarship, demonstrate the difficulty of representing the value of women's bodies in anything other than medical terms. The three feminist scholars who have analyzed the controversy—the two angered by the risk messages and one who felt the campaign was unfairly tamed—all use medical evidence as the stick by which to measure the ethicality of the program (did it unfairly scare women with uncertain statistics? did it misinform women by not providing the best evidence?). The possibility of valuing breastfeeding and promoting its practice outside of a medicalized discourse of its biological contributions to health does not emerge in these arguments.

The initial controversy over the scientific basis of the NBAC's risk messages emerged within the medical perspective of public health promotion and, in that context, demonstrates a shared belief concerning the scientific case for breastfeeding. The scientists and public health personnel behind the campaign tried to address a cultural consensus that refuses to perceive not breastfeeding as a risk to health. This cultural consensus—that replacement feeding does not risk babies' health and well-being—contributes to the scenario discussed in the previous chapter on West Nile virus. Risks to breastfeeding are easier to establish when the culture does not really believe in its value, is ambivalent about scientific claims about risks of replacement feeding, and fears other risks to health more substantively because they fit more readily into cultural patterns of risk selection.

Interestingly, there seems to be a consensus that breastfeeding is beneficial. The lack of consensus concerns the flip side of this positive belief—that not breastfeeding is risky. Most breastfeeding advocates would say this pattern exists because breastfeeding is perceived to be an optimal practice but that formula feeding is understood to be normal. My analysis in this chapter concurs with this view.

Negative Risk

During fall 2003, representatives of infant formula companies met with members of the American Academy of Pediatrics (AAP) at their annual meeting in New Orleans. They were upset about a forthcoming national campaign to promote breastfeeding, part of an overall strategy begun by David Satcher, the U.S. Surgeon General under Bill Clinton, and produced by the Ad Council in cooperation with the Department of Health and Human Services under the Bush administration.[1] Formula companies were concerned about the overall strategy of the Ad Council, which was to emphasize the health risks of not breastfeeding, rather than the standard method of highlighting the health benefits of breastfeeding. Breastfeeding advocates, who in the late 1990s began to stress the importance of representing nursing as a normal, rather than optimal, method of infant feeding, were pleased with this new approach to breastfeeding promotion on a national scale.[2] The start of the campaign was delayed over a year, however, as the original May 2003 launch date was set back repeatedly until a revised set of advertisements and public service announcements (PSAs) were released in June 2004. This delay was occasioned, at least in part, by objections placed by the president and executive director of the AAP (after their meeting with formula company representatives) with DHHS representatives concerning the scientific evidence supporting the negative risk message. The revised campaign still used the new strategy of highlighting the risks of not breastfeeding but did so with muted language, fewer statistics, and without mentioning specific illnesses like diabetes or childhood leukemia.[3]

The controversy over the promotion of breastfeeding—a public health goal enumerated in the DHHS's *Healthy People 2000* goals[4]—using negative risk information turned on both the representation of risk and the status of the scientific evidence concerning the dangers of not breastfeeding. Pro-breastfeeding pediatricians were furious that AAP leaders capitulated to formula companies because they feared losing the substantial funding offered to the organization by those corporations. Their anger depended on their understanding of current medical research on breastfeeding and its unqualified demonstration of the health deficits of not breastfeeding. The leaders of the AAP, who were not affiliated with the Breastfeeding Section of the organization, were less than enthusiastic about the medical evidence for the campaign's proposed claims. Then-president of the AAP, Dr. Carden Johnston, claimed in his objections to the DHHS that the science behind the Ad Council campaign was "just not solid yet, and you know how some of these breastfeeding enthusiasts can lack objectivity."[5] AAP executive director Dr. Joseph Sanders stated a concern about inculcating mothers' guilt if their nonbreastfed children "later developed leukemia or another medical condition," suggesting that it is better to emphasize the benefits of breastfeeding than the risks of not doing so.[6]

There is much to be said about the relationship of guilt to knowledge concerning issues of health and illness, and I discuss this relation in the next chapter.[7] Here, however, I want to focus on the relation between the rhetoric of risk and scientific evidence. On the one hand, those who argued that the negative risk message is inappropriate claimed that the medical evidence is not compelling enough to warrant this kind of approach. On the other hand, those who argued that promoting breastfeeding by stressing the risks of not breastfeeding saw the scientific case for human milk as very convincing if not incontrovertible. Furthermore, for supporters of the original campaign, belief in the benefits of breastfeeding is the same as believing in the risks of replacement feeding.

The quotation from Dr. Johnston demonstrates not only his distrust of the very evidence that many of his fellow pediatricians support but also his belief that breastfeeding supporters, whether physicians or not, can lack objectivity. Breastfeeding advocates who welcomed the Ad Council campaign felt that the new approach finally acknowledged the growing body of evidence revealing "dramatically different health outcomes for populations of breast and formula-fed babies, even when controlling for socioeconomic and other factors. The new ad campaign was designed to reflect this research and to catapult the issue of breastfeeding into the same category of public health concerns as smoking, car seat use, childhood vaccinations, and SIDS prevention."[8] That this body of evidence was cited by the AAP's own Breastfeeding Section in defense of the campaign demonstrates the irony of a professional health organization split over its own internal debates about the validity of biomedical findings.

Feminist Breastfeeding Controversies

The conflicting perspectives on the scientific evidence concerning the dangers of replacement feeding are particularly apparent in feminist interpretations of the Ad Council campaign. In a lengthy article about feminism and breastfeeding in the prominent women's studies journal *Signs,* medical historian Jacqueline Wolf details the delay and transformation of the campaign, arguing that it is a breastfeeding controversy "beg[ging] for feminist voices" because feminists should "be especially concerned when the nation's foremost health organizations use the concept of choice to deny women information." This argument depends on the reader's sense of anger that a professional medical organization could side with formula companies against health. Earlier in the article she spends three full pages putting together the scientific evidence for breastfeeding's contribution to infant and maternal health. The evidence includes the broad claim that "not getting adequate human milk as an infant seems to increase infant mortality and rates of serious chronic diseases and conditions in older children and adults. These include sudden infant death syndrome (SIDS), obesity, diabetes, asthma, cardiovascular disease, leukemia, and lymphoma." Refusing to set up the United States or other countries in the global north as safe havens for formula use, Jacqueline Wolf cites a 2004 study that "found that formula-fed infants [in the United States] were five times more likely to die before their first birthday than breastfed infants" and other research suggesting that different breastfeeding rates between black and white women "might account for the race gap in infant mortality at least as much as low birth weight."[9] By the time she gets to the Ad Council controversy, she has presented the scientific evidence and also discussed current low U.S. breastfeeding rates, the lack of support for nursing among medical professionals, breastfeeding in U.S. history, the decline of breastfeeding in the late nineteenth and early twentieth centuries, and the development of La Leche League in the 1950s, all with an eye toward convincing her feminist readers that breastfeeding should garner more attention from feminists, precisely because the evidence demonstrates its value to women and children. In Jacqueline Wolf's analysis it is the culture—including some members of the medical profession—that does not support the practice of breastfeeding. All of her arguments, then, rest on the value of the scientific evidence and its veracity. Without this foundation, her discussion would be about ideology, and not about how ideology interferes with logical and science-based public health goals and programs.

Philosopher Rebecca Kukla, in an article published in the feminist philosophy journal *Hypatia* at roughly the same time as Jacqueline Wolf's *Signs* article, presents a diametrically opposed interpretation of the Ad Council campaign, although she does not focus on the delay of its launch and its changed content but on the actual campaign that was released in June 2004. Arguing against the general presumption of the campaign, that mothers choose not to breastfeed at least in part because they do not have adequate information about the risks of formula feeding, Kukla is most convincing when she discusses other reasons why women do not nurse—lack of social support, inadequate accommodations for breastfeeding at work, discomfort as a result of being a sexual assault survivor, general hostility toward the sexuality of breastfeeding, for example. Yet her vociferous arguments against the campaign are bolstered by a representation of the scientific research supporting breastfeeding's contributions to health as equivocal and overstated, especially for women in the United States and other countries in the global north: "While breast milk is clearly (ceteris paribus) the healthiest food for infants, we know that babies in developed countries routinely thrive on infant formula. We also know that most of the negative health outcomes correlated with formula feeding are also correlated with low income, parental smoking, lack of access to regular primary care, and other markers of social vulnerability. Thus infant formula *per se* cannot be plausibly construed as posing a known risk of serious harm to infants." This and other similar statements ground her claims that the Ad Council campaign participates in a broader cultural project that aims to make women responsible for health outcomes that are beyond their control.[10]

The ideological project of breastfeeding promotion that the campaign participates in also, in Kukla's analysis, forwards a distortion of women's moral responsibility to their children.

Public service announcements that focus on how breastfeeding lessens the risk of [various diseases] serve to focus mothers' moral attention on these outcomes, rather than, for instance, on social, emotional, and familial vulnerability and insecurity. Against certain social background conditions, this moral focus can constitute a distortion in moral perception. When breastfeeding is not a livable, safe option for a woman ... telling her she is harming her child and denying its natural entitlement if she doesn't do it distorts her moral understanding. This understanding makes some mothers misplace blame and shame, misunderstand their moral responsibilities and priorities, and misconstrue what good mothering requires.[11]

Yet this moral distortion is only possible to detect if the risks of not breastfeeding are minimized, as Kukla suggests. Indeed, Kukla continually talks about the "benefits of breastfeeding," using this traditional language rather than the transformed rhetoric focusing on the risks of replacement feeding. This is because she disagrees with the negative risk approach, which emphasizes possible harms. She is right to argue that public health education campaigns are normative, presenting information in order to persuade individuals about proper behaviors. But she also implies a moral responsibility to health, in this text and in her book, *Mass Hysteria: Medicine, Culture, and Mothers' Bodies.* So it is only because breastfeeding, in her view, benefits health but does not cause a significant shift in health outcomes that her interpretation of the moral distortion of the campaign is plausible. In her view the distortions of the campaign harm the autonomy and integrity of mothers—because the campaign harms mothers' ability to make choices as a result of its potential to shame them or distort their moral capacity to reason—and thus its method of breastfeeding promotion is unacceptable to feminists (and others) interested in promoting women's ethical personhood.

Joan Wolf (no relation to Jacqueline Wolf), in an article that infuriated many breastfeeding advocates, echoes many of Rebecca Kukla's concerns and offers a scathing critique of the NBAC as a participant in an ideological war against American mothers. In "Is Breast Really Best? Risk and Total Motherhood in the National Breastfeeding Awareness Campaign," Joan Wolf does not even concede benefits to breastfeeding. She argues that the evidence for risks of not breastfeeding is so weak that it does not merit a national public health campaign: "Breast-feeding research, in which the results are inconsistent and fail to account for identifiable confounding variables, provided a shaky foundation for the NBAC and reveals the inevitable uncertainty involved in evaluating evidence for public health." Indeed, Joan Wolf claims that medical breastfeeding advocates are motivated by an unwarranted belief in the superiority of breastfeeding, suggesting that the Department of Health and Human Services developed the NBAC as a result of these "axiomatic" views.[12]

A significant proportion of feminist scholarship on breastfeeding is skeptical of most of the positive impacts of breastfeeding on the health of women and children in industrialized countries.[13] This trend dominated feminist thinking on the topic during the 1990s. Both Rebecca Kukla and Joan Wolf continue this trend, suggesting there is not enough good evidence for the risk messages of the NBAC. This critique implies that if there were better, more conclusive, more scientifically persuasive evidence, such a campaign might be warranted. Jacqueline Wolf, on the other hand, argues for a minority position in feminist conversations about breastfeeding, focusing on the issue of women's misinformation by medical authorities who are themselves beholden to external interests (formula companies).[14]

The status of evidence—its accuracy and its value—lies at the core of the feminist controversy over the NBAC and its meanings for women. The purpose of the evidence in each essay is to ground the arguments about the campaign that follow. Thus the biomedical evidence cited in the campaign has a rhetorical value for these scholars, who point to it as the cause of the campaign's ethical failures or as a rationale for feminist anger at the changes in the campaign forced by formula companies and conflicts within the AAP. Even Joan Wolf admits, in her response to Judy Hopkinson's commentary on her article, "My concern is less with the science per se than with the uses to which it has been put."[15] If, for Jacqueline Wolf, ideology gets in the way of a straightforward approach to the public health necessity of promoting breastfeeding, for both Joan Wolf and Rebecca Kukla ideology informs and motivates the NBAC, which enforces women's responsibility for infant and child welfare without acknowledging the social and economic circumstances of women's subordination and lack of power over their own lives.

I share many of Kukla's and Joan Wolf's concerns about the NBAC and its representations of motherhood, particularly in the video public service announcements, which featured pregnant women riding mechanical bulls or participating in logrolling contests, with the message "You wouldn't take risks before your baby is born. Why start after?"[16] Yet I am struck by the fact that their positions are made possible by presentations of the scientific evidence diametrically opposed to that of Jacqueline Wolf, who argued strenuously that women were misled by a weakened campaign after the AAP's complaints. The equivocation among physicians and public health leaders concerning the evidence for the risks of not breastfeeding allows Kukla and

Joan Wolf to argue that the campaign's true purpose is ideological. Joan Wolf devotes much space in her article to a discussion of "total motherhood," her term for the current "moral code in which mothers are exhorted to optimize every dimension of children's lives, beginning with the womb."[17] Although she never states it outright, she implies that the NBAC was primarily motivated by cultural commitments to total motherhood as an ideology that enforces unrealistic expectations on women and even encourages them to engage in behaviors that are against their best interests.

She would not be able to make this argument without claiming that the medical evidence concerning the replacement feeding risks is inconclusive. In this, Joan Wolf relies on the scientized framework of evidence-based medicine to define the value of breastfeeding. Of course, she is engaged in criticizing a public health initiative, as is Rebecca Kukla. Arguing against the medical evidence that provides the rationale for the NBAC is rhetorically effective. Joan Wolf argues in addition that public health campaigns must be scrupulous in their use of risk discourses, given that most people are terrible at assessing risk and the use of such discourses thus functions to scare individuals into prescribed behaviors. Articulating a negative risk message in the context of inconsistent evidence of a benefit to health is, in her view, unethical.[18]

Yet Jacqueline Wolf states unequivocally, "Women have the right to know that current research indicates that breastfeeding duration matters."[19] And Jane Heinig and Judy Hopkinson responded to Joan Wolf with claims that her evidence is wrong or misleading. Heinig and Hopkinson, both academic lactation researchers, also use evidence rhetorically. In their view, the evidence, while acknowledged to be somewhat inconsistent at times (given the difficulty of defining how much breastfeeding counts as breastfeeding and how it should be classified), demonstrates substantial advantages to breastfeeding. For them the evidence supports a risk-based public health message because it identifies significant risks to not breastfeeding. In this perspective, science provides evidentiary support for a rhetoric emphasizing, even exploiting, concerns about health risks, even though both Heinig and Hopkinson express reservations about the specific risk messages in the NBAC.[20]

Joan Wolf, by suggesting that the belief in the superiority of breast milk over infant formulas is "axiomatic," claims that there is "an overwhelming consensus that breastfeeding is the optimal form of nutrition for babies." She footnotes various medical societies (American Academy of Family

Physicians, American College of Obstetricians and Gynecologists, American Dietetic Association, among others) "officially recommending breastfeeding."[21] But this supposed consensus does not seem to be realized in practice by many physicians and other health-care workers. And there is no general *cultural* consensus that science identifies substantial health risks to formula feeding, and this is demonstrated by the controversies engendered by the NBAC itself. It appears that while there is strong and widespread understanding of the benefits of breastfeeding, there is no corollary acceptance of the risks of formula feeding.

By cultural consensus I mean a widespread belief in and adherence to an idea or set of ideas that are related to specific cultural practices. As an example, one might say that there is a significant cultural consensus that cars are an essential element of the American way of life, even in the face of rising oil prices and political crises in the geographical regions that provide much of the world's oil. Americans believe in their right to cheap gas even in the face of geopolitical constraints. The cultural consensus is not simply a matter of belief, however; it is evidenced in lifestyles, expressed through common cultural practices, and structured into the built environment. The materiality of the cultural consensus concerning automobiles is evident in the organization of suburbs, the lack of public transportation infrastructure in many American communities, and the scheduling of children's activities without regard to the individual effort required to assure their attendance.

With respect to breastfeeding, one can note that according to medical organizations, breastfeeding is understood to be the most appropriate and nutritionally beneficial mode of infant feeding, but simple observation indicates that there is no cultural consensus that such information trumps other factors influencing people's infant feeding decisions and practices. American citizens might believe that breastfeeding is best for infants, but practices indicate that this belief does not alter the general consensus that formula feeding does not confer enough risk to health to be concerned about it. The fact that rates of initiation of breastfeeding are relatively high (almost three-quarters of new mothers), while breastfeeding duration up to a year remains far more difficult (about one-fifth of mothers are still breastfeeding at one year), demonstrates that practice trumps belief when it comes to infant feeding. Indeed, because breastfeeding is presented so often as a superior practice, rather than the norm, it is possible that many Americans hold both views simultaneously. Breast is best but formula is (almost) just as good.

It is cultural consensus, rather than the verifiability or accuracy of scientific data, that determines what constitutes a plausible scientific rationale for social behaviors like breastfeeding. This is a critical lesson from Mary Douglas and Aaron Wildavsky's theory of risk selection. A cultural consensus is necessary to transform data into meaningful practices, political action, or even a change in scientific theories themselves. Cultural consensus guides the selection and perception of risks, and thus the understanding of the scientific evidence that ostensibly identifies and evaluates risks.

In this particular case, one's stance with respect to the representation of risk in the NBAC depends upon one's stance with respect to the scientific case for breastfeeding as a significant—or better, critical—contribution to health. If one believes in the evidence of a critical contribution to health, then it is much more difficult to argue against a negative risk approach. When health is at stake, forceful persuasion is perceived as necessary, at least within the context of medicalization. The current cultural consensus in the United States is close to the equivocal presentation of evidence that Rebecca Kukla provides, which can be presented as *breastfeeding is better, but for many women formula feeding may be preferable, and besides, babies thrive on formula anyway.*[22] The cultural tension over public health efforts to inform women of the potential harms of not breastfeeding emerges precisely because a cultural consensus about that particular interpretation of the scientific evidence has not coalesced.

Joan Wolf's article pushes the argument against breastfeeding promotion further; in analyzing it we can see what is really at stake in this entire discussion. The troublesome aspects of her discussion are not her ideas about total motherhood, nor her complaints about the NBAC's lack of an ethical basis in good evidence, nor her suggestion that breastfeeding advocates are so committed to breastfeeding that they lose all objectivity in assessing medical studies (although this last argument surely enraged certain researchers in the field). For me the main problem is that the article is pervaded by the sense that without the support of "consistent" evidence with "strong associations" concerning the specific health contributions made by breastfeeding, as a practice of mothering it does not have any value for women at all. By extension, mothers' bodies are not unique and have no contribution to make to their offspring's well-being. Indeed, any suggestion that mothers have a special relation to offspring gestated in and fed by their bodies is forestalled by her argument that singling out mothers as different and especially responsible for their offspring's health is improper and politically dangerous.

This difficulty demonstrates how mothers' bodies are devalued within medicalized modernity. The devaluation of breastfeeding in Joan Wolf's article is a result of the framing of the issue within medicine. This point is most clear when she argues that factors other than breastfeeding may be responsible for the improved outcomes of breastfed children found in some studies. This is the "confounding factors" argument (suggested by Rebecca Kukla as well when she uses the phrase *ceteris paribus,* or "all other things being equal") in which Joan Wolf suggests that many studies demonstrating a benefit to breastfeeding cannot separate associated factors—or, more specifically, factors not in breast milk itself—in analyzing the findings. Thus, she argues, it is not possible to suggest that breastfeeding itself promotes increased intelligence, as an example, since such outcomes might be "attributable not to breast milk but to behavior linked with breast-feeding, and bottle-fed children with attentive mothers and/or fathers would be equally likely to have higher scores on intelligence tests."[23] The idea that breastfeeding involves a package of behaviors whose component parts might never be able to be separated and verified scientifically does not seem to have occurred to her. Not all the contributions of breastfeeding to health can be measured through studies of breast milk; more than simply the components of breast milk itself matter in identifying the value of breastfeeding. Breastfeeding in Joan Wolf's representation is merely a mode of getting a substance—breast milk—into babies, and practices associated with it (such as holding, eye contact with baby, increased bodily contact overall, increased attentiveness to hunger cues, among others) are perceived to be inherently transferable to all instances of infant feeding.[24]

Thus, although Joan Wolf critiques the risk society's "pervasiveness of scientific authority and an endless production of data that either support or revise existing risk determinations," which leads to a "culture of fear" and dependence on expert authorities to parse the meanings of dangerous practices and substances, she herself uses a decidedly scientized argument to criticize medical breastfeeding studies and their findings. And she also suggests, in a rather offhand way, that breast milk itself is dangerous, given that chemical contaminants have been identified in it.[25] Given her skepticism about the research concerning the health contributions of breastfeeding and breast milk, it is startling to find her mentioning without caveat scientific findings whose impact on health is often thought to be equivocal, especially after she has challenged at length the scientific evidence for the risk of not breastfeeding, evidence that is accepted, in her own accounting, by many medical organizations like the American Academy of Family Physicians and the American College of Obstetricians and Gynecologists, among others.[26]

Joan Wolf's move to identify risks of breastfeeding demonstrates again the importance of Douglas and Wildavsky's theory of risk selection. In the preceding chapter I argued that it is far easier to identify risks to a culturally anomalous practice, especially when its benefits are equivocated publicly. Known risks, whether real or imagined, are more persuasive than ephemeral benefits, especially when to get such benefits one must behave in a manner inconsistent with cultural expectations and typical practices. Given cultural tendencies to fear microbial illness and the difficulty of breastfeeding as a practice for most mothers, worry about breastfeeding risks like West Nile virus dominates the news cycle, while fears about replacement feeding are routinely dismissed and publicly contested. The cultural devaluation of women's bodies and the belief that their bodies must be regulated in order to be adequate for gestation and lactation—an issue I develop more fully in chapters 8 and 9—provides ballast for this particular algorithm of risk and responsibility.

For many health-care providers and breastfeeding advocates, discussing and publicizing the medical evidence for the benefits of breastfeeding is a way of valuing women's bodies and their contribution to their children's health. Many feminists find the focus on scientific verification of women's embodied practices distasteful.[27] Joan Wolf and Rebecca Kukla interpret scientific evidence to refute the evidence base of the NBAC, within the medical model, and thus frame the controversy as an ideological conflict over women's roles and behaviors that is staged through a scientific argument about breastfeeding. In my view, their argument ends up devaluing women as mothers, even though it does point out how public health practices and policies are enmeshed in ideologies inimical to women's liberation.

Conclusion

Joan Wolf and Rebecca Kukla are right to question the rhetorical gestures of the NBAC, which target women's individual decision making without taking aim at structural impediments to breastfeeding and which identify "bad mothers" as a way of delineating proper maternal behaviors.[28] The campaign implicitly enforces an ideal of good motherhood that does not take social circumstances into consideration and that exploits women's vulnerabilities as mothers. Their critique of the NBAC gets at a larger question applicable to all social marketing public health campaigns: can individuals be educated to behave in ways that contribute significantly to health and well-being? What kind of message is effective in changing behaviors? What are the ethical bases of a risk-based message? How should governmental agencies promote practices identified as health-care priorities?

Other Ad Council campaigns have conveyed effective, risk-based messages. Many of us no longer allow friends to drive while intoxicated, most of us wear our seat belts, and we know that people are responsible for forest fires. Why is breastfeeding perceived to be different as a public health issue? Why shouldn't public health campaigns tell women (and others) what will happen with greater frequency if they do not breastfeed their babies? Joan Wolf points out that obesity-prevention programs involve some of the same moral imperatives as the NBAC, and she also argues they are based on similarly flawed scientific evidence. Again, the ethical argument against public health initiatives that rely on risk messages grounds itself in an argument about equivocal scientific evidence. Breastfeeding is perceived by some as different from other health-care priorities—not warranting a risk message with the invocation of dire consequences—because it lacks a cultural consensus confirming the scientific evidence about its positive health outcomes.

I agree with Rebecca Kukla that most women who do not breastfeed are aware that formula feeding is not as healthy as breastfeeding. Women refrain from breastfeeding because of a host of cultural, economic, and social-structural issues, not primarily because of a lack of information.[29] Kukla strongly condemns the Ad Council's overall strategy in the NBAC, which she argues "is built upon the presumption that women *have* the real choice to breastfeed but are too selfish to do so without manipulation."[30] But what do we make of the argument of the Ad Council and the Department of Health and Human Services, that focus groups suggested the negative risk approach as the most effective way to get the message across? Does this merely show that ordinary Americans like to blame mothers personally for behaviors that are determined, or at least heavily influenced, by social structure, cultural belief, and straightforward economic constraints? Kukla, Joan Wolf, and the leaders of the AAP in fall 2003 agree that blaming mothers is improper (although the AAP leaders' statements neglect to discuss the multiple social determinants impeding women's choice or ability to breast-feed), but Kukla never mentions guilt, while the doctors trot out this worn-out rationale for presenting breastfeeding's contributions to health as "benefits" in the old risk scenario.

Infant formula manufacturers, women's rights organizations, leading pediatricians, and some feminists worry that mothers might feel guilty if their infant feeding choice were connected to negative health outcomes.[31] This unseemly alliance demonstrates a cultural consensus concerning the impropriety of making mothers feel guilty. It is connected, I think, to the argument that the science behind breastfeeding advocacy is equivocal. Joan Wolf's discussion clarifies this issue significantly, since her argument about the inappropriateness of the NBAC's so-called fear message explores the scientific case for breastfeeding specifically in relation to public health ethics, suggesting that only ironclad causal findings should motivate risk-based public health campaigns. In the next chapter I examine the relation of risk to guilt in greater detail.

Breastfeeding advocates are tired of the way that cultural ambivalence about nursing continues to undermine their efforts on behalf of women and babies, and, as Jacqueline Wolf shows, not all feminists believe that ide-ologies subordinating women overdetermine the message of public health campaigns concerning breastfeeding. Better evidence will not, however, change a debate that is displaced from its primary context—the social sphere—and argued through scientific discourses and findings. What an-gered some feminists about the NBAC was its exploitation of antiwoman tactics (using the image of "bad mothers" to encourage women to behave as "good mothers") to promote a practice that is difficult for most women to engage for more than a few months. Indeed, many feminists see such tactics as themselves risky to women's survival and well-being, as they suggest a willingness to turn women against one another in an effort to achieve a sta-tistical public health target.

I don't see that the NBAC was unusually reprehensible in this regard. Rather, it seemed to me to be a run-of-the-mill campaign that neglected to think through the political consequences of its message. In getting the cul-tural consensus wrong, it misjudged the meaning of medical evidence con-cerning formula feeding for most people. Its purpose was to change the cul-tural consensus toward one that would recognize and select the risks of replacement feeding, but its creators misrecognized or failed to account for the distance between knowledge and practice in the cultural construction of risk. Knowledge—as evidence, statistics, or other forms of information—does not automatically transform attitudes or practices if the cultural context, in terms of both belief and materiality, does not lend itself to change.[32]

What concerns me most about the NBAC was the almost total lack of human bodies in the campaign: few breasts on display and even an absence of people entirely in the poster series.[33] In addition, I am struck by how the value of breastfeeding in general is assessed predominantly in relation to medical evidence. The most culturally influential discourses concerning breastfeeding are either completely medicalized or emerge from a kind of New Age/total motherhood amalgam that essentializes and idealizes maternity overall and breastfeeding in particular. Neither of these, it seems to me, gets at why breastfeeding should be a concern for feminists, who should be able to step outside of the cultural conflicts over women's bodies that are enacted in breastfeeding controversies instead of participating in them.

Such a gesture would allow us to understand how the framework of medicalization displaces the controversy into terms that can putatively be settled by evidence. This is, of course, the technological-objective approach to risk management, the standard bureaucratic approach on which the NBAC itself was based. But controversies over women's bodies are rarely evidence based. Risks are selected, or not selected, because the cultural context creates a consensus of "sense" that dictates what will and will not be perceived as dangerous. The United States is a society that depends on the easy provision of infant formula to allow women access to the public sphere, to confirm sameness between men and women, and to disavow any distinctive value to the maternal body. Getting infant formula to be perceived as a risk in a such a context is a tall order indeed. It should be no wonder that the original risk message was so easily muted, nor that the creators of the NBAC resorted to a message playing on a familiar cultural script of mother blame.

CHAPTER 7

Guilt

IN A CONTROVERSIAL 2006 *New York Times* article about a U.S. Senate proposal to require warning labels on cans of infant formula, "Breast-Feed Or Else," guilt makes a prominent appearance. After first introducing the National Breastfeeding Awareness Campaign, the article focuses on a mother who "couldn't" breastfeed and felt terrible guilt about it. Then the discussion turns to the difficulty of nursing in the context of paid employment and the few, if any, social support mechanisms to help breastfeeding mothers at work. Ellen Galinsky, president of the nonprofit Families and Work Institute, weighs in with "I'm concerned about the guilt that mothers will feel. . . . It's hard enough going back to work." And yet the article goes on to offer an extensive and positive presentation of scientific evidence in favor of breastfeeding, making the title "Breast-Feed Or Else" seem more inflammatory than descriptive of the content and overall message. Interspersed in the discussion of the science of breastfeeding medicine is the story of another mother, this one a woman who gave up her career at the birth of her first child and breastfed all three of her children for extended periods, not leaving them except for the birth of another.[1]

Thus "Breast-Feed Or Else" presents the reader with two mothers, one guilty and purportedly unable to breastfeed and the other a fountain of milk who, it seems, can't do anything but breastfeed ("It's a whole lifestyle," she says). Guilt is presented in the context of an innate inability to breastfeed and in the context of most U.S. mothers' work situations, both of which are, in fact, socially produced circumstances that could be rectified through better breastfeeding management by the mother and changes to U.S. laws concerning maternity leave.[2] It is true that, in the absence of such changes, many women do feel guilty that they do not or cannot breastfeed, especially when public health campaigns focus on educating women about the contribution that breastfeeding makes to health and the potential harms of infant formula. Yet this makes it all the more startling that Ellen Galinsky, president of the Families and Work Institute, focuses on the guilt mothers might feel rather than the way in which emerging scientific research on breastfeeding should impel legislators to extend maternity leave and support nursing mothers. What makes guilt the initial response to information that breastfeeding makes crucial contributions to infant and maternal health? Why is maternal guilt so publicly accepted as a reason not to question certain infant feeding practices?

Predictably, the Infant Formula Council did not agree that the scientific evidence warrants warning labels, as reported in the article. Interestingly, many feminists responding to "Breast-Feed Or Else" on the Sociologists for Women in Society listserv argued similarly, suggesting that the scientific evidence ignores social factors that may compromise research claims and that causal links between breast milk ingestion and improved health are tenuous. These academics, who dominated the listserv response to the article, read the campaign for infant formula warning labels as another piece of a larger social project to make motherhood more difficult and punish mothers who don't live up to a particular domestic standard or who are unable for economic reasons to successfully breastfeed. For these academic feminists, the scientific evidence serves as an ideological gambit to make women feel guilty about their choices as mothers.[3] In her 2006 *Signs* article, discussed in the previous chapter, Jacqueline Wolf demonstrates that objections to the NBAC raised the issue of maternal guilt in the context of challenges to scientific evidence.[4] This latter point is crucial to the discussion here, because (as I argued previously) if the science was incontrovertible, then there would be no plausible excuse (at least in the context of public health) not to offer the information, even if it made women feel guilty.[5] Dr. Suzanne Haynes, senior scientist in the Office of Women's Health, a division of the Department of Health and Human Services, suggests that infant feeding is "the only field of public health, except perhaps physical activity, where there is never talk about the risk."[6] So the strategy to maintain the status quo, which proscribes talk of risk in relation to infant feeding, needs both the specter of guilt and the suggestion that evidence concerning the risks of not breastfeeding is equivocal. The question here is why this particular strategy is shared by some feminists and all infant formula companies. After all, it's a bit odd to find activist and academic feminists agreeing with representatives of large multinational corporations about a practice that is economically linked to the corporations' well-being.

One answer is that this apparent alliance is a result of a feminist argument gone awry and accepted by mainstream American culture, which accepts the guilt argument in lieu of making substantive changes to the material circumstances of mothers' lives. Everyone can claim that they are pro-mother if they bring up the question of maternal guilt. No one wants to make mothers feel guilty. Yet are mothers actually less guilty (and do they feel less guilty) if they don't have accurate information about their practices as mothers? Jacqueline Wolf argues that feminists have always stood for accurate biomedical information, noting that in the mid-1970s the Boston Women's Health Book Collective "urge[d] women to 'do something about those doctors who were condescending, paternalistic, judgmental, and *noninformative.*'"[7] But with this argument we are back at the quandary of the scientific case for breastfeeding, its evidentiary status, and its rhetorical function in specific discursive situations.

There are no large-scale public complaints about risk information and the inculcation of guilt with respect to sudden infant death syndrome (SIDS), for example, even though millions of babies have survived sleeping on their stomachs (the now proscribed sleeping position for young infants). This is because, except in marginal circles, Americans don't publicly challenge the scientific evidence on which this particular medical advice is made. There is no cultural consensus that the evidence is equivocal, even if individual parents decide to contravene the advice based on personal experience or familial tradition. Of course, there is no industry that stands to benefit from invoking maternal guilt as an unfortunate result of disseminated scientific research concerning SIDS. Formula companies invoke the specter of maternal guilt because it is in their best interest and it is a discourse with cultural currency. Guilt beats the evidence concerning the risks of formula use every time.

The guilt is thought to result only from certain kinds of public health strategies—telling women that breastfeeding is best is not seen to promote guilt in the same way that telling women formula feeding is a potentially harmful behavior that increases a child's risk of developing juvenile diabetes (as an example) is perceived to.[8] So the articulation of the problem of guilt is not only dependent on an equivocal presentation of the scientific case for breastfeeding; it also relies on an understanding of risk discourse within public health campaigns. Ultimately, the question of guilt—why it is raised as an issue with respect to breastfeeding, whether it is a legitimate concern in this context, and how it has come to be an agreed-upon limit to the kinds of information offered to women about infant feeding—is related to risk as an emerging and powerful discourse within medicine and, in particular, contemporary public health strategies.

What is the worldview supported by the lack of consensus concerning purported health risks of formula feeding? Assuming that the scientific evidence of these risks is as compelling and plausible as the scientific evidence of other highly publicized risks to health, is there a consensus that mothers find the barriers to breastfeeding too difficult to surmount? Such a consensus would have to be accompanied by the belief that the health contributions of breastfeeding are simply not worth the extensive effort in order to constitute a true denial of formula risks. Certainly American citizens find the risks of poor nutritional habits difficult to overcome, but this does not stop major public health agencies from repeatedly trying to combat obesity and the effects of eating too much junk food. Is the invocation of guilt with respect to infant feeding simply an excuse, a way of obscuring a more fundamental link between formula feeding and foundational beliefs and institutions of the culture?

There are those who believe that all public health strategies that target individual behaviors are problematic insofar as they use guilt to motivate change. I discussed this briefly in the previous chapter concerning Joan Wolf's objections to perceived ethical lapses in the NBAC. In "Risk as Moral Danger: The Social and Political Functions of Risk Discourse in Public Health," Deborah Lupton argues that all public health discourses that identify "lifestyle" risks and emphasize the "negative outcome" of particular risk behaviors result in an "inducement of anxiety and guilt in those who have received the message about risks but do not change their behavior." She suggests that this public health approach "might be said to be unethical." In this view, inculcating guilt is a flawed method of alerting people to potentially risky behaviors, especially when public health "emphasizes lifestyle risks" and thus "serves as an effective Foucauldian agent of surveillance and control that is difficult to challenge because of its manifest benevolent goal of maintaining standards of health [and thereby] draw[ing] attention away from the structural causes of ill-health." Thus, "risk discourse as it is currently used in public health . . . targets the body as a site of toxicity, contamination and catastrophe, subject to and needful of a high degree of surveillance and control."[9] In this view, the response that negative risk

information about formula feeding might make mothers feel guilty is a response that should be extended to other public health campaigns that identify risky behaviors in the promotion of health. Feminists who voice concerns about pro-breastfeeding campaigns often are resisting what they
perceive to be an ideological move to bring the maternal body into greater
cultural regulation through breastfeeding. These are some of the critics
who state unequivocally, with apparent social support, that it is improper to
make mothers feel guilty about infant feeding behaviors.

Yet why is breastfeeding an anomalous example of public resistance to
public health promotion? Why don't we hear scores of complaints that recurrent messages about the health risks of being overweight will make the
obese feel guilty? That how babies sleep—in bed with family members, as
an example, rather than alone in a crib—is a family matter rather than a
medical issue?[10] Why does infant feeding seem to be one lifestyle practice
that people agree shouldn't be targeted by risk discourses because of how
easy it is to make mothers feel guilty if they cannot or choose not to breastfeed? One answer to these questions might be that certain messages make
mothers feel guilty because the risky behavior identified is out of mothers'
hands, that it is not really a lifestyle risk, and thus that it is something they
are victimized by rather than responsible for. The media's seeming emphasis on women's innate inability to breastfeed, without any discussion of how
most cases of insufficient milk are caused by poor management rather than
biological incapacity, would support this interpretation.

But this answer doesn't get to the core issue addressed by Mary Douglas
and Aaron Wildavsky, which is that risks are identified by a particular culture because they are risks that are perceived to threaten the culture's
worldview and the institutions upon which the culture depends. Lupton's
analysis operates on a more comfortable level for most of us, asking
whether we are being too strenuous, as a society, in targeting certain life
practices for guilt-inducing health promotion campaigns, as if health is the
province of individuals and the result of willpower. Douglas and Wildavsky
ask why we think certain aspects of our lives are risky in the first place.

They point out, "Causality in the external world is generally treated as
radically distinct from the results of individual perception." Because of this,
in the general perception,

risk is [perceived to be] a straightforward consequence of the dangers inherent in the physical situation, while attitudes toward risk

depend on individual personalities. When particular risks are objectively ascertainable, it follows that the gap between the expert and the lay public ought to be closed in only one direction—toward the opinion of experts: the lay public must be taught the facts; the scientific message must be clearly labeled.[11]

This is a description of the technical-objective approach to risk; it coincides with the approach of the NBAC itself. Yet many public health promotions fail not because of a bungled scientific message but as a result of the intractability of habit. Douglas and Wildavsky point out that habits are developed in the context of human communities that provide their meaning and also inform individuals' sense of risk.[12] Habits, as sedimentations of cultural belief and institutional investment, mitigate against perceiving certain dangers as risks.

In the muddled politics of the NBAC's delay—in conjunction with news articles like "Breast-Feed Or Else" and feminist arguments about the problems of health promotion that ignores the realities of women's lives—we see not only crass maneuvering by formula companies but a more generalized cultural resistance to the message that formula is a risky infant feeding method. Statistics on rates of breastfeeding in 2005 indicate that while about 70 percent of mothers breastfed right after birth, 36 percent were still breastfeeding at six months but only 14 percent were doing so exclusively as recommended by the AAP.[13] Mothers may begin breastfeeding but do not seem to resist the early shift to replacement feeding; it does not seem to be perceived as a risk to infant health and well-being. Formula feeding is not selected by most Americans as a risk worth paying attention to; it does not threaten a core value or institution of the culture. Indeed, one could make the opposite argument, that breastfeeding is a risk because it represents a threat to basic foundations of American life.

In public controversies about infant feeding in the United States, guilt operates rhetorically to justify the cultural resistance to seeing formula as a risk. The routine use of infant formulas, supported by the belief that replacement feeding does not confer significant health risks on mothers or babies, supports core aspects of the social formation in the United States and coheres with key cultural beliefs. While other wealthy countries with different, and more generous, social provision for mothers also see guilt invoked in debates about infant feeding, one would need to study their cultural systems to understand how its articulation functions in relation to core institutions and beliefs. My suspicion is that the injunction not to make mothers feel guilty about their behaviors is a key achievement of feminism across much of the global north, but it has become an easy rhetoric of equality that is often not matched by concrete changes in attitudes about mothers. Making mothers feel guilty may not be approved of, but they certainly remain responsible for infant health and welfare in most instances.

A number of beliefs and institutions support the guilt model. American culture is invested in sameness between men and women. In addition, core cultural ideas about adulthood idealize autonomous individuality and represent dependence as a negative quality or relation. Caring for infants is a highly medicalized and thus regulated practice. As a result, to feed one's baby with one's body brings that body into the realm of medical scrutiny in ways that are constraining to reigning models of liberation and independence. Finally, the abandonment of breastfeeding is historically associated with modernization, largely because shifts in family arrangement, labor force participation, and public norms of embodiment impel changes in women's social roles that affect their reproductive behavior and maternal practices. All of these factors work together to sustain the credibility of the guilt discourse, which itself supports the contemporary social formation by suggesting that infant feeding decisions are personal and independent of the cultural paradigm that determines them. In the concluding paragraphs of this chapter, I focus on the economic rationale that maintains the use of guilt as a rhetoric against breastfeeding promotion.[14]

Even though there are myriad popular discourses to the contrary, sameness between men and women is a basic tenet of American society because the economy depends on it. The core institutions of the culture depend on a growing capitalist economy with a large and flexible labor force. The labor force must not be allowed to make demands on employers or the government, a creed in the culture that is perhaps more extreme in the United States than in most other nations in the global north. Formal equality is required by capitalism, which nevertheless demands the ability to discriminate between workers in order to maintain a pool of low-wage workers. Indeed, the system as it is now encourages discrimination against women because mothers do leave and return to the workforce more than men.[15]

Almost all of the public discourses concerning differences between women and men focus on women's supposedly innate inferiority to men (difficulty with higher order mathematics, for example) or prove women's purported investment in monogamous heterosexual relationships. In other words, the discourses about sexual difference work with the economic commitment to sameness to enforce discriminatory treatment of women in employment and other sectors of civic life.

Mothers thus constitute a group of workers against whom employers can legitimately discriminate with lower wages and less job security, even though such discrimination may not be directed specifically or purposely at mothers. Instead, such discrimination is built into a system that does not recognize mothers' special needs. Mandated maternity leave with guaranteed return to work at the same or equivalent position would end this form of flexible discrimination routinely used against women. As Gerald Calnen points out, "Feeding decisions tend to be contingent upon employment decisions, rather than vice versa. The results of the National Survey of Family Growth indicate that most nursing mothers do not breastfeed and maintain employment concurrently." While the decision to breastfeed does not seem to be affected by maternal employment unless the mother will return to work within six weeks of the birth, the duration of breastfeeding appears to be significantly affected by employment.[16]

The guilt model maintains the sameness of the parenting relation by supporting practices that allow mothers to act like fathers in the society at large (through waged labor and participation in civic culture as autonomous individuals) but not feel guilty. That is, women can use the guilt discourse in order not to feel deficient as women for living their lives as men have traditionally lived theirs. This analysis demonstrates the key form of social organization maintained by a particular risk selection—contemporary labor force participation by women and the attendant outsourcing of child-care and child-rearing practices from the home, with the added employer practices of discriminating against women who leave the labor force intermittently to care for children—and explains the lack of concern about other risks, namely, formula feeding, even when these have been widely publicized.

The guilt model, while espoused by many feminists, ensures that women cannot make maternity matter as a statement, or experience, of sexual difference. In the United States, equality won in the equality-versus-difference debate, such that some feminists refuse to support maternity leave in favor of gender-neutral parental or family leave.[17] (By some accounts, the United States has the worst maternity support legislation in the global north.)[18] There is no mystery to why education level is one of the best indicators of breastfeeding initiation and duration (maternal age is another significant indicator).[19] Breastfeeding for longer than a few months means going against the cultural norm, and generally women with plentiful resources are more likely to succeed at culturally anomalous behaviors. Resources offer a buffer between an individual and social censure, economic discrimination, or familial resistance.[20] Education and age are often key factors in making those resources a reality.

Addressing mothers' guilty feelings about feeding decisions through reference to scientific evidence of breastfeeding's contributions to health would mean taking action to allow all mothers to breastfeed. Practically, trying to make sure that all babies are breastfed for at least a year, the AAP's recommended minimum duration, would necessitate changes to the economic structure by mandating guaranteed, extended, and paid maternity leave for all mothers. Thus, the economy's structure, which depends on being able to treat women like men, would be difficult to maintain if the society as a whole were to acknowledge the contributions that breastfeeding makes to health, especially long-term breastfeeding. The fact that the U.S. government consistently whittles away at welfare supports for poor women, most of whom are mothers, without much social protest, demonstrates the lack of widespread cultural support for any kind of social provision for mothers, let alone support for breastfeeding.

It seems to me that the scientific evidence of breastfeeding's contribution to health is as good as any other scientific evidence about health. I cannot agree with scholars like Joan Wolf who suggest that breastfeeding researchers are unable to be objective about the data that they produce. It seems to me that in exploring a culturally anomalous practice and defending its value in biological terms, breastfeeding scientists are working against cultural norms and thus liable to be more, rather than less, careful about their findings. Where they may err is in understanding why their findings do not have the cultural impact they imagine should result from publicizing them. The reason the scientific case for breastfeeding does not resonate with the general public—and with some experts who are themselves qualified to evaluate it—has nothing to do with its actual value as evidence. The problem is really that all the evidence in the world will not convince people whose worldview depends on not seeing formula feeding as a risk.

Formula manufacturers' investment in this blindness is self-evident: it promotes their bottom line. Mothers collude with formula companies' perspectives because to do so allows them to accommodate infant feeding to modern expectations of women's public roles and embodied behaviors.

Some feminists apparently fall in line with formula manufacturers and many mothers because they tend to see the breastfeeding advocacy as support for domestic femininity rather than as a call for enhanced freedoms for mothers. These feminists do not, as a group, see the denial of medical evidence for breastfeeding's contributions to health as a problem of misinformation; they are more likely to perceive scientific evidence about breastfeeding's benefits as an improper use of science to circumscribe and limit women's choices in modern societies.[21]

Breastfeeding advocates have difficulty promoting maternal nursing because the perceived risks of breastfeeding itself are high. In a culture that identifies the exchange of bodily fluids with significant risks to health, breastfeeding can only proceed as a highly mediated, medically supervised practice, a situation that leads to great difficulty getting appropriate information concerning routine breastfeeding management. During the 1990s, a series of media reports in the United States linked breastfeeding with infant death, highlighting the apparent difficulty of knowing if one's child is getting enough milk if it breastfeeds.[22] Breastfeeding is seen to conflict with women's sexual roles and sexual embodiment, both of which are becoming more and more public. Ironically, nursing in public, which would allow breastfeeding women greater social mobility, is often very difficult for women because of the risk of exposure, which they fear will be perceived as sexual.[23] In addition, many women experience breastfeeding as risky behavior because they feel themselves constantly at risk of not having enough milk, a psychological situation that can, in fact, lead to a diminishment of milk supply.

Most significant, to my mind, is the fact that most women work in contexts where being able to express their milk and save it for their baby's later consumption is not an option or at least is incredibly difficult.[24] Breastfeeding is simply not possible for most women to sustain in the context of waged employment, not in the current cultural, political, and economic circumstances of the United States. For this majority of American mothers, breastfeeding is experienced as a risk to their livelihood, and the suggestion that formula feeding incurs health risks for babies is met with counterclaims that making mothers feel guilty is wrong. No wonder it seems more plausible to worry about West Nile virus.

CHAPTER 8

Pollution Taboos and Pregnancy Advice

TOXIC CHEMICALS in the environment are a focus of concern for the risk society, one example of more general worries about the effects of modern industrialization on people and the planet. Lawrence Buell notes, however, that "toxic discourse . . . arises *both* from individual or social panic and from an evidential base in environmental phenomena." Noting that "toxic concern dates from late antiquity," Buell asserts that contemporary "toxic discourse is both always immoderate and yet always being reinforced by unsettling events," a fact that demonstrates its power *as a discourse* to inaugurate and sustain a palpable level of concern and crisis in the citizenry. Advocating a doubled approach to toxic discourse, one that "fuses social constructivist with environmental restorationist perspectives," Buell concludes (in part) that "evidence accumulates of the emergence of toxicity as a widely shared paradigm of cultural self-identification."[1] Concerns about contaminants during pregnancy, a growing trend in the management of gestation and motherhood in the United States, bear out this claim.

Buell identifies pastoralism as a genre shaping the forms of toxic discourse; pastoral values represent "the conviction that the biological environment ought to be more pristine than it is, ought to be a healthy, soul-nurturing habitat." Buell further points out that the use of the pastoral ideal emphasizes the notion of an individual right to clean air and water, among other requirements.[2] In the context of pollution fears of pregnancy, we will see that mothers' bodies are the represented environments that endanger a gestational pastoral ideal, and that the attention toward pregnant (and, increasingly, breastfeeding) women ignores mothers as persons with histories, constrained by circumstance, and responsive to multiple demands on them. That is, maternal bodies as the potentially toxic environment for fetuses and breastfeeding infants are rendered as if they could be separated from the dirty world in which all of us find ourselves.

Of course, purity issues historically have been targeted at the mother-to-be and her relation to the unborn she carries. In addition, there is a lengthy history of examining breast milk to determine if it is "good." Current trends in breast milk biomonitoring may be simple extensions of this practice. Yet today there are increased concerns about impurities or dangerous substances that threaten infants through their mothers' milk; these concerns have to do with fears that mothers endanger their infants through the everyday practices of living in a contaminated world. Scientific discourses and technological practices like biomonitoring and the measurement of chemical "body burden," discussed in the next chapter, are sophisticated ways of separating mothers off from the rest of the community as special people whose bodies must be controlled in order to be safe for their children. In this way new technoscientific practices come to operate much as pollution taboos have functioned historically: sequestering women, confining them to particular behaviors, regulating their bodies.

Yet modern cultures generally enforce their taboos through discipline rather than outright rules; this is a key claim in Foucault's approach to modernity. The advice book is an important venue for disseminating medical ideas about pregnancy, encouraging women to regulate their own experience in accordance with established, expert views. Pregnancy advice books advance the social project of medicalization, inculcating in women themselves medical attitudes about their embodied experiences and subordinating other kinds of information (and other sources) about pregnancy. This chapter addresses concerns about contaminants and mothers' bodies as they are expressed in pregnancy advice books. As my primary example I use the most popular and prominent pregnancy guidebook in the United States today, *What to Expect When You're Expecting*.[3]

What to Expect exemplifies the genre of lay medical advice that instructs American women in the normative expectations of motherhood. Of singular importance appears to be what goes into their bodies, so that what comes out (babies, breast milk) is regulated, safe, and pure.[4] My discussion here addresses the book's implicit expectation that maternal bodies need to be pure in order to be good; in the next chapter I analyze that expectation with respect to both its religious connotations and its refusal of breastfeeding itself as a model for the relation of the maternal body to toxins and, more generally, the environment. Like Buell, I analyze this toxic discourse about pregnancy with the understanding that toxic chemicals in the environment present a threat to human well-being *and* that, as a discourse, it operates "as an interlocked set of topoi whose force derives partly from the anxieties of late industrial culture, partly from deeper-rooted habits of thought and expression."[5]

To situate this chapter's arguments in the context of the book's overall framework of modern medicalization, I begin with a discussion of how the dissemination of ideas in the advice format represents a strategy of disciplinary biopower. The particular toxic discourses I examine here are framed by the advice format and its regulating functions in contemporary American culture.

Advice and Modernity

In a small study of women from the upper Midwestern United States, Denise Copelton argues that mothers-to-be use pregnancy advice books to compensate for inadequate or incomplete information from medical caregivers, to understand their own embodied experiences according to medical perception, and to evaluate symptoms and problems that occur during pregnancy. She suggests that women have come to rely on these guidebooks more heavily than they do friends or family for information about pregnancy and motherhood, subordinating local knowledge to the expert knowledge available in published books. While the guidebooks offer women medical information that can empower their relations with medical caregivers, Copelton concludes that because the books "enabled women to normalize their experience of pregnancy and reinterpret their experiences according to dominant medical understandings," they contributed to the "further medicalization of pregnancy."[6] She points out that obtaining and avidly reading pregnancy guidebooks has itself become a normative element of the pregnancy experience in the United States, suggesting that seeking information from professional experts and incorporating it into daily practices is a fundamental element of modern maternity in the global north.

Obtaining and putting into practice medical knowledge is a strategy meant to address risk in a social context that relies on expert systems and abstract knowledge to secure safety and identify culturally appropriate behaviors. Anthony Giddens's concept of disembedding and the consequent need to engender trust outside of immediate social relations comes to mind here. For Giddens, the extraction of individuals from traditional social relations is a cornerstone of modernity. Disembedding requires new modes of trust that force people to rely on expert systems, rather than individuals that they know personally, in most aspects of daily life. Through this process people come to trust professional discourses and experts unknown to them with greater frequency than they trust individuals in their families or immediate social circles. There results a kind of thinning-out of social relations in favor of professionalized knowledge.

The pregnancy advice book thus emblematizes modern maternal experience, insofar as it represents how women are thought to best equip themselves to be mothers: gaining knowledge and interpreting their own experiences by reading books. As Copelton suggests, the guidebooks have a disciplinary function as well, normalizing the experience of pregnancy into a medical model and inculcating in women themselves the regulatory practices expected by medical professionals. These books are mechanisms of modern discipline in a Foucauldian sense. Indeed, they seem perfect examples of how individuals create within themselves regulatory norms required by the social formation. Written ostensibly to offer information as a way of dispelling the mysteries of pregnancy and reducing risks (by offering women information about what constitutes a serious symptom of something gone wrong and what is normal in pregnancy), the pregnancy guide demonstrates how to regulate individuals into certain behaviors in the absence of more direct social control or the dissemination of information through local contacts. Becoming a modern maternal subject is, in part, a function of becoming the subject of expert medical knowledge. The pregnancy guidebook exemplifies this mechanism of modern biopower.[7]

Historian Barbara Duden would probably see the pregnancy advice book as a mechanism subordinating the phenomenology of pregnancy (and women's personal power to name their experience) to medical knowledge.[8] But it seems to me that the more significant point of focus is the function of these books in modern societies: they replace information about pregnancy and childbirth that flowed otherwise, from people one knew intimately and through direct observation.[9] This is one reason why so many pregnancy advice books take on a chatty tone and are formatted as direct answers to specific questions (as *What to Expect* is), as if the reader were in conversation with the author(s): the books substitute for an actual interlocutor who would be the traditional source of knowledge. In the disembedded social contexts of modernity, book knowledge substitutes for local knowledge. This is why the pregnancy advice book provides an important source of information about contemporary pregnancy: it is the repository of norms, values, and beliefs guiding women's experience and informing their self-perceptions. In addition, it represents fundamental elements of modern social relations, specifically the importance of expert systems in the discipline of modern subjects.

The use of information as a strategy to reduce pregnancy risks is an element of the more general medicalization of social life. This is not to say that information does not reduce risk, but rather to point out that the focus on information and education has other effects as well. As Copelton remarks, "Despite its many positive benefits, sociologists argue that medicalization expands the social control functions of medicine."[10] Significantly, the focus on information, a hallmark of public health campaigns that rely on social marketing (rather than, for example, infrastructure enhancement), emphasizes personal responsibility and agency in the fight against disease and the avoidance of health risks. Personal knowledge—and the presumed ability to act on such knowledge—replaces community responsibility as the primary mechanism of improved health outcomes.

This kind of approach to public health is evident in a recent *Washington Post* series on pregnancy and maternal mortality in Sierra Leone, a country where a woman's chance of dying in childbirth is one in eight. Pointing out that "the underlying cause" of this abominable statistic is "simply life in poor countries: Governments don't provide enough decent hospitals or doctors; families can't afford medications," author Kevin Sullivan goes on to say, "A lack of education and horrible roads cause women to make unwise health choices, so that they often prefer the dirt floor of home to deliveries at the hands of a qualified stranger at a distant hospital." While Sullivan continues with the comment, "Women die in childbirth every day, according to people who study the issue, because of cultures and traditions that place more worth on the lives of men," we see that in his view, if women could learn to make wiser choices, if they could choose the stranger in the hospital over the less professionally educated local midwife, many lives would be saved. In a subsequent article, Sullivan quotes a "British-trained director" of a hospital in Koinadugu, a rural district of northeastern Sierra Leone, who believes that "many [women] don't fully understand the risks [of pregnancy and childbirth], and are daunted by the costs and distances they need to travel for care."[11]

In these examples, women's understanding of their condition and its potentially deadly risks are embedded in infrastructure issues of significant proportion: lack of good roads, tremendous expenses associated with medical care, unavailable medical care, and the need to trust professionals rather than neighbors. These causes of high maternal mortality result from Sierra Leone's poverty, which also affects the lack of a social structure to support modern prenatal care. Obviously, there are many interventions that could improve maternity outcomes in Sierra Leone; since its maternal mortality rate is so high, one imagines that anything could help. But I wonder why maternal decision making is emphasized in these generally well-balanced articles. Why talk about women's "unwise choices" when it seems that there are so few good ones to make?

Indeed, in "A Mother's Final Look at Life," Sullivan demonstrates that Fatmata Jalloh and her sister Batuli consistently made decisions that seem reasonable, given their circumstances: when Fatmata began complaining of back pain, they thought to go to the clinic where she was "registered for prenatal care" but believed the half-hour walk would be too difficult. Instead, they decided to see a neighborhood nurse with experience delivering babies. Fatmata delivered soon after her arrival in the nurse's home, and all seemed well until a number of hours later when she began hemorrhaging. Her husband found a car to take her to the hospital, but she had already lost too much blood. Given the time-frame offered in the article, it seems that if they had decided to go to the clinic in the first place, Fatmata might have given birth by the side of the road. Of course it is a problem that the local nurse "had no medication or equipment to stanch the hemorrhaging." (Sullivan reports that she said, "I don't do complications here.")[12] But it is not clear that, in the absence of numerous other interrelated transformations in the country—including improved local and national infrastructures—expectant mothers like Fatmata Jalloh could make better choices than the ones she made.

The focus on education, and on the choices education is thought to offer, is an example of modern faith in knowledge. But such faith depends upon other facets of modern life that the articles highlight as dangerously missing from Sierra Leone—adequate and affordable public transportation to health clinics, financially accessible medical care, good roads and public water supplies. The list could continue. My point in analyzing these recent articles about maternity in one of the poorest countries in the world is not meant to criticize attempts to raise levels of maternal education and women's understanding of the risks of pregnancy and childbirth. My point is to demonstrate how much faith people from the global north hold in abstract knowledge systems and professional strangers, and how important it is to transmit that faith to others in order to improve health outcomes worldwide, since global biomedicine is built on a foundation of these beliefs.

Pregnancy advice books are a way of inculcating and reinforcing this faith in expert knowledge and information from strangers. They are a primary element of the modern experience of pregnancy, because they incorporate solutions to the dilemma of the disembedded individual who needs trustworthy information from experts to manage a personal experience that is now regulated through medical institutions. In this way they are a primary instance of ideology, an enactment of ideas that enforce social and material relations at the core of modern social formations. Pregnancy advice books are part of a social apparatus that maintains these relations for subjects already constituted through the modern social formations of affluent societies.

In the next section of the chapter, I examine how *What to Expect* represents the problem of chemical contaminants during pregnancy, focusing on how expectant mothers are imagined as decision makers able to control their environments.

Contaminants and Additives

In my copy of *What to Expect When You're Expecting*, the second edition, published in 1991, the advice about pesticide exposure initially conveys a rather relaxed attitude toward the problem, meant to calm expectant mothers.

> The fact is that all of the environmental factors that are not within your control when you're pregnant—a job that has you sitting in front of a video terminal, a hometown that's polluted with carbon monoxide, incidental brief exposures to paint fumes, hair dyes, insecticides—have far less impact on the outcome of your pregnancy than the factors you have complete control over, such as getting good, regular medical care, eating an excellent diet, and not drinking, smoking, or taking nonprescribed drugs once you found out you're pregnant.[13]

Then I read "it's generally safer to live with [bugs] than to eliminate them through the use of chemical insecticides, some of which have been linked to birth defects." That seems to suggest that insecticides are dangerous and should be avoided. Further, the authors state, "Stay out of the apartment for a day or two if that's possible, and ventilate with open windows for as long as practical. The chemicals are potentially dangerous only as long as the fumes linger." However, the risk message gets more confused: "If you have been accidentally exposed to insecticides or herbicides, don't be alarmed. Brief, indirect exposure isn't likely to have done any harm to your baby."[14] Finally, in the last section of this chapter, the subtitle, "What It's Important to Know: Playing Baby Roulette," seems to suggest the most dire perspective.

In the third edition of *What to Expect* (2002), the authors retitled this last section so that it reads "What It's Important to Know: Putting Risk in Perspective." This welcome change of message involves no substantive change in the discussion, however, nor in the earlier material about insecticides. Perusal of Canadian physician Gideon Koren's *The Complete Guide to Everyday Risks in Pregnancy and Breastfeeding* offers similar information, although perhaps more straightforwardly: "It is probably best to avoid [pesticides], if possible. If the interior of your home must be sprayed, stay out of the home two to three times longer than recommended by the pesticide manufacturer. Have someone open the windows after spraying, in order to ventilate the area well."[15]

What to Expect focuses, ultimately, on choices and maternal agency: "During pregnancy you will be challenged to make intelligent decisions in dozens of situations, weighing risk against benefit. Keep in mind that an occasional wrong choice isn't likely to affect your pregnancy, though repeated ones might."[16] The calculus of risk, then, is arrayed against a perspective on pregnancy that emphasizes mothers as thinking subjects—which might seem to be a good thing, until we realize that mothers' thinking is, in this text and others like it, consistently represented as a weighing of options concerning the fetus inside her. The notion of herself as a body with its own needs and perspectives fades away. Good pregnant mothers make the right choice (for the fetus) most of the time, the "intelligent decision" in the "dozens of situations" they are confronted with. Good pregnant mothers weigh risk against benefit. The entire experience of pregnancy, it seems, is in the control of mothers who are risk calculators in the extreme. Rather than promoting maternal agency, this figuration of mothers-as-underwriters suggests a kind of straitjacket of maternal choice, wherein the experience of pregnancy both entails and ignores the self/other dichotomy that defines it as an existential condition.[17]

This thinking risk-calculator of pregnancy eats every day, and much of the anxiety about maternal choice is funneled through issues concerning weight gain and diet. After learning about substances to fear and avoid in the chapter "Throughout Your Pregnancy," I read about what to put into my body in "The Pregnancy Diet," information that is extended throughout the book in subsequent chapters, in sections with titles like "Chemicals in Foods" and "Eating Out." The advice in *What to Expect* is typical of the ruling "low fat/high fiber" regime of the late twentieth century, with added information about increased protein intake for pregnancy. There is a decided emphasis on efficiency in eating: of paramount importance is getting the right nutrients into one's body without adding too many "empty" calories that just add fat to the mother's body and do nothing for the developing fetus. (A food is not efficient if its caloric component is high in relation to its nutritional contribution.) With a section on "guilt-free cheating" (really, what's the point?), the chapter on diet represents a rather standard, if idealized, view of what pregnant women should eat, replete with the doublespeak Helena Michie and Naomi Cahn have identified as a feature of the text's diet advice. As an example, in a small boxed section on "Playing Protein Catch-up," the authors give some tips about getting in extra protein at the end of the day, "if you do ever find yourself a half or even a full serving short at the end of the day." After suggesting three possible snacks—egg salad on whole wheat crackers, a "Double-the-Milk shake," or cottage cheese—they advise against ready-made high-protein supplements because "they could contain ingredients that are unsafe during pregnancy . . . [and may result in] taking in *too much* protein."[18]

The chapter following "The Pregnancy Diet," entitled "The Second Month," includes more information about food, addressing concerns about occasional fast food intake and additives and chemicals in foods, in addition to questions about food safety. While in this chapter Eisenberg et al. write that pregnant women don't need to worry much about cholesterol ("pregnant women . . . are in an enviable position as far as bacon, egg, and steak lovers are concerned"), the authors also advise that sodium nitrite and sodium nitrate are "UNSAFE in the amounts typically consumed or very poorly tested." In other words (and this is just one example), a food additive found in almost all readily available lunch meats, cured meats, bacon products, and hot dogs is considered by these authors to be unsafe for pregnant women. Moreover, with respect to "eating safe," they recommend that all "ready-cooked meats" like hot dogs or bologna be heated to 165 degrees Fahrenheit prior to eating.[19] Readers are encouraged to read food labels intensely and to be careful of a wide variety of ethnic cuisines, or at least portions of those cuisines that do not comply with the standards of the prescribed low fat/high fiber diet.

It's not just that heating corned beef before making a sandwich is a pain in the neck, or that nitrite/nitrate-free hot dogs are hard to find; nor is it just that women are being advised to account for every bit of food and drink that enters into their bodies. Pregnancy advice books like *What to Expect When You're Expecting* demonstrate precisely how pregnant women are imagined as the ideal subjects of our contemporary concern about what goes into our bodies and how the ordinary foods and dietary experiences of our culture are feared as dangerous to our health. This is not to say that they are *not* dangerous, but merely to suggest that we hold pregnant women to a kind of idealized standard about their bodies and their health. And it would be easy to say, "Well, if those foods are dangerous, pregnant women should stay away from them. After all, it's not that hard." But with hot dogs, and lunch meats, and even bacon, we are speaking about foods central to the diets of many American men and women. It is not just the fact that this advice requires extra care toward health from pregnant women, it is that the advice demands culturally anomalous behaviors toward food and eating.[20]

American attitudes toward alcohol consumption during pregnancy—and, more recently, during breastfeeding—represent another example of this tendency to isolate mothers through expectations of purity.

Drink

Comparison between industrialized countries is instructive with regard to attitudes about pregnant women and alcohol. Information on the Web site of the British Nutrition Foundation offers a clear yet relatively relaxed view of alcohol consumption during pregnancy.

> Drinking alcohol during pregnancy can damage the unborn child, so pregnant women may prefer to avoid alcohol. The Department of Health advises that to minimise the risk to the unborn child, women who are trying to become pregnant or are at any stage of pregnancy should not drink more than 1 or 2 units of alcohol once or twice a

week, and should avoid heavy drinking sessions. One unit is a small glass of wine, a half pint of ordinary strength beer, lager or cider, or a single 25ml (pub) measure of spirits.[21]

American advice on this matter tends toward absolute abstention from alcohol, at least during pregnancy and also, in recent publications, during breastfeeding as well. *What to Expect* has this to say: "although you shouldn't worry about what you drank before you were pregnant, it would be prudent to abstain for the rest of your pregnancy—except for a celebratory half glass of wine on a very special occasion."[22]

With respect to breastfeeding and alcohol consumption, in *The Complete Guide to Everyday Risks in Pregnancy and Breastfeeding* author Gideon Koren writes, "While ample evidence indicates that drinking alcohol during pregnancy poses a severe and avoidable risk to the fetus, the risks of drinking alcohol while breastfeeding are not well defined." He then goes on to suggest that because there has been no safe level of alcohol in breast milk established, "the safest choice is to avoid exposure to the nursing infant." To aid mothers, he developed a chart indicating the number of hours to wait after imbibing, dependent on a woman's weight and the number of drinks ingested (fig. 1).[23] Rebecca Kukla would argue that Koren's chart is a "technic" designed to "terrorize" women "with extremist rhetoric concerning the risks of alcohol, drugs, and other substances that they may be tempted to ingest. Doctors and pregnancy guides regularly tell women that no amount of alcohol can be acceptably ingested during pregnancy, even though researchers have been unable to find any detrimental effects of alcohol consumption among pregnant women who drink lightly to moderately, as part of a healthy lifestyle rather than as self-medication."[24]

In *Message in a Bottle: The Making of Fetal Alcohol Syndrome,* medical historian Janet Golden suggests that the decision by public health experts and administrators to advocate total abstinence from alcohol during pregnancy has never made good sense, given the evidence that fetal alcohol syndrome (FAS) is caused by excessive alcohol ingestion by addicted (i.e., alcoholic) mothers while pregnant. What is striking about her findings is that the "core principle of teratology—that individual fetuses vary in their vulnerability to particular agents and thus there can be no absolute safe level of exposure" offered health workers a rationale to regulate the alcohol consumption of all pregnant women without necessarily helping those specific women with alcohol consumption problems, that is, those most likely to

Mother's Weight kg (lbs)	No. of Drinks (Hours : Minutes) 1 drink = 340 g (12 oz) of 5% beer, or 141.75 g (5 oz) of 11% wine, or 42.53 g (1.5 oz) of 40% liquor.											
	1	2	3	4	5	6	7	8	9	10	11	12
40.8 (90)	2:50	5:40	8:30	11:20	14:10	17:00	19:51	22:41				
43.1 (95)	2:46	5:32	8:19	11:05	13:52	16:38	19:25	22:11				
45.4 (100)	2:42	5:25	8:08	10:51	13:34	16:17	19:00	21:43				
47.6 (105)	2:39	5:19	7:58	10:38	13:18	15:57	18:37	21:16	23:56			
49.9 (110)	2:36	5:12	7:49	10:25	13:01	15:38	18:14	20:50	23:27			
52.2 (115)	2:33	5:06	7:39	10:12	12:46	15:19	17:52	20:25	22:59			
54.4 (120)	2:30	5:00	7:30	10:00	12:31	15:01	17:31	20:01	22:32			
56.7 (125)	2:27	4:54	7:22	9:49	12:16	14:44	17:11	19:38	22:06			
59.0 (130)	2:24	4:49	7:13	9:38	12:03	14:27	16:52	19:16	21:41			
61.2 (135)	2:21	4:43	7:05	9:27	11:49	14:11	16:33	18:55	21:17	23:39		
63.5 (140)	2:19	4:30	6:50	9:17	11:37	13:56	16:15	18:35	20:54	23:14		
65.8 (145)	2:16	4:33	6:50	9:07	11:24	13:41	15:58	18:15	20:32	22:49		
68.0 (150)	2:14	4:29	6:43	8:58	11:12	13:27	15:41	17:56	20:10	22:25		
70.3 (155)	2:12	4:24	6:36	8:48	11:01	13:13	15:25	17:37	19:49	22:02		
72.6 (160)	2:10	4:20	6:30	8:40	10:50	13:00	15:10	17:20	19:30	21:40	23:50	
74.8 (165)	2:07	4:15	6:23	8:31	10:39	12:47	14:54	17:02	19:10	21:18	23:50	
77.1 (170)	2:05	4:11	6:17	8:23	10:28	12:34	14:40	16:46	18:51	20:57	23:03	
79.3 (175)	2:03	4:07	6:11	8:14	10:18	12:22	14:26	16:29	18:33	20:37	22:40	
81.6 (180)	2:01	4:03	6:05	8:07	10:08	12:10	14:12	16:14	18:15	20:17	22:19	
83.9 (185)	1:59	3:59	5:59	7:59	9:59	11:59	13:59	15:59	17:58	19:58	21:58	23:58
86.2 (190)	1:58	3:56	5:54	7:52	9:50	11:48	13:46	15:44	17:42	19:40	21:38	23:36
88.5 (195)	1:56	3:52	5:48	7:44	9:41	11:37	13:33	15:29	17:26	19:22	21:18	23:14
90.7 (200)	1:54	3:49	5:43	7:38	9:32	11:27	13:21	15:16	17:10	19:05	20:59	22:54
93.0 (205)	1:52	3:45	5:38	7:31	9:24	11:17	13:09	15:02	16:55	18:48	20:41	22:34
95.3 (210)	1:51	3:42	5:33	7:24	9:16	11:07	12:58	14:49	16:41	18:32	20:23	22:14

Fig. 1. Breastfeeding and alcohol consumption chart from *The Complete Guide to Everyday Risks in Pregnancy and Breastfeeding,* by Gideon Koren, MD, FRCP (C), 206. (Copyright Gideon Koren, 2004. Published by Robert Rose Inc. Printed with permission.)

give birth to babies affected by FAS. Indeed, the decision to "emphasi[ze] broad-scale public health education, rather than programmatic efforts to help severely alcoholic women through specialized inpatient programs, social service support, and prenatal care, meant that those at greatest risk of bearing affected babies received the same attention and resources as those least likely to have such children." She adds, "Rates of FAS did not decline and the syndrome ultimately became a marker of maternal misbehavior rather than an indication that new measures were needed to help alcoholic women."[25] Because alcohol had long been thought to be good for pregnant women, and because drinking was an ordinary aspect of middle-class American life in the 1970s and 1980s, it took some time before the general populace agreed to the public health guidelines concerning alcohol consumption during pregnancy. Golden notes that the first warning from the National Institute on Alcohol Abuse and Alcoholism, in 1977, simply suggested that pregnant women limit their alcohol consumption to two drinks per day. In 1981, however, a new warning was released advising pregnant women away from all alcoholic beverages.

This attitude, which requires that mothers-to-be and breastfeeding mothers behave in culturally anomalous ways with regard to what passes from them to the fetus, is evident in other discussions in Koren's *Complete Guide to Everyday Risks of Pregnancy and Breastfeeding.* The text as a whole is concerned with environmental contaminants and medicines that either go through the placenta to the developing fetus or through breast milk to nursing babies. While the overall message concerning medicines and breastfeeding is reassuring, in that the advice suggests that "most medications are excreted into breast milk in very small quantities [meaning] that typically, your baby will receive very small amounts of the drug," it is clear that discussion of the issue is necessary because it is normal to take both prescription and over-the-counter medications, sometimes quite a few in various combinations.[26] Thus it is precisely the conditions of modern biomedicine that, at least in part, cause us to be extra cautious about what gets to babies through their mothers' bodies, even as it is medicine itself that helps us to determine medicinal teratogenicity and/or other problems resulting from the action of mothers' bodies as chemical conduits. The need to be vigilant about "everyday risks" is emblematic of the risk society, in which routine risks are necessary and feared because they are central to the conditions of modern life.

Risk and Pollution: A Conclusion

There are actually two cultural trends that come together around these expectations of maternal behavior during pregnancy: pollution rituals concerning pregnancy and measures to control risks in terms of Ulrich Beck's notion of "reflexive modernity." Pregnant women are likely to be subject to a culture's pollution taboos in particular ways.[27] In the context of contemporary society, in which environmental contamination is a routine worry that is simultaneously produced by the very advances that have brought us to the (post)modern moment and in which medications and industrially prepared foods are standard components of daily living, pollution taboos are expressed through what seem to be logical concerns about what pregnant women eat and drink and what environmental hazards they are exposed to.[28] The attention to environmental contaminants (or alcohol abuse or drug use) seems reasonable as part of normal living in the risk society, but these are particular ways of understanding the maternal body as always in danger of being polluted and thus needing to be regulated so that matter stays in its rightful place. After all, pregnant women live at the margins of acceptable personhood, literally in touch with what Mary Douglas calls a "transitional area" or "person in a marginal state."[29] The "logic" of these concerns relies on the cultural context in which they are selected and recognized as legitimate concerns. In broader cultural analysis, we can see that they function as pollution taboos like any other pollution taboos—they serve to demarcate proper social boundaries through body symbolism, and they operate to establish and maintain perceptions of order and matter in its place. Thus the targeting of environmental contaminants—a concern emerging from the conditions of industrialized modernity—is both a constitutive element of the risk society and also an indication that modern cultures select risks in the same ways and for the same reasons as nonmodern cultures: to identify dirt and other impurities that threaten the cultural system from within. To repeat a quotation from Lawrence Buell, toxic discourse is "an interlocked set of topoi whose force derives partly from the anxieties of late industrial culture, [and] partly from deeper-rooted habits of thought and expression."[30]

In addition, as Anna Lowenhaupt Tsing argues, "new perinatal vigilance . . . is an agenda that isolates female reproductive experience from every other aspect of women's lives, requiring that pregnancy be a transcendent

moment that can carry every woman outside the complexity of her particular history."[31] Australian scholar Helen Keane writes, with respect to advice about complete abstention from alcohol by pregnant women,

> The faith in education demonstrated by public health FAS discourse
> is premised on a view of the mother-to-be as a rational and au-
> tonomous agent able to decide what is best on the basis of reason and
> knowledge and then convert this decision into appropriate action.…
>
> Messages like this construct pregnant women as free to choose
> between different actions and behaviours to secure their own well-
> being and the health of their babies. They treat both the action of be-
> coming pregnant and behaviours such as abstaining from alcohol
> and eating a balanced diet as matters of pure individual choice. The
> pregnant woman is lifted out from her particular social positioning,
> the world in and through which she lives, and she appears as an ab-
> stract, strangely disembodied figure unbounded by any constraints
> to her agency.[32]

Both Keane and Tsing suggest that discursive and material practices disembedding women from historical circumstances and making possible expectations of total rational behavior erroneously imagine women's power.
Keane puts it this way: "The pregnant woman is embedded in social relations and discourses which both limit her behaviours and actions and make
them possible. Her (embodied) subjectivity is a product of her movement
amongst these multiple discourses and relationships of power, not the
starting point of her actions in the world."[33]

The requirement for gestational purity distinguishes pregnant women
from the rest of us and makes them a cultural anomaly.[34] If pregnant
women accede to requirements that they restrict their diets, their environments, and their daily activities to protect the unborn, then they conform to
the moral demands of the public that they behave better than the rest of us,
demonstrating their fitness as mothers through their sacrificial commitment to the other within. Yet they also behave as we wish we could, or believe we should, in the context of broad social fears about the effects of
modernization on bodies and the natural world. In the industrialized
world, women become mothers through a highly codified and medically
regulated experience of pregnancy, an experience that tries to mold them
into the kind of mothers who make deliberative choices about what goes

into their bodies so that what comes out of those bodies—babies, breast milk—is pure and healthy, the determined result of rational decisions and planned, minimized risks. They are subject to wide-ranging anxieties about the fate of human bodies in the social world, and must demonstrate through their embodied practices their goodness, which qualifies them to be mothers.

To behave differently as a pregnant woman is to tempt fate, to invite punishments in the guise of congenital defects, higher risks of cancer, and increased infant morbidity and mortality. The mechanism of punishment here is not altogether different from other, nonscientific systems of belief. Modern pollution beliefs suggest that particular illnesses are the result of contamination by toxic chemicals in the environment, the result of not being careful enough (either as individuals or as a culture) to safeguard health. Again, this is not to state that certain illnesses or disorders are not caused by environmental contaminants. What I am arguing is that pollution beliefs are supported by science just as they are supported by superstitions or other belief systems. They demonstrate a need to describe all causes of death or illness and to do away with morbidity and mortality as things that happen without known cause. Modern pollution beliefs are pollution beliefs all the same, and while industrialization offers newly dangerous modes of pollution, it does not seem to transform common cultural responses to these threats.

CHAPTER 9

Contamination and the Sacred Maternal Body

THIS CHAPTER concerns representations of human milk and mothers' bodies in environmentalist discourses about chemical contaminants, a primary instance of what Lawrence Buell identifies as "toxic discourse." Breastfeeding advocates worry that biomonitoring of breast milk—the use of breast milk to study chemical body burdens across populations—will inhibit women from nursing. Environmental advocates want to use rhetorically powerful images (such as toxic breast milk) to goad governments and international bodies to action on limiting the use of toxic chemicals and regulating their environmental impact.[1] These policy controversies between breastfeeding advocates and environmentalists arise in the context of expectations of maternal purity evident in public debates about pregnant women and their diets, fetuses and the wombs they inhabit, and breastfeeding women and their sacred roles. This chapter asks us to wonder what would an examination of toxic chemicals in the environment look like if it did not use the figure of the pure mother as its antithesis and goal. That is, how would environmental toxins in breast milk be figured if the maternal body was not viewed through what Lawrence Buell calls "the rose-colored lens of pastoral-utopian innocence"?[2] After all, the body of the breastfeeding mother is always-already corrupt, a body that is of the world and thus implicated in its filth as all of our bodies are.

Impure Mothers

Sandra Steingraber has written extensively about environmental contamination and, more recently, about the contamination of breast milk and its significance for the breast–bottle controversy. Steingraber's work is compelling and fascinating, yet also troublesome. Even though she supports breastfeeding while identifying the significant danger to infants from contaminated breast milk, she does so only by representing maternal nursing as a "sacrament" that should be protected. By linking the impurities in the breast milk of modern mothers to the violation of a sacred relation, Steingraber makes explicit the obscured expectation that maternal purity stands against a corrupted, sexual, bad maternity.

Steingraber's *Living Downstream: An Ecologist Looks at Cancer and the Environment* contains nine distinct passages in which breastfeeding or breast milk is mentioned. Let me offer a few as examples.

> Childhood cancer in Los Angeles was found to be associated with parental exposure to pesticides during pregnancy or nursing.
>
> When painted onto [turtle] eggs, PCBs turn red-eared sliders from male to female. Moreover, this happens at very low concentrations—levels comparable to the average level of PCBs now found in the breast milk of women living in industrialized countries.
>
> First, we see why infants are at special risk: residues of fat-soluble pesticides contained in the food eaten by nursing mothers are distilled even further in breast milk. In essence, breastfeeding infants occupy a higher rung on the food chain than the rest of us. In many cases, human milk contains pesticide and other residues in excess of limits established for commercially marketed food.
>
> Organochlorine contaminants are not easily expunged from our tissues. Their sharp decline in concentration over the course of breastfeeding, therefore, represents the movement of accumulated toxins from mother to child. It signifies that during the intimate act of nursing, a burden of public poisons—insect killers, electrical insulating fluids, industrial solvents, and incinerator residues—is shifted from one generation to the tiny bodies of the next.[3]

In the entire text of *Living Downstream,* Steingraber never mentions that alternatives to breast milk are industrial products and thus contribute to the pollution problems she investigates in the book. Instead, she offers us the following information: "By 1976, roughly 25 percent of all U.S. breast milk was too contaminated to be bottled and sold as a food commodity."[4]

What we learn from *Living Downstream* is that breastfeeding is a dangerous activity, that artificial infant formulas are highly regulated substances that ensure protection from environmental contamination, that infants are beings whose position in the food chain (at the top) places them at particular risk of contamination from their mothers' bodies, that nursing is an intimate activity that is secretly fraught with danger. What should be an intimate, healthy, loving practice is instead the transfer of poison "from one generation to the next." These figurations are based on scientific evidence, but also convey deep suspicion of what comes from the mother's body, especially since it comes through a relation of intimacy and assumed protection. Partly, this is an effect of the reiteration of the problem of breast milk and breastfeeding without an analysis of the contribution of infant formula manufacture to environmental contamination. But we shall also see that when Steingraber addresses breastfeeding in a more balanced fashion, arguing for it despite the environmental risks, she can do so only by invoking it as a "sacrament" between mother and child.

As an example, in *Having Faith: An Ecologist's Journey to Motherhood*, Steingraber discusses the difficulties of bringing breast milk contamination into public consciousness: "On the one hand we have the chemical adulteration of human milk. On the other is the bodily sacrament between mother and child. Can we speak of them both in the same breath? Can we look at one without turning away from the other?" She argues that we "need to insist that breastfeeding is a sacrament of motherhood that cannot be reduced to a risk-benefit equation—even if we did have all the data to create one. By placing breastfeeding in a human rights context, we avoid stultifying breast-versus-bottle discussions that urge us to either shut up and nurse or switch to formula if we're so worried about toxic chemicals." Yet certainly "placing breastfeeding in a human rights context" does not mandate that we treat the practice as a sacrament and thereby celebrate (and enforce) the pure intimacy of maternal-infant bonding. Even if we want to claim a "toxic-free future" as our goal, we might hesitate to demand pure breast milk as a human right. As Penny Van Esterik points out, few considerations of environmental toxins in human milk situate the mother in context, as the target of a variety of environmental, economic, social, and cultural forces that together create the present state of her body.[5]

Breastfeeding is perceived as a sacrament in particular cultural contexts and within specific social relations. To use *sacrament* to define its value socially (beyond the medicalized perspective on its values that Steingraber offers earlier) is to return us to the tradition of "Maria Lactans" that Fiona

Giles has pointed out is one trend in the iconography of sacred nursing.[6] While many people will rally behind sacraments as things needing protection from the ravages of modern, industrial society, sacraments can also be cloistered experiences, protected through regulation and surveillance.

The risk-benefit analysis can be avoided or challenged in other ways, for example, by arguing that women have a right to breastfeed and not to worry about toxic transfer. It seems reasonable to suggest that women have the right to not be perceived as responsible for environmental conditions out of their control. It may be that advocates want to argue for more balanced information about mothers' bodies—information that does not point to the evidence of contamination as its source.[7] If advocates choose to argue for breastfeeding as a human right, the argument should be staged without drawing on the language of the sacred. The conceptual purity of religious discourse is inviting, but the problem of environmental contamination and toxic chemicals in breast milk resides in the more troublesome realm of politics.

Steingraber uses religious rhetoric juxtaposed against medical evidence and discourse: "Surely . . . the toxic contamination of breast milk—to the degree that it routinely violates laws governing contaminant levels in commercial foodstuffs and threatens a woman's ability to produce sufficient milk to feed her child—is also a violation of this sacred communion. The presence of toxic chemicals in breast milk compromises its goodness and lowers its capacity to heal, to promote brain growth, and orchestrate the development of the immune system."[8] One reason the religious discourse so successfully argues the case for medicine—that is, the use of references to the sacred to describe a "goodness" that in the next sentence is described in relation to healing, brain growth, and the immune system—is that breast milk is aligned with purity in the advocacy literature. Breast milk is pure because it doesn't need to be mixed with anything, can be left out longer than formula without spoiling (if it's been expressed), and is unadulterated. One doesn't worry about spoilage of breast milk because it is usually ingested at the point of production, unlike infant formula, which should be consumed within a certain time or discarded. Breast milk is also a living substance that contributes to the health of the infant who imbibes it, not just the infant's growth (this is the medical argument). Thus, breast milk purity is aligned with the medical view of its superior biological profile. This language allows a slippage into purity in the other sense, the religious sensibility that mothers are really madonnas and it is up to society to ensure their purity. Thus, what seems like an argument for ecological well-being ends up articulating an ideologically confining vision of motherhood.

Yet breast milk is effective biologically in part because it is not pure, that is, because it responds to viruses and bacteria. Breast milk harbors antibodies and other antiviral properties, but these are effective only insofar as the mother has an infection or has had one. Its antibacterial qualities are likewise dependent on the mother's current colonization by bacteria. We cannot really imagine that human milk has ever been free of contamination. While humans have not always lived under the specifically polluted environments of industrialized societies, humans have always created toxic chemicals ingested by mothers, at least since the advent of fire. At a purely commonsense level, the notion of pure human milk is a fiction, one that misrepresents the action of the mother's body in contemporary society and looks back toward an imagined past that is also misrepresented. And since reproduction for humans is still conducted sexually (assistive reproductive technologies notwithstanding), breast milk never comes from a pure body in this sense either. The discourse of purity can be understood, at least in part, as an attempt to ward off the meanings of the sexual acts that precede childbirth and breastfeeding, and thus to make a fetish of breastfeeding as a pure activity against its own sexual meanings.[9]

Of course, the advocacy discourse of purity emerged, in the middle of the last century, as a refutation of the prevalence of practices like swabbing the nursing mother's nipples with rubbing alcohol before allowing the baby to nurse, as if breasts, like bottles, needed sterilization before they were ready for the infant. It is also an argument for breastfeeding against the standardization represented by infant formulas: breast milk is always there, ready and waiting, pure from the source, rather than constituting an industrial product that needs to be evaluated and tested. In this way, "purity" can also be rhetorical and political, articulated as part of a strategy to enhance mothers' value and to support breastfeeding against the assaults on maternal competence that encouraged its abandonment.

Body Burdens

Steingraber's comment concerning the 25 percent of breast milk that is too contaminated to be sold as a commodity is disturbing precisely because the analogy turns the milk into a commodity for the purposes of comparison. We can see this same magical perspective on the potential toxicity of breast milk articulated by Florence Williams, who declares that "if human milk were sold at the local Piggly Wiggly, some stock would exceed federal food-safety levels for DDT residues and PCB's."[10] Now, of course, mothers can send their expressed breast milk to be analyzed as if it were a food product. Williams sent her own breast milk to be tested for polybrominated diphenyl ether (PBDE) flame retardants, a process called biomonitoring.

Biomonitoring is a way of determining the personal chemical body burden of individuals in a given society and can be used to understand the population burden when studied in groups of people. Some environmental activists argue that it is an effective way of "bring[ing] otherwise remote policy debates to a very personal level."[11] Yet biomonitoring treats human bodies as if they were industrialized products, perhaps an inevitable result of living in environments so infused by industry and its chemical creations that we cannot separate ourselves either physically or nominally from those processes. Biomonitoring seems a clear example of our collective discomfort with the processes of modernization that make contemporary life different from previous historical periods. It also represents a predictably modern remedy for such discomfort—regulation. Surveillance of individuals is figured as a remedy to solve a problem endemic to modernity.

In addition, the role of breastfeeding and breast milk in environmentalist debates over chemical body burdens provides an example of how imaginary constructions of maternal purity affect policy debates that concern women's bodies. But these debates also concern the actual use of breast milk to determine and publicize environmental contamination. Breastfeeding advocates are wary of projects using breast milk to determine chemical body burdens because they are afraid that such projects will convince large numbers of women that breast milk is a dangerous substance. Advocates also believe that the use of breast milk in these ways contributes to perceptions of women's bodies as toxic and the source of contamination; they promote approaches to chemical contamination that target industry, rather than women's bodies, as the source of the problem.

The uses of breast milk in scientific projects—even if such projects are targeted for the social good—change the meanings of breast milk by treating it like a scientific object. Advocates' work to mitigate the effects of breast milk biomonitoring on breastfeeding practices demonstrates awareness of this problem, as the historical tendencies toward modernization lead to the abandonment of breastfeeding across populations. Bringing back breastfeeding as an ordinary mode of infant feeding in the global north has needed the strong support of public health and medical institutions. The success of such endeavors is mitigated by the fact that breastfeeding now only occurs in these countries under the supervision of medical personnel and as a highly medicalized practice. Using breast milk to measure chemical body burdens in this context seems like a logical thing to do, especially if one is concerned about the chemicals one's baby ingests, because it follows the general regulatory pattern of the experiences of pregnancy and well-baby care. Given the disciplining experiences of pregnancy in industrialized countries like the United States, this is a concern instilled in mothers before they give birth.

This section of the chapter treats the ambivalences and difficulties of biomonitoring and the discourses of breastfeeding advocacy that claim the value of human milk in the face of its obvious infiltration by toxic chemicals. In it I examine how advocates and environmentalists represent the problem of chemical contamination of breast milk, identifying specific rhetorical patterns in the presentation of the issues. Instead of focusing on the ways in which advocates and environmentalists differ in their representation of breast milk contamination and its meanings, however, I look at similarities in the way both groups address this problem. Other scholars, notably Penny Van Esterik, have analyzed both rifts between breastfeeding advocacy groups and environmentalists on this issue and the problem of media risk communication that is unbalanced and inflammatory. Instead I am interested in exploring the shared effects of portrayals of breast milk biomonitoring as a necessary activity that signals problems with the environment and that may promote the abandonment of breastfeeding, although this is not their intended purpose. Such an approach allows me to demonstrate that even those accounts that are sympathetic to breastfeeding and support its contributions to health participate in discourses of risk that play upon the themes already discussed in this book: the importance of maternal regulation during pregnancy, the tendency to emphasize the risks of breastfeeding rather than the risks of not breastfeeding, and the ambivalence generated by impure maternal bodies.

Advocates and environmentalists tend to identify the chemical contaminants found in breast milk but then emphasize its unique contributions to health when discussing its value in infant feeding. They share a desire to safeguard breastfeeding even as breast milk is identified as a conveyer of contamination. Yet the rhetoric used to present the problem demonstrates the difficulty of this balancing act—just knowing the number of chemical contaminants in breast milk is a humbling lesson in acknowledging the dangerous permeability of human bodies. It's hard to accommodate this knowledge and also accept breastfeeding without fear of the involuntary effects of breast milk toxicity. That there exists a background expectation of pure mothers and a belief in breastfeeding as a sacramental activity affects the way any representation of the toxins in breast milk trades on fear and may influence individual practices.

Breast milk is used in biomonitoring because it is relatively easy to collect (as opposed to other kinds of tissue and excretory samples) and because its fat content makes it an ideal medium to use to identify bioaccumulative chemicals. La Leche League International (LLLI) and the International Lactation Consultant Association (ILCA), both point out that using breast milk in biomonitoring is not meant by environmental groups as an assault on breastfeeding, but they emphasize that such practices may have the effect of raising concerns about the safety of nursing. In its media release "Breastfeeding Remains Best Choice in a Polluted World," La Leche League announces, "Any substances found in human milk because of this routine testing are a reflection of the exposure in all humans living in that particular area and not a statement about breastfeeding." ILCA's "Position on Breastfeeding, Breast Milk, and Environmental Contaminants" notes, "Unfortunately, it is possible that the concerns expressed by environmental groups may be sensationalized or misinterpreted by the media and cause undue concern among breastfeeding mothers."[12] However, the problems posed by the discourses of environmental groups concerning breast milk contamination are not only (or even primarily) the result of sensationalizing by the media. Rather, the difficulty is evident in the rhetoric of these groups as they try to articulate the hazards of chemical contaminants in breast milk at the same time that they present information about the benefits of breastfeeding.

Communication of pollution risks is fraught with problems. As Pascal Milly argues, with reference to concerns about PCB contamination of the traditional foodstuffs of the Far North Canadian Inuit, both the pollutants and the "risk communication failures" migrate from the industrialized South to "the most vulnerable people in Canada." That is, people whose overall good health depends on the ingestion of traditional or "country" foods, including breastfeeding their young, learn about high PCB body burdens in their communities as a result of researchers' attempts to measure the spread of the chemical and its effects on various groups.[13] The fear, of course, is that the information about chemical body burdens will change the very practices on which the community's health depends, even if it is those practices that lead to relatively high levels of toxins in the body. This is the primary fear of breastfeeding advocates who see too much attention being paid to toxic chemicals in breast milk. Environmental groups try to support breastfeeding as beneficial to health, and even as a safeguard against the possible effects of environmental contaminants, but the rhetorical complexities of their multiple political goals undermine this support.

For example, an extensive report for the Environmental Working Group (EWG), *Mothers' Milk: Record Levels of Toxic Fire Retardants Found in American Mothers' Breast Milk,* discusses findings from several studies, including one the EWG itself conducted, concerning the high levels of PBDEs in the breast milk of American women. The levels in U.S. women appear to be the highest in the world. After stating that in utero exposure to toxins like PCBs appears to be much more dangerous than any exposure through breastfeeding, the authors of the report write, "Despite the numerous benefits associated with breastfeeding the detection of PBDEs in breast milk signals dangerous exposures to the developing fetus and baby. . . . In-utero transfer and breastfeeding are suspected as major sources of PBDE levels in infant serum. . . . The evidence that young children are especially exposed and uniquely vulnerable to these toxic chemicals heightens the need for action to limit exposures." This section is directly followed by a sidebar titled "Breast Milk Is Still Best." A similar rhetoric is used to promote breastfeeding in the context of environmental contamination.

> Evidence of the accumulation of chemicals in women's bodies and breast milk may prompt mothers to question the safety of their breast milk as a food for their baby. *However,* the evidence is clear: Women should breastfeed their children and continue to do so for as long as possible.
>
> *Even though* breastfed infants are exposed to higher levels of chemicals over their first few years of life, they have lower levels of childhood cancers, breast cancer and other illnesses believed to be linked to chemical exposure.
>
> *Despite* evidence that breastfeeding can protect against subtle health effects caused by in-utero chemical exposures, we should still be cautious with our children's exposure to chemicals.
>
> In all but the most extreme circumstances, then, breast milk re-

mains the best food for babies. *Yet* we cannot ignore the increasing burdens of persistent contaminants in the bodies of mothers and children.[14]

The qualifying terms, which I have emphasized with italics, demonstrate the difficulty of conveying concern about the findings of contaminants in breast milk in conjunction with a promotion of breastfeeding as an appropriate mode of infant feeding. Each statement about the contribution that breastfeeding makes to health is preceded or followed by a qualifier concerning contaminants and their deleterious effects.

The political goals of environmentalists' rhetoric concerning the severity of the contaminants include inciting fear and anger in individuals so that they will act to end the use of such contaminants. People who respond in this way might find it difficult to accommodate knowledge of the chemicals in mothers' bodies and breast milk with the understanding that "even so" breastfeeding is best. After all, some of these people are the very mothers who have been cautioned against ingesting certain kinds of fish because of their high levels of mercury. The absolutism required of mothers during gestation (no alcohol, no cured meats, etc.) encourages mothers to be alarmed about *any* possible source of contamination.

The EWG does include a short section called "Concerns with Infant Formulas" that highlights problems associated with the use of tap water to mix powdered infant formulas (the least expensive and thus most common form), with the lack of fatty acids in formula, and with potential excess levels of manganese in both dairy and soy preparations. And yet it may be easier to accept potential risks attendant to formula use rather than those involved in breastfeeding, given that infant formula is recognized as an industrial product and, because of that, regulated. Purity is not necessarily expected from infant formulas as a matter of course, although predictability and standardization are, two attributes that may be seen as preferable to the lack of standardizability inherent in breastfeeding.[15]

Moreover, as I argued in the chapter on the U.S. National Breastfeeding Awareness Campaign, the American public is far more likely to identify specific risks of breastfeeding than general risks associated with formula use. There is an established cultural consensus on this matter, evident in the widespread agreement that making mothers feel guilty about not breastfeeding is bad. There is no widespread sentiment that making mothers feel nervous about breastfeeding by publicizing the contaminants in breast milk is a problem. The LLL media release and the ILCA position paper both acknowledge the importance of understanding maternal concerns about environmental contamination and provide information about how to personally avoid excess exposures. They do not express dismay that the issue is addressed or that mothers should not know this information for their own good, which is how the guilt argument works in the breast–bottle debate.

The LLL media release, other breastfeeding-friendly texts that deal with concerns about chemical contaminants, and environmentalist reports all make specific recommendations concerning personal practices that can lessen exposure to environmental toxins. For example, the British Web site BabyCentre includes the following list of actions.

- Limit your exposure to household paints, glues, furniture strippers, nail polish, petrol fumes. . . .
- Eat further down the food chain. . . .
- Eat organic if possible. . . .
- Avoid baked or fried foods made with animal fats, and eat fresh rather than processed foods where possible. . . .
- Avoid fish liver oil food supplements, such as cod liver oil. . . .
- Avoid incinerator discharge if you can. . . .[16]

The media release from La Leche League includes "10 Simple Steps to Help Reduce the Level of Chemicals in Your Body," and even the EWG report *Mothers' Milk* has a list of things that "parents and concerned consumers [can] do" about exposure to PBDEs, which is longer than the list of things that the U.S. Congress should do to reduce population exposure in general. (It is notable that their list includes the exclamatory recommendation to "Breastfeed your child!")[17]

The emphasis on personal behaviors that might decrease exposure to dangerous chemicals is both practical and troubling. As LLL notes, "It is impossible to reduce exposure to all chemical elements." It is true that individuals can, theoretically, do much to reduce exposure: for example, recent studies have shown that children fed organic food reduce their personal body burden dramatically in just a few months. Yet the list of specific actions that individuals can take personalizes what is clearly a widespread social problem, and it also presupposes an individual who has significant control over numerous aspects of her life. Just the simple suggestion to "eat organic when possible" raises the related issues of expense and access. When LLL remarks that "those in the work force [should] attempt to avoid occupational exposure to chemical contaminants and seek to improve workplace chemical safety standards for all employees, especially pregnant and lactating women," it is clear that they are suggesting an enabling strategy (take charge of your situation and do something positive for others!) but perhaps also overestimating women's power to regulate their work environments or make changes that affect themselves, let alone others.[18]

It is hard not to see the hallmarks of modernity—and the expectation that women are all modern in the same way—in these discussions. Women are presented as powerful and empowering, able to transform industrial practices through activism. Individuals become the focus of exposure reduction, and personal responsibility for body burden is the default expectation. Yet Penny Van Esterik points out, "The belief that individuals are responsible for their personal health is particularly disturbing in the case of breastfeeding and chemical contaminants. Breastfeeding does not exist in isolation from . . . the processes of globalization that tolerate, or even encourage industrial pollution." She questions the focus on breasts and breastfeeding in the environmentalist discussions of body burden and the effect of toxins on human bodies, suggesting that this emphasis—to the exclusion of other imagined foci, like testicles and semen—demonstrates a cultural tendency to figure women's bodies as "risky environments" and to identify problems in those bodies with "a fear of total system breakdown." Noting that "women are blamed for exposing their children to contaminants, poisoning themselves and their children, downloading contaminants from their bodies to their children's bodies," Van Esterik implies that without a feminist understanding of the way women's bodies are portrayed in the debates about environmental toxins, the effect of biomonitoring processes that rely on excretions from women's bodies—excretions that already tend to be perceived suspiciously within and across cultures—will be further distrust of breastfeeding as an ordinary practice of biological maternity. Thus while the information from various organizations suggests specific ways to avoid exposure to contaminants, women cannot escape the burden of responsibility for being the environment for their fetuses and infants, and thus for seeming to be the source of contamination of their children.[19]

There is another representational issue that emerges in these toxic discourses about human milk. Some advocates use the figure of the "canary in a coal mine" to accentuate the significance and semiotics of the maternal body in these debates. For example, Jack Newman, reknowned physician and breastfeeding advocate, writes, "The fact that there are pollutants in breastmilk can be likened to the situation of the canary in the coal mine."[20] The "canary in a coal mine" analogy works to solidify the perception of women's bodies as instrumental—and thus as experimental subjects. After all, the canary is the dispensable animal that alerts coal miners to the existence of poisonous gas. The canary analogy also suggests women as vulnerable, sensitive victims, highlighting the subjugating impact of expectations of maternal purity on mothers.

Van Esterik includes a section titled "Woman as Canary: The Sentinel Gender" in the conclusion to *Risks, Rights, and Regulation* but does not discuss the figure. By suggesting that women act as "sentinels," standing watch or guard, Van Esterik transforms the passive meaning of the canary. This figuration heralds a more active role for women, in keeping with the idea of women as neoliberal agents who actively seek to know their body burden and discipline themselves to be pure. This is clearly not her intention. But the notion of a canary in this context is anything but active. After all, the canary's job is a passive one: to wait in the hope that toxic gases don't kill it.

Conclusion

Reading through reports on contaminants pervasive in the environment and, consequently, in human bodies and human milk is terrifying. It is meant to be an agonizing experience, goading the reader to action, preferably of a political sort. But I find the discourses about contamination and body burden to be paralyzing, as I surf various Web sites for information about the ten most toxic fruits and vegetables and the ten least toxic. What do I do when I learn that apples, which my son eats with his lunch almost every day, are number two on the "most toxic" list, behind peaches, my daughter's favorite summer fruit? How worried should I be? Is it worth it to buy organic apples and peaches, which are at least twice as expensive as the nonorganic varieties in my local grocery store? How do I know what "worth it" means, since in my immediate family no one has ever had cancer, the disease most commonly associated with exposure to environmental toxins? When I go to a Web site that will identify personal body products that do not have known toxic chemicals in them, or ingredients thought to be carcinogenic, the products that are listed for me are made by companies that I am not familiar with and are certainly not available on the shelves of my local drug store or supermarket. I don't want to become a person whose relationship to the environment—to my own environment—is paranoid or obsessive-compulsive. But I don't know how to respond to the information about environmental contaminants in my own body without feeling that an obsessed and somewhat paranoid posture is the only way to come close to a safe lifestyle.[21]

These are classic dilemmas of the risk society. There are no knowledge practices adequate to compensate for risk discourses that we are in contact with every day. It does not seem possible to account for the actual contaminants that we encounter in the ordinary activities of living, nor to escape their penetration of our bodies and lives. Pregnant and lactating women are special targets of these risk discourses because of their special status as the physical caretakers of the young, but their bodies also exemplify the permeability that fears of chemical contaminants concern. After all, toxic contaminants seep into our bodies through its permeable orifices and tissue. Mothers' bodies demonstrate this permeability, the lack of rigid body boundaries, in the very physiology of maternity.

For many women, technocratic approaches to their pregnancies help to manage the feeling of lack of control that accompanies such a life-changing (and body-altering) process. While many women I know have commented on the ridiculous rigidity of the "Pregnancy Diet" in *What to Expect When You're Expecting,* others are clearly enthusiastic about a regimented practice of eating that promises to be best for the baby and to help mom not gain too much weight. The regulatory practices of maternal care could only become standard practice if most women were willing to sacrifice their freedoms in exchange for the promise of a better baby and a safer experience overall, including better birth outcomes. That many of the regulatory practices don't actually result in better birth outcomes is less significant than the fact that the engagement of such practices, like fetal monitoring during labor and delivery, is thought to signal potential dangers and thus avert disastrous outcomes.[22] Of course, it is also quite possible that stringent instructions about behavior are largely accepted in the breach; this is one implication of Janet Golden's study of fetal alcohol syndrome. Discursive acquiescence to technocratic authority does not necessarily indicate complete compliance or, even in cases of compliance, agreement.

The regulatory premises of biomonitoring are similar to those generally accepted disciplinary practices of maternity that have few positive outcomes on health but are required anyway. It is not clear how much knowing what one's body burden is at an individual level contributes to health or improved outcomes for babies and children. It seems prudent to avoid exposure to known carcinogens, just as it seems prudent to use as few harsh chemicals in the course of an ordinary life as we possibly can. But the meanings of biomonitoring and the use of breast milk as a substance with which to measure body burdens are bound up with the logic of maternal regulation in obstetric care. That is, the logic of biomonitoring and the meaning of breast milk in its practices follow from the logics of maternal regulation and discipline, which go beyond prudence and depend on unrealizable expectations of maternal purity.

Biomonitoring is clearly an important way of tracking the extent of chemical infiltration of human populations in order to assess the overall consequences of environmental contamination. Understanding population exposures is a public health responsibility in the age of industrialization. But the personalizing logic of the risk society encourages a particular attention to pregnant and lactating bodies that turns motherhood into a risk endgame, in which every action a mother takes is registered through a risk-benefit algorithm. This attention is an effect of the desire to use maternal bodies as examples of modernity gone wrong, but because such use relies on the implicit expectation of maternal purity, mothers themselves are placed in the terrible position of being identified as the source of toxins that "naturally" move from the environment to their babies through the permeable conduit of their own bodies.

Biomonitoring practices that use breast milk to determine chemical body burden act as another medical technic to both fetishize and devalue the maternal body, even as they are engaged for the purpose of identifying dangerous environmental toxins and their effects on human health. This is because such practices cannot escape a contemporary cultural context in which the transfer of substances from mother to fetus and baby is highly regulated and scrutinized. Breastfeeding is disciplined through monitoring technologies so that its potential dangers are codified and made into data sets. The discourses of the environmentalist movement identify breast milk as biologically safer and better for infants than formula, but it is still the language of science that determines whether mothers' milk is good enough for the pure babies whose innocence is corrupted by the ravages of modernity as they infect/affect maternal embodiment. As Rebecca Kukla would argue, the unruly mother is still an imagined danger to her infant, and the fetish mother is held out as the idealized pure mother whose milk is kept away from contaminants through strictly circumscribed behaviors that, in effect, would isolate mothers from the mainstream of American life if they were to be followed. Mothers are left with a semiparanoid sense of failure that their children will become ill because of what nourishes them from their bodies, a sensibility that can all but erase the empowerment that might come from confidence in the nutritive and emotional role of em-bodied motherhood. It is difficult to see the advantage of such a paradigm to the lived realities of most mothers.

PART 3

Breastfeeding and Global Public Health: Denial, Choice, and HIV/AIDS

CHAPTER 10

MTCT

THE TERM *AIDS* was first used in July 1982, but approximately one year previously, Elizabeth Glaser (wife of 1970s television star Paul Michael Glaser) gave birth to the couple's first child, a daughter, Ariel, in Los Angeles. On bed rest for the final three months of her pregnancy, Glaser hemorrhaged after the birth and was transfused with donated blood at the West Hollywood hospital where she delivered. In 1985, four-year-old Ariel became sick with diarrhea and other ailments whose cause was not determined until she was tested for HIV. Ariel, her mother, and her younger brother Jake were all HIV-positive, but Ariel had AIDS. According to the story Elizabeth Glaser tells in her memoir, *In the Absence of Angels,* her doctors believed that Ariel became infected with HIV through her mother's breast milk; Jake's infection was presumed to have occurred during gestation or the birthing process.[1]

Elizabeth Glaser's story exemplifies the tragic ironies of breastfeeding in the age of HIV/AIDS. She entered into motherhood during a period of renewed interest in breastfeeding on the part of American women but was infected with HIV through the routine hospital practice of transfusion for postpartum hemorrhage. It was not until 1985 that the blood supply in the United States would be routinely tested for HIV.

In the last quarter of the twentieth century, breastfeeding in the United States surged back from its lowest rates in the modern period. Increased rates of breastfeeding over this entire period were somewhat uneven, with the late 1980s and early 1990s representing a dip in an otherwise uphill climb in initiation rates. Anne Wright and Richard Schanler attribute the initial "resurgence of breastfeeding in all major segments of society [to] the pervasive influence of the natural childbirth movement of the 1960s and 1970s, with its effects on the standard management of childbirth," noting also the impact of changing emphasis in the U.S. Department of Agriculture's nutrition program for Women, Infants, and Children (WIC) toward greater support of breastfeeding. Pointing out that most national and international efforts to promote breastfeeding occurred after the 1970s, they suggest that these may have influenced the increases in rates of breastfeeding initiation in the later 1990s.[2] In 1989 the U.S. surgeon general, C. Everett Koop, made positive public statements about breastfeeding following the formation of a workshop devoted to the issue, and in 1994 the American Academy of Pediatrics formed its Task Force on Breastfeeding, later to evolve into a formal section of the organization.[3]

During the decade that HIV/AIDS emerged to public awareness, first in the United States and then internationally, the breastfeeding movement was becoming a strong presence in global public health. Breastfeeding advocates were just getting global policy initiatives to protect and support maternal nursing off the ground when it was determined that HIV existed in breast milk and could infect infants and children through breastfeeding. At the time, the evidence base of breastfeeding medicine (as it is now called) was not well developed and was viewed skeptically by many in the medical establishment.[4] Many of the public health debates concerning recommendations with regard to breastfeeding and HIV transmission have at their core divergent opinions about the contribution that breastfeeding makes to health and the ability of scientific research to quantify this contribution. As a result, strong supporters of breastfeeding have seemed, from the perspective of the AIDS prevention movement, to be ignoring the significance of HIV transmission through breastfeeding. Breastfeeding supporters argue that the opposite can be said of AIDS public health efforts that ignore the contributions breastfeeding makes to the health and well-being of infants and children worldwide.

This background conflict informs public health debates around breastfeeding and HIV transmission. In this chapter I introduce the basic history of global breastfeeding initiatives in the last quarter of the twentieth century, discussing their development in relation to emerging public health guidelines concerning mother-to-child transmission (MTCT) of HIV. I include information about MTCT and discuss the public health debates about how HIV-positive mothers in the global north and south should feed their babies in light of scientific findings. I also introduce denial as a concept used to criticize mothers and their decisions, and discuss its relation to AIDS denialism, which challenges the scientific research on HIV as the cause of AIDS. Breastfeeding advocacy and research in the context of maternal HIV infection exist in problematic tension with AIDS denialism. Mothers, of course, live out their lives in relation to the discourses that evaluate their behaviors and judge their motivations. Representations of HIV-positive mothers reveal the political and biological terrain on which denial signifies, proliferates, and participates in the unfolding of global AIDS tragedies.

Pediatric AIDS and the Global Breastfeeding Movement

The 1980s was an important period for breastfeeding advocacy, and it wasn't until late in the decade that global public health policymakers began to consider the implications of maternal HIV infection on breastfeeding. In the United States, the lowest rates of breastfeeding occurred around 1970, when fewer than one-quarter of American babies were fed with their mother's milk. As infant formula companies expanded their markets to the global south, a variety of international groups became involved in trying to protect and support breastfeeding. A worldwide boycott of the Nestlé corporation began in 1977, targeting the largest global infant formula manufacturer for its manipulative and egregious attempts to enlarge its markets into the global south, where poor mothers face a number of obstacles in the safe use of artificial baby milk. In 1981 the World Health Assembly (WHA) passed the International Code of Marketing of Breastmilk Substitutes. Of 122 nations voting, the United States was the only vote against the Code (three other countries abstained).[5]

In addition to combating the influence of infant formula manufacturers, breastfeeding advocates realized that significant infrastructure issues were contributing to declining breastfeeding rates worldwide, including shifts toward hospitalized childbirth, women's increasing entry into capitalist labor markets, and modernization in general. Processes of modernization disrupt customary familial practices and the transfer of traditional knowledge within communities in favor of supervision by experts and trust in technocratic systems. Increasing attention to the structured contexts in which new mothers might learn about and receive support in breastfeeding management became more and more significant to global efforts to promote maternal nursing, in addition to including breastfeeding in national health-care goals and projects. In 1989, the World Health Organization (WHO) and the United Nations Children's Fund (UNICEF) came out with a joint statement including the "Ten Steps to Successful Breastfeeding," which later became the core of the Baby Friendly Hospital Initiative (BFHI, launched by a WHO/UNICEF partnership in 1991). The Innocenti Declaration, adopted in 1990 by ten UN agencies and thirty-two countries, called for "national breastfeeding policies and . . . appropriate national targets for the 90s."[6] It also established exclusive breastfeeding for the first four to six months of an infant's life as the optimal method of infant feeding.[7]

At the same time as these international initiatives concerning breastfeeding were discussed, developed, and launched, AIDS emerged as a significant public health threat, first identified in the United States but soon after understood to be a global phenomenon. By the late 1980s, there was evidence that postnatal pediatric HIV infection could occur through breastfeeding, although neither the actual risk nor the mechanism was clearly understood (and they continue to be debated). At the time breastfeeding supporters around the globe were gearing up for the second Nestlé boycott in 1988, an international meeting on HIV and breastfeeding had already been held by WHO (in 1987). The recommendation coming out of this meeting stated, "in places where infection and malnutrition were the major cause of infant death, women should be advised to breastfeed irrespective of their HIV status."[8]

A consensus statement was issued in 1992 that included a version of this recommendation, which remained official WHO/UNICEF policy until 1997, when WHO, UNICEF, and UNAIDS issued a policy statement that effectively changed the existing recommendation of full support for breastfeeding "in places where infection and malnutrition were the major cause of infant death" to one of "informed choice." While the 1997 policy did state that "as a general principle, in all populations, irrespective of HIV infection rates, breastfeeding should continue to be protected, promoted, and supported," it also stated that HIV-positive mothers should be counseled about "the benefits of breastfeeding, on the risk of HIV transmission through breastfeeding, and on the risks and possible advantages associated with other methods of infant feeding."[9] Further development of this policy in 2000–2001 added what are called the AFASS criteria—that if replacement feeding was found to be affordable, feasible, acceptable, sustainable, and safe, HIV-positive mothers could be counseled against breastfeeding their infants.[10]

Another wrinkle in this developing history is the fact that researchers in Durban, South Africa, in an ongoing study with initial published results in

1999 and 2001, suggested that exclusive breastfeeding seemed to confer similar preventive advantages with respect to HIV transmission as exclusive formula feeding. That is, in the late 1990s, just as public health guidelines were moving away from wholehearted support for breastfeeding in resource-poor contexts with high rates of HIV infection, some research began to suggest that transmission of HIV was the same for both exclusive breast-feeders and exclusive formula feeders. Breastfeeding supporters have heralded these studies, discussed below, as demonstrating that international policy groups were too quick to abandon full support for breastfeeding in populations with high HIV prevalence among childbearing women.[11]

Breastfeeding Transmission of HIV

The current state of research on the transmission of HIV from mothers to fetuses and infants is constantly changing, as is all medical research with respect to HIV/AIDS. In addition, there are so many individual small-scale studies about the efficacy of various interventions that it would be impossible to survey the entire field with confidence. In this section I provide a general overview of the issues, with some discussion of the medical controversies at the core of debates concerning infant feeding and HIV transmission.

In 2005, "[only] 9% of pregnant women in low- and middle-income countries were offered services to prevent transmission [of HIV] to their newborns."[12] By 2006, the global estimate of pregnant women treated with antiretrovirals had significantly improved, to 23 percent, but this still means that most women around the globe are not being offered antiretroviral treatment to help prevent HIV transmission during gestation or labor and delivery, which are crucial periods for transmission of the virus.[13] The following discussion must be read in this context—one in which understanding and treatment protocols seem to be no match for the lack of resources necessary to meet existing need.[14]

Most pediatric AIDS is caused by vertical transmission during gestation or labor and delivery, with the perinatal period as the most dangerous. Without maternal antiretroviral prophylaxis or therapy, the vertical transmission rate "varies from approximately 20 to 30 percent."[15] Research has suggested an increased risk attributable to breastfeeding (postnatal vertical transmission) around 15 percent, but the actual risk for individual mother-infant pairs varies according to a number of factors, including the mother's viral load and her breast health during nursing. Recommendations concerning infant feeding in populations characterized by high seroprevalence and extreme poverty must "balanc[e] the competing risks" of formula feeding and breastfeeding.[16] These competing risks involve the difficulty of replacement feeding in resource-poor contexts (lack of adequate water supply, lack of refrigeration, difficulty maintaining sanitary conditions, etc.) compared to the chance of infecting the infant through customary nursing.[17]

Customary nursing is not the same as exclusive breastfeeding, which is a mode of breastfeeding defined through a medical model. Researchers hypothesize that HIV infection of the infant during breastfeeding occurs through disturbances in the baby's digestive system, which allow the virus to pass into the bloodstream. These disturbances are caused by the addition of foods or drinks, including water, to the baby's diet of human milk. Human milk by itself does not normally cause digestive difficulties and is associated with healthier mucosal lining of the gut. Mixed feeding, which defines the norm of customary nursing around the world, is probably the most dangerous form of feeding for infants of HIV-positive mothers, because it puts babies in contact with HIV at the same time that it disturbs their digestive system, making them susceptible to infection.[18]

In 1999, researchers in South Africa first provided evidence that exclusive breastfeeding for the first six months conveyed similar risks for HIV infection as exclusive replacement feeding with infant formula. These data offered breastfeeding advocates some hope that the HIV pandemic would not wholly displace the important work of the Nestlé boycott and related breastfeeding advocacy activities in resisting routine replacement feeding in the global south.[19] Current World Health Organization policy concerning infant feeding in the context of maternal HIV infection, confirmed in a technical consultation in October 2006, suggests that mothers must make infant feeding decisions based on their individual circumstances.[20] This is the policy that used to be known as "informed choice," language that does not appear in the consensus statement of the 2006 technical consultation.[21]

Of course, mothers always make decisions based on their individual circumstances; it is curious that the WHO guidelines enshrine this obvious fact in public health policy. The guidelines are meant to support public health workers as they advise pregnant and newly parturient women about their HIV status and its effects on their infant feeding practices. In this way, the WHO guidelines on infant feeding in the case of maternal HIV infection are meant to assist public health workers who had been accustomed to promoting breastfeeding with almost all of their clients. Since the development of the AFASS criteria, these counselors have had to assess the feasibility of replacement feeding for each mother, yet the AFASS criteria are often very difficult to evaluate in specific cases, as I discuss at greater length in the final chapter.[22]

Louise Kuhn, Zena Stein, and Mervyn Susser comment that they "are aware of no published studies of interventions to make formula feeding safer" in resource-poor contexts. Their bleak assessment, that "truly informed choice is seldom a reality," given that "no choice can assure the prevention of HIV transmission while insuring the good health of the child," demonstrates the difficulty of creating public health guidelines in contexts where lack of infrastructure exacerbates uncertainties in scientific knowledge.[23]

Current policy and practice in the United States is to legally enforce replacement feeding when the mother is HIV-positive.[24] In these contexts, lack of precise knowledge about the transmission rate of HIV through breastfeeding is obviated by the relative safety of providing replacement feeding for infants of HIV-positive mothers. For example, U.S. Centers for Disease Control (CDC) advice to HIV-positive pregnant women is very clear: get medical care, take your medicine, get to the hospital early during labor, don't breastfeed, give your baby her medicine, and keep your baby's appointments with her doctors.[25] South African researcher Anna Coutsoudis and colleagues note that public health programs based on avoidance of breastfeeding and antiretroviral drug treatment (during labor and delivery and after birth for the infant) have reduced mother-to-child-transmission of HIV to below 3 percent in industrialized countries and some middle-income countries like Thailand and Brazil.[26]

In the resource-poor contexts of the global south, research is more mixed concerning replacement feeding for the babies of HIV-positive mothers, largely because of significantly increased morbidity and mortality of nonbreastfed infants.[27] In presenting evidence that attempts to balance competing risks to infant health, Kuhn, Stein, and Susser suggest that "formula is favored over the breast when infant mortality rates are at the lower end of the distribution, say less than about 70–80 per 1000 live births" when a 14 percent postnatal transmission rate is assumed, or less than about 40 per 1,000 live births when a 7 percent postnatal transmission rate is assumed. Assuming a 21 percent transmission rate, formula would be favored with a mortality rate of less than 100 per 1,000 live births.[28] The uncertainty around the actual transmission rate for HIV through breastfeeding causes some uncertainty in the recommendation. Basically, and from the perspective of breastfeeding advocates, in contexts where infants die in high numbers breastfeeding will still be protective of most babies even though some will contract HIV through maternal nursing. Advocates argue that research supporting exclusive breastfeeding through adequate counseling and infrastructure support demonstrates that breastfeeding will ensure the survival of more children overall than emphasis on formula provision for HIV-positive mothers.[29]

From the perspective of breastfeeding advocates, not breastfeeding by HIV-positive women offers a more definitive benefit for infants where infant mortality rates are low, generally more common in high- and middle-income countries. However, policy recommendations do not seem to account for differences in resources among women in the global north, or differences in infant mortality rates between groups or classes of people in industrialized nations.[30] In the United States, the CDC suggests that "you can get help buying baby formula if you need it" but does not direct mothers to appropriate agencies to find that help.[31]

Infant feeding choice in the context of HIV infection means something entirely different from what many, perhaps most, women in the global north have understood as the answer to the question "breast or bottle?" Some researchers have commented that the practices women are perceived to choose are themselves not adequately understood, as breastfeeding itself is often, even in scientific studies, neither quantified nor specifically defined.[32] White and Kuhn, Stein, and Susser note that customary breastfeeding is really mixed feeding (the provision of culturally approved infant foods along with breastfeeding), which, as I discussed above, is the most dangerous feeding practice for HIV-positive mothers and their infants.[33] Thus, in advocating exclusive breastfeeding for HIV-positive mothers in resource-poor contexts with high infant mortality rates, public health officials are not advocating for what was once the ubiquitous practice that is now corrupted by infant formula manufacturers. These manufacturers only exploited an already existent practice by encouraging mothers to purchase an infant food commodity to provide along with breast milk, as a replacement for traditional food supplements.

However, the introduction of breast milk substitutes fed through bottles as a culturally approved food itself seems to change the cultural balance that used to favor predominant breastfeeding, which is why breastfeeding advocates work against the free provision of infant formulas to HIV-positive women. They argue for cup feeding of infant formulas, where necessary, for the same reason. Breastfeeding advocates are afraid of what they call "spillover effect," a concern about replacement feeding being perceived as the preferred method of infant feeding for all women, and not just those who are HIV-positive.[34] Spillover of replacement feeding practices in resource-poor contexts would mean increasing infant morbidity and mortality due to not breastfeeding. But exclusive breastfeeding, a method promoted by medicine in the global north as the approved mode of breastfeeding for HIV-negative women, and by some in the global south as the approved mode for HIV-positive women, may have other, unintended side effects of its own.

Medicalization

One side effect of the public health response to mother-to-child transmission of HIV may be the medicalization of breastfeeding for everyone. For example, the publication *Infant Feeding Options in the Context of HIV* details the following information for "recommended feeding practices for women who are HIV negative or who do not know their HIV status."

> Exclusive breastfeeding for the first six months and the prevention and treatment of breast conditions . . . should be recommended practices for all mothers who are HIV negative or who do not know their status. These "safer breastfeeding" practices are optimal for the health of the mother and her infant and may reduce the risk of transmission among infected mothers who do not know their status. *Widespread promotion of these practices as a cultural norm may prevent them from becoming stigmatizing behaviors associated with HIV infection.*[35]

There is no doubt that stigma avoidance is involved in infant feeding decisions where HIV is a factor. Public health debates involve discussions of the cultural acceptability of replacement feeding, acknowledging that in some contexts a mother must breastfeed her infant in order to avoid punishment or to establish herself as the mother of the child.[36] Here, however, stigma avoidance is used conceptually to bolster a specific kind of breastfeeding promoted by medicine in response to HIV infection. The medically approved form of breastfeeding is to be promoted as the cultural norm in order to make sure that it is not associated with the stigma-producing condition of HIV infection. That is, exclusive breastfeeding should be performed by all mothers so that it becomes the cultural norm and HIV-positive women will not stand out as different if they feed their children this way, as opposed to various customary practices of mixed feeding. This is clearly an instance of medicalization. Significantly, in this instance medicalization is engaged precisely for its normalizing effects: the promotion of exclusive breastfeeding (a medical norm) will normalize the practice for all mothers, preventing some from being singled out as HIV-positive.

My comments are not meant to deny the biological benefits of exclusive breastfeeding to the infants of both HIV-positive and HIV-negative mothers. Public health workers focus on the ways in which basic social activities, like breastfeeding, can be managed to improve health. The application of scientific knowledge to routine aspects of daily living, like clean water and refrigeration of certain foodstuffs, has saved countless lives.[37] The milk of HIV-positive mothers does contain human immunodeficiency virus, and breastfeeding by HIV-positive women does infect some infants.[38] Certainly, mother-to-child transmission through nursing must be addressed and needs a medical response.

Yet one potential side effect of public health responses to the HIV pandemic may be the transformation of infant feeding practices worldwide, making them conform all the more tightly to a medical model. Medicalization is a constituent element of modernity, transforming individual and collective experience by bringing more and more activities under the purview of medicine as a disciplinary institution. Common social practices are redefined through medicalization, losing their personal and cultural meanings in order to accommodate new significations determined by scientific frameworks. Because breastfeeding is a biosocial practice linked to other aspects of material life and their meanings, it has had an important role in local cultural meaning systems.

The HIV pandemic did not initiate the medicalization of breastfeeding in the global south. This phenomenon began when infant formula manufacturers began to aggressively market their products to poor women in poor countries without adequate public health infrastructures to handle the increased morbidity of their formula-fed infants. In other words, the medicalization of breastfeeding occurred, in part, as a reaction to the commoditization of infant feeding globally, which began early in the twentieth century but intensified in the second half. In the United States and other industrialized countries, medicine has been the primary supporter of increased rates of breastfeeding initiation and duration since the 1950s. Organizations like La Leche League, begun as a peer group of concerned mothers, rely on a medical model and medical evidence of breastfeeding's contributions to health. But HIV/AIDS has changed the public health focus in the global south from more breastfeeding to exclusive breastfeeding, and its potential side effect is the increasing medicalization of breastfeeding worldwide. This means that medical meanings of breastfeeding may come to predominate over local, culturally embedded significations, with consequences that are not clear at present. If the example of the United States is representative, some possible consequences include increased commoditization of breastfeeding itself, perceptions by mothers that their infant feeding practices are scrutinized and judged by strangers, and intensifying attention to mothers' practices as choices that are either affirmed or repudiated by scientific evidence.[39]

Breastfeeding is not always about health or immunity or nutrition, intelligence or development or disease prevention. Yet, to take the United States as an example, "modern mothers" in the global north are often so immersed in modern medicalized perceptions of breastfeeding that it does not seem odd to configure it that way, to imagine exclusive breastfeeding as the natural method because it is promoted by medicine as the right way to nurse. After all, most women in the United States learn to breastfeed from medical professionals and accede, albeit at times ambivalently, to medicine's signifying power to define the practices of good mothers. But breastfeeding traditions are local, and influenced as much by cultural demands as biological ones. While public health agendas may necessitate transforming local and varied breastfeeding practices in order to safeguard infant wellbeing worldwide, it would be wrong to suggest that medical prescriptions are natural and can be mandated without losses. Iatrogenesis is the known consequence of medicalization.

Mothers in Denial

"In the whole AIDS epidemic, no question is more heartbreaking and confounding than this: Why would a mother choose to condemn her baby to death?"[40]

This sentence is the opening gambit in a *New York Times Magazine* feature article on AIDS in South Africa, published in August 2006, a week before the International AIDS Conference in Toronto. The mother in question decided not to take nevirapine as prophylaxis during childbirth to prevent HIV infection of her baby.[41] According to the article, South African mothers by the thousands refuse antiretroviral prophylaxis during labor because they will not admit to being HIV-positive. Tina Rosenberg, the author of the article, represents this decision as a death sentence for the baby and wonders what kind of mother would do such a thing.

Anna Lowenhaupt Tsing has identified this particular rhetorical construction in an article appropriately titled "Monster Stories."

> Again and again I found the women's specific history eclipsed by a broader question: What kind of a woman could endanger her own offspring at the moment of birth, the moment which should most excite her maternal sentiments? This question generated its own answer: Only a person completely lacking in parental—and human— sensibilities could commit such an act. To those who considered their cases, these women were, as one prosecutor put it, "unnatural," "bizarre," and "without basic human emotions."[42]

While Tsing's research focuses on young women who hide their pregnancies and give birth alone, often hiding or neglecting the newborn, the basic pattern of representation is the same. The question "what kind of mother would do such a thing?" is a rhetorical question in the most literal sense, since the answer is a foregone conclusion: the wrong kind of mother, a mother who does not properly love her child. As Moland and Blystad point out, "Mother's love is presumably a universal phenomenon and is an implicit condition in numerous health promotion and disease prevention programs targeting children." While they believe that maternal love is in fact a crucial element of child health promotion programs, they also question "whether [relying on it] is effective and acceptable in the absence of treatment and support to secure the health and the survival of the mother."[43] HIV-positive mothers in the global south are among the most vulnerable women in the world and, as Moland and Blystad demonstrate, deserve greater understanding of the cultural and economic conditions that constrain their decisions.

Despite her forbidding beginning ("Why would a mother choose to condemn her baby to death?"), Rosenberg writes a relatively sympathetic piece on the difficulties of achieving goals for HIV treatment in South Africa. The opening statement about mothers is meant to stress how significant denial is in the social response to the AIDS epidemic in South Africa. There are numerous barriers to treatment access, and the stigma of admitting to HIV infection is very high. Rosenberg notes that disclosing a positive status to one's partner can result in physical violence. She also suggests that there are plenty of things that Americans are in denial about concerning their health—smoking, breast lumps, trans fats—an important concession that it is not only "those Africans" who refuse to deal with health risks (although Americans are not represented as having any denial about HIV/AIDS). She even identifies patient noncompliance as a responsibility of the medical profession and not just the individual: "when a pregnant woman chooses to keep the nevirapine tablet in her pocket, the real failing belongs to the health system, which did not consider what would help her to follow medical advice."[44] Yet through the rest of her article Rosenberg rarely talks about the startling and sensationalized dilemma she presents as her opening—the HIV-positive mother who refuses the ARV prophylaxis that is believed to protect her newborn baby.[45] It sets a tone and establishes a perspective that haunts the article's researched arguments.

Most of the piece concerns taboos around HIV infection and various public health strategies to attract teens and other vulnerable groups to more open discussions about sexual behavior and safe sex practices. When she does address mothers, Rosenberg continues the troubling vein she began with. Describing a nurse's strategy "that sometimes helps," she describes a basically manipulative gesture: "If an H.I.V.-positive woman does not want to take the nevirapine, Molotsi thrusts a piece of paper and a pen toward the woman, essentially making her take responsibility for her decision. 'Would you really like your baby to have the virus?' she asks. 'If you don't take the pill, you will have to sign.'" This strategy, while no doubt often successful, is essentially coercive, using the woman's own fear of being revealed as HIV-positive to "encourage" her to take medication she has refused. That Rosenberg looks on the strategy with such approbation suggests the extent to which she sees mothers who refuse biomedical treatment as basically irrational. Indeed, she writes that HIV is a disease "that primarily hits the notoriously irrational young."[46]

The assumption that humans behave rationally with respect to clearly articulated professional advice concerning health and risk is central to modern biomedical strategies for improved health and well-being. Rosenberg ends her article with the following statement: "Without attention to the social, psychological, and cultural factors surrounding the disease, we are throwing away money and lives. Twenty-five years into the epidemic, we now know how to keep people from dying of AIDS. The challenge for the future is to keep them from dying of stigma, denial and silence."[47] Here we see that knowledge about health and illness comes from biomedicine; ignorance is a part of the "social, psychological, and cultural factors surrounding the disease"—it is integral to the "stigma, denial, and silence" that cause death. Medicine brings life; cultural factors are deadly.

I heard this discursive construction over and over again at the 2006 International AIDS Conference in Toronto; racism, gender inequality, and poverty were loudly proclaimed to be the global "drivers" of the epidemic, but biotechnical strategies like male circumcision and microbicides represented solutions. Indeed, at one session the chair opened the discussion by suggesting that scientists needed to counter the ideological obstructions of politicians; that is, good science should challenge the "bad attitudes" that impede the progress of medicine to address and treat disease.[48]

It is true that policies resulting from "bad" attitudes have impeded the fight against HIV, including the George W. Bush administration's restrictions on aid to organizations that did not have a stated policy against prostitution, its preference for abstinence-only approaches to HIV/AIDS prevention, and the Russian government's refusal to countenance needle-exchange programs in a country where the main behavior fueling the epidemic is intravenous drug use (to name only a few examples). Indeed, the history of HIV/AIDS in the United States was initially one of repeated attempts to get the attention of the government to adequately recognize AIDS as a public health issue and appropriately fund prevention, treatment, and research efforts.[49] But it is also true that culture is not simply the negative context from which stricken individuals must be extricated in order to save them with the ideologically neutral technologies of contemporary biomedicine. Biomedical culture, as I like to call it, actively constructs behavior that contravenes its principles as irrational—that is, mothers who do not take nevirapine are understood to be acting irrationally only within a narrowly circumscribed definition of rational behavior, generally understood as compliance with medical norms and expectations. The power of biomedical culture is its significant claim on improved health and well-being, but its technical success does not alter the fact that its claims are made on the basis of shutting out and denying other claims to truth, well-being, and signification.

The mother who refuses nevirapine—that barbaric, "other" mother who is represented in the *New York Times Magazine* as the quintessential African AIDS mother—emblematizes the viral mother. As described earlier, the viral mother is imagined through the development paradigm of the global north, in which individual choice and subservience to medical expertise are the hallmarks of good mothering. The viral mother chooses her bad behavior out of a panoply of possible behaviors marked by their adherence to medical norms. Her children are construed as innocent victims of her behavior, which is understood to be irrational if it does not cohere with the logic of biomedical advice. The viral mother of the global south is the logical descendant of the Nestlé mother, who was duped into formula feeding by rapacious multinational corporations bent on widening their market share through duplicitous strategies targeting women in areas of the world where replacement feeding was not safe. In the global south, both are understood to be victims of their resource-poor contexts and their own ignorance—the viral mother because she is invested in cultural paradigms that resist the knowledge produced by modern biomedical practices, and the Nestlé mother because she was convinced by global industry posing as purveyors of that very knowledge.

Mothers are victimized by poverty, by gender inequality, by racism, and by the lack of adequate medical care and contemporary medical technologies in resource-poor settings. The material realities of women's lives are directly affected by global inequities and imbalances of power. In the context of women's lives, culture and biomedicine are not separate but intermingled (if, at times, contradictorily), because biomedical perspectives are themselves culturally inflected. Women do not deny or ignore medicine and treatment solely as a result of ignorance or irrationality. Their responses are logical in their own contexts and attentive to specific material and rhetorical realities. It is only through an acknowledgment of the cultural embeddedness of biomedicine in particular attitudes toward life and the body (attitudes developed in the global north, primarily, and thus embedded in its cultural contexts) that we can hope to understand what appears to be repudiation of what biomedicine offers as a response to HIV/AIDS.[50]

Conclusion

Ironically, the AIDS pandemic has been a primary cause of new modes of empowered activism among those afflicted. Yet HIV-positive mothers do not seem to be able to capitalize on forms of "therapeutic citizenship" that have allowed people living with AIDS around the world to become "empowered HIV activists and advocates, either for themselves or for their children." Anthropologists Blystad and Moland argue that this is because

> the conceptual incongruity between notions of fertility and life on the one hand and notions of death and dying on the other hand, or more concretely between motherly love, nourishment and care on the one hand and threats of immoral sexuality leading to a deadly infection on the other ... [are] incompatible notions ... visibly manifested in the bodies of these young HIV positive women. . . . It is the young vulnerable mother who has to carry the burden of these incompatible notions.

In addition, they point out that most prevention of mother-to-child transmission (PMTCT) programs do not involve sustained ARV treatment for mothers, "the number one trigger for empowered AIDS activism."[51]

HIV-positive mothers are vulnerable in the material and phenomenological sense described above, as a result of their special relation to their offspring, but also in the discursive contexts that frame others' views of them. HIV transmission through breastfeeding remains largely misunderstood as a public health problem outside of experts in the public health community. Even among the experts there are ongoing debates about appropriate actions to prevent transmission and safeguard the health of children around the world. These conflicts are addressed more fully in the final chapter. All of the chapters in this part of *Viral Mothers* illuminate two important conceptual frames that constrain public perceptions of HIV-positive mothers and global breastfeeding advocacy, as well as professional views of the public health response to maternal HIV infection in the global south. These frames are *denial* and *choice*. Denial operates as a judgment on mothers at the same time that it circulates globally—in the form of denialism—as a resistance to hegemonic scientific theories about AIDS. Choice operates as the obverse of denial, in that it signifies active reason in response to a problem. Both terms, and the conceptual frames they refer to, represent the effects of modernizing paradigms on mothers' practices; analyzing them alerts us to the intractable dilemmas of knowledge and circumstance in the face of HIV.

CHAPTER 11

Denialist Rhetorics

HOW DO YOU tell the dissenters from the quacks?

This is a central question of denialism. The temptation is to say that we tell the dissenters from the quacks by examining the evidence and determining the truth. Dissenters have legitimate claims to make using novel forms of argument and new interpretations of evidence, while quacks are cranks, fighting the status quo without any evident factual basis and certainly without regard for the truth as others see it. One might learn from a dissenter; in any event, it's worthwhile to engage them in conversation. Quacks, on the other hand, are better left alone, as debating with them dignifies their arguments, lending credence to illogic, bias, and empty claims.

AIDS denialists are quacks. This, at least, is the view of the authors of "denialism blog," an excellent Web site that identifies and defines various forms of denialism. The authors define denialism as "the employment of rhetorical tactics to give the appearance of argument or legitimate debate, when in actuality there is none. These false arguments are used when one has few or no facts to support one's viewpoint against a scientific consensus or against overwhelming evidence to the contrary. They are effective in distracting from actual useful debate using emotionally appealing, but ultimately empty and illogical assertions." As a "ground rule," "we don't argue with cranks. Part of understanding denialism is knowing that it's futile to argue with them, and giving them yet another forum is unnecessary."[1]

I am sympathetic to this position; a few years ago, I refused to attend an AIDS denialist presentation on my campus. Yet in examining denialism in the context of science studies, I think it is more difficult to discern an absolute distinction between a quack and a true dissenter, between a denialist and a science skeptic. Indeed, any form of science denialism presents an instance of the core concerns of science studies. Denialism questions the nature and value of scientific evidence and the authority necessary to determine "scientific facts." It is easy to dismiss AIDS denialists as quacks or cranks, especially when one can find errors in their scientific reasoning or places where they present false information. But identifying their beliefs as pseudoscience does little to illuminate the persuasive power of their explanations and the reasons why many people abandon or disregard the mainstream scientific consensus to agree that HIV is not the cause of AIDS.[2] Further, studying denialism demonstrates the rhetorical features of all knowledge, by which I mean that knowledge and truth never stand on their own as self-evident but must be argued for as pertinent, factual, and valid forms of information.

AIDS denialists contend that there is ongoing scientific controversy concerning HIV as the cause of AIDS, thus situating their challenge to scientific orthodoxy within normal scientific discovery and the routine revision of prior beliefs and theories. Many AIDS denialists go further, suggesting that some sort of conspiracy among scientists and governments is at work in maintaining agreement around HIV as the cause of AIDS. In South Africa, AIDS denialism became a way to repudiate non-African approaches to the disease, as well as to refute emerging theories about an African origin to HIV, a situation I discuss in more detail in the next chapter. While I would not go so far as to say that AIDS denialists are self-consciously rhetorical, they do seem to acknowledge the contested and argumentative contexts of scientific knowledge, while those responding to them often suggest that existing scientific evidence has the authority of uncontestable truth. In charging that AIDS denialists engage in explicitly rhetorical argumentation (and by that most mean semantic and empty), their refuters suggest that scientific knowledge stands above or beyond the cultural contexts in which it is produced and has no relation to the language in which its value is represented.

Yet despite this tacit acknowledgment of the contestatory contexts of scientific knowledge production, denialist rhetorics seem to offer a certainty that can be tempting when there is real scientific uncertainty, which is the case with public health guidance concerning infant feeding in instances of maternal HIV infection. Mother-to-child transmission of HIV provides numerous uncertainties to the scientific and public health communities, and translating research into policy in this arena has proved particularly difficult given the multiple determinants of infant morbidity and mortality in the global south. Adopting AIDS denialist positions has been one response by some breastfeeding activists. Understanding the historical challenges of global breastfeeding activism is helpful in interpreting this strange relationship, although such understanding does not excuse the questionable politics implied in it.

My aim is to untangle the denialist rhetorics with reference to maternal HIV infection. Denialist arguments often function as disruptions to good faith efforts to understand what to do with conflicting biomedical evidence and clinical experience.[3] But I also seek to understand how denialism, as it has played a role in structuring debates around infant feeding, frames the way we think about mothers' actions. Denialist discourses often represent mothers as victims of a rapacious medical profession, intent on furthering its own goals as an institution at the expense of individuals. As we saw in the preceding chapter, denial is a way of representing mothers whose decisions do not cohere with biomedical perspectives. To be "in denial" is a way of characterizing a person's behavior as refusing to acknowledge reality as others see it. It is a way of identifying the motivation for decisions that are perceived to be faulty or against common sense. Yet to claim that there are clear-cut decisions that are obviously best for HIV-positive mothers in all circumstances ignores not only the scientific and policy controversies at issue but also the specific decision-making contexts for women around the world. Identifying the rhetoric of denialism and detailing how it influences public perceptions of mothers are steps toward imagining the complexity of real-life decisions and practices for HIV-positive women. Instead of pointing fingers at those in denial, we might begin to understand the logic of decision making for subjects in diverse circumstances, with different perspectives on health, well-being, and the promise of modern biomedicine.

Nevertheless, it is important to underscore the repugnance of AIDS denialist positions and repudiate their effects. Denial of HIV as the cause of AIDS leads people to accept bogus treatments or to engage in questionable practices that have little or no efficacy against the infection. Official state-supported AIDS denialism led to the deaths of millions, by some counts, in South Africa. Acceptance of the viral cause of AIDS holds out hope for treatment and, if not cure, the maintenance of HIV as a chronic illness rather than a "death sentence." From a purely pragmatic perspective, the scientific consensus concerning HIV as the cause of AIDS provides both a theory and a set of practices that have changed the life prospects of millions of infected people around the globe.

One can be a biomedical skeptic and still accept the germ theory of disease. Understanding the cultural construction of HIV does not mean abandoning HIV as a meaningful and real viral entity. As Paula Treichler suggests, "the use of the concept *cultural construction* intensifies the responsibility to make choices."[4] In many ways, the existence of AIDS denialism sets in bold relief the consequences of believing in what the denialists call the scientific orthodoxy of HIV/AIDS: the possibility of partial treatment through antiretroviral drugs that, while not without side effects, offer a stay against opportunistic infection for a majority of patients. As the current narrative truth of AIDS causality and treatment possibilities, HIV is the best story available. Choosing it is not only an effect of cultural contexts, it is an ethical imperative when the horizon of possible choices is limited and bleak.

Introducing AIDS Denialism

Denial is a situated response to AIDS, to motherhood, and to the promise of biomedicine. AIDS denialism—defined as opposition to the idea that HIV is the cause of AIDS and including refutation of retroviral treatments as a legitimate response to the epidemic—is perhaps matched by an equally virulent "breastfeeding denialism," which many claim leads to the premature death of millions of children each year.[5] This assertion is not meant to countenance AIDS denialism, but to put the representation of "mothers in denial" in proper perspective.

Stanley Cohen's book *States of Denial: Knowing about Atrocities and Suffering* is the quintessential reference for sociological and psychological approaches to denial, especially those that influence political denials or wrongdoing. Cohen is specifically interested in denial of knowledge or the suffering of others. Denialism, a term not found in *States of Denial,* can be a form of "official denial," in Cohen's analysis a state-sponsored or institutionalized response of not knowing. But denialism does not map directly onto denial as a concept. Denialism organizes itself self-consciously as being against what is known as the truth, either historical or scientific truth for which there is felt to be strong evidence. In this chapter and the next, I am interested in linking perceptions of individual denial (usually portrayed as psychological or defensive in nature) to denialism as a rhetoric, that is, to denialism as it is constituted in discourse.[6]

AIDS denialism is a rhetorical gambit based on cultural skepticism about scientific and biomedical institutions and their believability. Mimicking other denialist positions (like those concerning global warming and evolution), AIDS denialists float conspiracy theories about a monolithic "AIDS science orthodoxy" that does not admit iconoclastic positions or investigators and vigilantly polices its territory to exclude contrary interlopers. But my claim that AIDS denialism is a rhetoric is not just based on its use of misleading, biased, and false statements. AIDS denialism demonstrates the rhetorical nature of all scientific knowledge and shows how necessary cultural consensus is in establishing the truth of scientific ideas. In this sense, AIDS denialism truly is a form of scientific controversy, even though those who refute its claims try to prove that it is a form of pseudo-science, demonstrating that scientific controversies are also cultural controversies.

Challenging AIDS denialist statements with verified scientific findings is the routine response, but such challenges do not really address the core of the denialist strategy, which is to cast doubt on the accepted science of HIV/AIDS. Because the challenges and counterchallenges often utilize highly technical language, it's very difficult for laypeople to parse the distinctions between the positions, a factor I discuss in the following chapter. To claim that denialism operates rhetorically is to locate its strength and persuasiveness in specific communicative contexts. Identifying and exploring the rhetoric of AIDS denialism reveals skepticism about the factual grounding of scientific findings, the contexts of scientific research, and the disinterest with which scientists are thought to go about their business. In other words, AIDS denialism demonstrates a relatively widespread skepticism about the believability of biomedical science as it is practiced globally and as the origin of objective truths about health and disease. The cultural bases of this skepticism vary as to context.

Identifying denialism as a rhetorical strategy is important in two ways. First, isolating the stylistic and persuasive structures of denialist arguments demonstrates the constitutive features of denialist discourses. The fact that denialism persistently uses such features makes it relatively easy to mark those discourses and interlocutors who are not arguing in good faith but attempting to disrupt the truth-seeking functions of scientific endeavor. That such features are consistent across denialist arguments leads to the second significant impact of understanding the rhetoric of denialism: it is precisely because denialism offers a consistent and readily identifiable mode of argumentation that it can be adopted (and adapted) to suit a variety of purposes. In other words, its rhetorical capacities are well suited to appropriation.[7]

In the end, denialism is about refuting what most others think of as common knowledge or accepted truth. Exploring denialism is about understanding how certain beliefs that seem illogical to some are completely rational and believable to others, even as such explorations can identify the kinds of beliefs that do, indeed, kill. In the discussion that follows in this chapter and the next I show that the knife cuts both ways. Biomedical responses are not themselves successful refutations of denialist claims, because the logic of denialism is not scientific but based on cultural skepticism. AIDS denialism asserts truth claims against the normative understanding of AIDS, but uses the language of science rhetorically, thereby making successful counterchallenges in scientific terms extremely difficult. More and better science is not effective as an antidote to this strategy, but articulating a cultural consensus about acceptable responses to the epidemic is. The challenge of AIDS denialism is a cultural challenge and thus must be met with cultural arguments.

Knowledge Production in Science and the Case of HIV/AIDS

In an article entitled "AIDS Denialists: How to Respond," John S. James, editor and publisher of *AIDS Treatment News*, lists "seven deadly deceptions" that characterize AIDS denialist arguments.

1. HIV is harmless (or does not exist), and AIDS is not contagious—so sexual and other precautions are unnecessary.
2. The HIV test is unreliable—so don't get tested.
3. AIDS drugs are poisons, pushed by doctors corrupted by the pharmaceutical industry—so don't take any of them . . .
4. Viral load and CD4 tests are useless—so don't use them.
5. AIDS deaths would have gone down [after the introduction of highly active antiretroviral treatments, or HAART, in 1996], even without new treatments—so you don't need medical care.
6. AIDS is over, or never existed, or only affected small risk groups—so there is no important need for medical research on AIDS or HIV, or for AIDS services.

7. The free speech of dissenters has been suppressed—so you can't believe anything you hear.[8]

James distinguishes denialists from dissidents, suggesting that "there can be many kinds of AIDS dissent" but that denialists are not arguing in good faith within a scientific controversy but attempting to promote "bizarre medicine, telling people with a major illness to reject care entirely." In advising readers how to respond to denialist charges, James states that "back-and-forth debate format is not especially useful here, because it tends to turn on technical points, asking readers to make their own decisions on the scientific merits of the issue, which most people are not prepared to do." In other words, counterarguments that use scientific data to refute AIDS denialist claims are not efficacious in the real-world contexts in which laypeople manage decisions about health, illness, and medical care. James does assert that "we will need an in-depth, well-referenced document explaining the issues to health-care and AIDS service professionals, and also to patients and anyone else who wants this detailed information," a statement that reveals his belief that in the end scientific information will be instrumental in thwarting the denialists' aims.[9]

According to science studies scholars, scientific controversies are never decided entirely within the domain of science using factual evidence in an absolute and pure manner to dispel disbelief. In this perspective, all scientific controversies are also cultural controversies, argued in the domain of science but never apart from social relations or cultural contexts. There are various ways to argue that science is culturally constructed, depending on disciplinary and theoretical frameworks, but most positions hold that "facts" themselves must be argued into existence and are not really facts until accepted as such by a quorum of authorized individuals. This issue is particularly important in understanding AIDS denialism as it emerged from what Steven Epstein has called the "causation controversy."[10]

Before 1996, when evidence of the success of highly active antiretroviral treatments (HAART) against HIV was presented at the International AIDS Conference in Vancouver, there was an active dissent to the theory that HIV causes AIDS.[11] Exploring this dissent fully is beyond the scope of this chapter, but in reviewing the work of three prominent AIDS scholars we can begin to understand the cultural dimensions of consensus making in science. The twelve years of scientific dissent concerning the existence of HIV (roughly from its discovery in 1983–84 to 1996) demonstrate how scientific controversy can be sustained when there is no clear medical response to an identified illness. In the period after 1996, ARV treatments targeting HIV began to curb rates of AIDS in the global north, and dissemination of ARVs in the global south became a pressing public health mandate. It appears that what we now call AIDS denialism emerged from AIDS dissent when the facts of HIV coalesced in scientific circles. Instead of constituting an alternative scientific position, this position became, from the perspective of established AIDS scientists, the belief of quacks or cranks.

To understand denialism, then, we must consider the controversies over the causation of AIDS—not to rehash old debates and invoke dead questions, but to more fully comprehend the controversies themselves as cultural struggles over meaning and authority. This section of the chapter does not present a comprehensive overview of the causation controversies. Rather, in it I briefly describe pertinent arguments from the work of Steven Epstein, Paula Treichler, and Cindy Patton, each of whom approaches the consolidation of knowledge around HIV as the cause of AIDS from a slightly different angle within the larger field of science studies. Situating denialism within the controversies that once defined its positions as dissent is a first step toward identifying the rhetoric of denialist arguments, which is the subject of the next section of the chapter.

In *Inventing AIDS,* Cindy Patton focuses, in part, on the rise of virology in addressing AIDS once the virus (HIV) was isolated and determined to be the cause of AIDS. Since AIDS defined a set of conditions caused by impaired immunity, immunologists initially enjoyed authority over research concerning this new disease state. Patton writes, "In the early 1980s, immunological interpretations of AIDS emphasized the relationship between environmental management and internal bodily breakdown." This interpretation focused on gay lifestyle, which included "immune overload due to drugs, 'fast' living, an excessive exposure to semen . . . or simply too much sex."[12] Yet "when virologists analyzed the same AIDS epidemiological studies which immunologists saw as evidence for a social or environmental cause of AIDS, they saw instead evidence of a sexually transmissible pathogen." Although, as Patton notes, to this point "a pathogenic disease of the immune system [had never] been conceptualized," "in AIDS a compromise occurred between competing systems of explanation; etiological agent and immune system breakdown theories were brought into line via the discovery of an agent which 'attacked,' or more accurately, disarmed the immune system." Patton argues that "greater technological and financial commitments (and potential rewards) of virology linked data and dollar to become the dominant way of thinking about AIDS."[13]

One consequence of the victory of virology was that "immune system support therapy researches took a back seat or were abandoned to non-Western therapies." This is in part because "biomedical research was oriented toward a virologic model, seeking a 'magic bullet' along the lines of AZT." Writing in the later 1980s, Patton remarks, "Virology's assumption that a virus can simply be eliminated or blocked has mis-directed research efforts for nearly three years, denying thousands of people potential therapies [i.e., immune-boosting therapies] which could have prolonged or improved the quality of their lives."[14]

Cindy Patton's discussion of the way in which the identification of the cause of AIDS as a virus affected medical approaches to its treatment is similar to Paula Treichler's more extensive commentary on the cultural construction of HIV. Treichler's purpose is less critical than explanatory, in that she concentrates on the ways in which we can claim and understand HIV as a cultural construction, a named entity produced through struggles over meaning, scientific practice, and symbolization. For her, HIV/AIDS is a case that demonstrates the cultural construction of scientific objects but does not discount their reality. Instead, she demonstrates Latour and Woolgar's claim that "*reality* [is] discursively . . . the set of statements considered too costly to modify."[15] Using Bruno Latour's notion of the scientific "black box," those concepts whose tortuous paths to truth no longer have to be acknowledged or even known because they are now "facts" without necessary history or cultural context, Treichler describes how "HIV has come to seem natural, inevitable, and taken for granted as the cause of AIDS," a situation that "mark[s] this construction of reality as the hegemonic position from which AIDS research and treatment are typically understood."[16] In part, this occurs through the bracketing of culture as that which impedes scientific discovery rather than the context through which all scientific activity takes place.

For Treichler, HIV is a constructed reality, but a reality nonetheless: "Both fabrication and fact, HIV has become, in short, a reality that is too costly to give up." An example of its construction is the history of its names. Describing this history, Treichler notes that names make the thing signified seem "coherent" and "unified," and they "establish entities for the public as both socially significant and conceptually real." Ultimately, "the existence of

HIV and AIDS as unifying signifiers now makes it possible to proceed *in discourse* as though the questions have been resolved." Naming thus confers a solidity to entities referred to, even though "manifestation in writing reveals the presence not of an object but of a sign."[17] In a reference to the semiotician Charles Peirce, Treichler indicates a belief in the infinite recursion of meaning deferred through symbolization. Reference is always to another symbol (or sign), so that "the referent" is never an object but always something that stands in for it. This is what Treichler means by "in discourse," above. Language makes it seem as if the real is there and referred to, but it also covers over and conceals the real through its very performance. For Treichler, then, the discursive history of HIV demonstrates its fabrication as well as its reality, and dissent must be understood through the perception of knowledge and facts as cultural constructions that establish the real as we know it.

Steven Epstein provides the most comprehensive account of AIDS dissent in the period prior to HAART in *Impure Science,* his discussion of the causation and treatment controversies concerning HIV/AIDS. A sociologist engaged in science studies, Epstein shows how HIV became identified as the cause of AIDS. He then follows the history of controversy between the dissenters and the "AIDS orthodoxy" through the early 1990s, focusing on the fight for scientific credibility and the relation of scientific inquiry to the public activism characteristic of AIDS controversies. Like Treichler, Epstein is interested in how knowledge is produced. But his methodology is firmly in science and technology studies. Rather than focusing on the phenomenology of HIV as a cultural construction, he addresses the actors engaged in the construction and then the interactions in claims about knowledge and authority.

In a moment of summing up, Epstein writes, "The construction of belief about the causes of AIDS, and the dynamics of controversy, cannot be understood through an analysis of the 'scientific field' as traditionally understood—as a self-contained arena in which credentialed researchers are the only important actors. Rather, a highly public and somewhat 'open' field has been the site of incessant struggle, negotiation, cooperation, and interaction among a variety of individuals, institutions, and organizations."[18]

Epstein demonstrates that both the dissenters and the mainstream AIDS scientists held divergent views of what constituted evidence of HIV's role in causing AIDS. Both sides felt that the other was acting in bad faith: "From Duesberg's standpoint, the defenders of orthodoxy were always 'moving the goalposts' whenever its predictions were proved false; from the vantage point of the dominant position, the dissenters were forever cooking up newer and stricter criteria of proof that their opponents were then expected to meet."[19] (Peter Duesberg is a prominent AIDS denialist and professor of molecular and cell biology at the University of California, Berkeley.)[20] Presciently, Epstein cautioned, "Most likely there is no scientific test that would settle the causation controversy to the satisfaction of all sides. *A different sort of proof probably would spell the end of the controversy, however: if the AIDS establishment were to succeed in finding an impressively successful antiviral drug or vaccine, it is unlikely that anyone would continue to pay much attention to the dissidents.*"[21] Post-1996 AIDS research, after the rollout of HAART and subsequent successes with a variety of drug regimens, does tend to ignore the AIDS dissenters who do not believe that HIV causes AIDS. The most vociferous of these are usually termed *denialists*.

Interestingly, Epstein's discussion of the AIDS dissident scientists demonstrates that, in general, they hold onto what Patton identified as the earlier immunological view of an assault on the immune system from "lifestyle" behaviors like drug use and supposedly excessive sexual activity. The refusal to believe that HIV caused AIDS is, in part, a refusal to accede to the virologists' definition of the disease as caused by a single pathogen. Much of the attack on Duesberg and other AIDS denialists continues to be that they are not virologists (or retrovirologists) and thus cannot understand the science involved.[22] In the denialist era, when treatments that diminish viral load and improve patients' CD4 counts (an important marker of the immune system's viability) seem to prove the viral account of the disease, those who disagree appear to be against established science and, accordingly, the "truth" about AIDS.

From the perspective of 2009, when the international discussion about HIV/AIDS concerns the global scale-up of treatment and whether to treat everyone who tests HIV-positive (regardless of CD4 count) with antiretroviral drugs in order to diminish transmission, the causation controversy seems like ancient history. HIV is surely a fact that we cannot afford to give up. And yet AIDS denialism continues as a force questioning the established science of HIV, attacking both the knowledge produced by scientists studying HIV disease and the overall funding apparatus that draws together national governments, international pharmaceutical corporations, and international public welfare organizations like the World Health Organization and UNICEF, as well as private philanthropies like the Gates Foundation, in a common project that the denialists believe is wrong-headed. Denialism is a continuation of the causation controversy in the ARV era. While Epstein, citing René Dubois, suggests that "it can be dangerous to infer medical etiology 'backwards' from treatment effectiveness," the science establishment has "black-boxed" HIV as the cause of AIDS, bolstered by the treatment effectiveness of antiretroviral drugs in combination therapy.[23]

Given that the establishment of treatment effectiveness has weakened their claims, it is germane to ask how denialists make their arguments and establish their credibility. In large part, they continue to question the validity of research results based on concerns about study design and the formulation of research questions that predispose researchers to conform to established ideas. Part 1 of Epstein's *Impure Science,* concerning the causation controversy prior to 1996, offers an extensive discussion of these methods. But because the causation controversy is now seen by many to be a historical, and thus closed, issue, current denialists are apt to question what they call establishment science and the financial incentives for scientists to adhere to what they call the AIDS orthodoxy. Indeed, while some dissenters continue to pursue unorthodox scientific theories about AIDS causation, many denialists raise the specter of conspiracy theories in arguing their case for a nonviral cause of AIDS. Denialists seek to return to the scientific moment before HIV became the way to identify the cause of AIDS, the name of an entity they variously claim does not exist, has not been isolated, or could not possibly cause the syndromic consequences indicative of AIDS. They rail against the domination of particular views against dissenting, iconoclastic voices, arguing that politics, and not science, has cemented the case for HIV. In so doing, they come to be seen as antiscience quacks, intent on causing doubt and interfering with the important search for truth exemplified in the normal routines of basic research and publication by peer review.

Arguing Denialism and Arguing Back

The technical arguments of AIDS denialists—as well as arguments directed back at them—are difficult to follow. As John James suggests, refuting denialism often depends on the explanation of the details of scientific experimentation techniques to nonscientists. Even careful explanation can be complex and opaque to nonscientists, as it must parse the language of science and the protocols for research in order to refute the rhetorical strategies of AIDS denialists. One such strategy is the argument that HIV/AIDS human subjects research is itself dangerous and rigged by pharmaceutical companies to push their products.[24] This is one used repeatedly by journalist Celia Farber in her March 2006 *Harper's* magazine article, "Out of Control: AIDS and the Corruption of Medical Science." This article garnered a significant rebuttal, authored by Robert Gallo (the American discoverer of HIV) and other prominent scientists and AIDS treatment activists and journalists, available on the Internet through the South African AIDS Treatment Action Campaign (TAC) and the Web site AIDStruth.org. In this section of the chapter, I examine Farber's *Harper's* article in detail, as well as the rebuttal of Gallo et al., in order to illuminate the rhetoric of AIDS denialism.

Gallo and his colleagues name four different kinds of error in Farber's article: those that are (1) *misleading* (implying a false fact), (2) *false* (stating directly a false fact), (3) *unfair* (implying "sinister motives" without evidence), or (4) *biased* (neglecting facts that do not support her ideas). Each error is identified by the page and type, and a sometimes lengthy counterargument is provided by the authors to refute Farber's claims. This attack on AIDS denialism is against its "rhetoric," implying a negative definition of rhetoric as language use that manipulates the reader through the use of lies and misleading statements. This is a typical representation of rhetoric as what Wayne Booth calls "rhetrickery."[25] Such a perspective on rhetoric itself denies the rhetorical aspects of all language use, even scientific statements, and attempts to align scientific "truth" with evidence that is beyond language and thus culture.

The analysis of denialism that I offer treats all language use as rhetorical. To give an example of Farber's argument and the rebuttal by AIDS scientists and others, let me offer a quotation from the beginning of "Out of Control."

The objective of the trial, PACTG 1022, was to compare the "treatment-limiting toxicities" of two anti-HIV drug regimens. The core drugs being compared were nelfinavir (trade name Viracept) and nevirapine (trade name Viramune). To that regimen, in each arm, two more drugs were added—zidovudine (AZT) and Lamivudine (Epivir) in a branded combination called Combivir. PACTG 1022 was a "safety" trial as well as an efficacy trial, which means that pregnant women were being used as research subjects to investigate "safety" and yet the trial was probing the outer limits of bearable toxicity. Given the reigning beliefs about HIV's pathogenicity, such trials are fairly commonplace, especially in the post-1994 era, when AZT was hailed for cutting transmission rates from mother to child.[26]

Gallo and his coauthors have the following to say about this particular paragraph, specifically pointing out Farber's comment that "the trial was probing the outer limits of bearable toxicity."

> PACTG 1022 compared ARVs, that had already been found to be safe and effective for treatment in the absence of pregnancy, in pregnant women. All drugs used in the trial had been shown in previous trials to benefit people with HIV. This is why the FDA has registered them. The PACTG 1022 trial happened to find higher than expected toxicity of nevirapine in very specific circumstances. Even here, toxicity was sufficiently rare as to be outweighed by the likely benefits of nevirapine use. The FDA revised its nevirapine recommendations on the basis of this trial. Nevirapine remains an important antiretroviral medicine whose benefits outweigh its risks.
>
> Nevirapine (or a drug, efavirenz, used instead of it) has been shown in an analysis of clinical trials to slow disease progression, particularly in patients with low CD4 counts.
>
> Safety trials are obviously associated with a calculated risk, but they are permitted when the expected benefits are considered to outweigh this risk. Would Farber suggest that no clinical trials be conducted whatsoever?[27]

It's important to understand that in this article, Farber represents "Joyce Ann Hafford," a "single mother," as dying after giving birth to her second child. Farber suggests that Hafford's death was a result of her being enrolled in this clinical trial after a positive HIV test during her pregnancy. Farber states specifically, "Joyce Ann Hafford was thirty-three years old and had always been healthy. She showed no signs of any of the clinical markers associated with AIDS." In addition, while her HIV test was positive, Farber writes that "Hafford was tested only once [an anomalous procedure], and she did not know that pregnancy itself can cause a false positive HIV test."[28] This last point was also refuted by Gallo and his colleagues.

In essence, Farber's claims about the kind of clinical trial Hafford was enrolled in are embedded in a narrative that charts an innocent woman's death at the hands of the AIDS biomedical machine (elsewhere in the article described by Farber as "a global, multibillion-dollar juggernaut of diagnostics, drugs, and activist organizations"). Gallo and his colleagues label this particular kind of error misleading, since they understand Farber to be purposefully misrepresenting the ARVs in the study, primarily concerning their clinical toxicity. Careful reading of Gallo et al.'s discussion of the misleading representation demonstrates that the scientists and their supporters are attempting to counter the idea that the risk in the trial was unwarranted, due to previous studies that had shown drug efficacy and the known risk of not treating pregnant women with ARVs.

Yet it seems to me that the sentence in Gallo et al.'s rebuttal that reads "The PACTG 1022 trial happened to find higher than expected toxicity of nevirapine in very specific circumstances" stands out. Even a knowledgeable reader might ask if Joyce Ann Hafford's death was one of these "specific circumstances." The portion of the rebuttal cited above is a defense of the scientific method and of clinical studies in general. Because of that it does not actually address directly the claims made by Farber that Hafford was a victim of an ill-conceived or badly conducted clinical trial.

Those claims are addressed throughout the rest of the thirty-five-page rebuttal document. Even with the critique I just offered, it's hard to imagine someone reading this lengthy text closely and coming away with a positive appreciation for Farber's claims, given the specificity of the scientific information and the careful exposition of Farber's methods of misinformation. But Farber's overall rhetorical strategy is not necessarily to make specific claims that individually stack up to scrutiny. Her basic goal seems to be to cast doubt in as many different ways as she possibly can. For example, she argues:

- the HIV test was untrustworthy
- the clinical trial was problematic from the start
- the patient wasn't advised properly
- negative outcomes from the study were hushed up
- researchers already knew about potential toxicities
- whistle-blowers were punished
- the definition of AIDS is different in different places and thus not properly scientific
- many studies of HIV/AIDS drugs don't follow proper double-blind protocols
- AIDS dissident scientists are routinely ignored
- global conspiracies support AIDS research
- researchers have never proven that HIV causes AIDS

The approach is scattershot. All the careful exposition in the world does not stand much of a chance against this kind of rhetorical tactic, because the ultimate point is to cast just enough doubt so that readers will lose faith in any statement about HIV/AIDS made by mainstream scientists or public health officials. Only one bit of seemingly reasonable data or argument amid this welter of information is necessary to make doubting AIDS a more viable response than trusting doctors and global health policymakers.

This rhetorical strategy is an important marker of AIDS denialist discourse. Henry Bauer's recent book, *The Origin, Persistence, and Failings of HIV/AIDS Theory,* similarly launches a number of challenges to the "AIDS orthodoxy," including:

- HIV does not appear to be a sexually transmitted infection
- the frequency of positive HIV tests does not measure the prevalence of infection
- HIV does not appear to be a blood-borne infection
- the definition of AIDS has changed over time so statistics are not comparable over time
- scientific investigations into racial disparities in HIV prevalence are racist
- racial disparities in the frequency of positive HIV tests have a genetic basis
- a positive HIV test result is a "marker of physiologic stress"
- pure HIV has never been isolated
- not all people who test positive for HIV become ill, and some who do test positive subsequently convert to seronegative status
- anal intercourse can introduce sperm into the bloodstream, which might be the cause of positive Western blot HIV tests in gay men
- there is no established proof that HIV causes AIDS
- there is lots of proof that HIV does not cause AIDS, primarily in the lack of correlation of relevant statistics
- AIDS in Africa (and perhaps the Caribbean?) is something entirely different from AIDS in the United States and western Europe[29]

Bauer also argues that the funding structure of scientific inquiry contributes to the silencing of dissident voices. While claiming that his work on

HIV/AIDS does not rely on conspiracy theories, he nevertheless suggests that scientific inquiry has been bureaucratized to such an extent that unorthodox challenges to reigning scientific consensus are impossible: "Bureaucracies don't know how to change their stance, bureaucracies don't like to be contradicted, bureaucracies will never willingly admit that they have been wrong about anything."[30] Bauer is arguing that how science gets done—through large-scale funding efforts provided by governments—inhibits the true free circulation of ideas, and especially the consideration of unpopular ideas that challenge the status quo. He believes that scientists and government funding agencies together maintain a fraudulent theory concerning the origin, spread, and treatment of HIV/AIDS, reinforcing his opinion that contrarian views do not have a chance of overcoming the wall of scientific and governmental consensus on the matter. The implication is that evidentiary controversies within AIDS science are obscured by an unacknowledged conspiracy that squashes dissent.

From the perspective of the so-called mainstream AIDS scientists, the deniers do not present valid scientific evidence to challenge established theories about the relation of HIV to AIDS or the epidemiology of the pandemic. Yet while epidemiologists Tara Smith and Stephen Novella believe deniers "seek to undermine the very philosophy of science itself, to distort public understanding of the scientific process, and to sow distrust of scientific institutions," many of the denialist rebuttals are filled with graphs, charts, and scientific arguments about plausible statistics and meaningful evidence.[31] Bauer is certainly in this latter group.

Bauer's work displays another rhetorical similarity to both denialist arguments and the so-called AIDS orthodoxy. He consistently cites as evidence for his arguments the work of Peter Duesberg, Harvey Bialy, and other AIDS deniers, creating a closed circle of citation that diminishes the impact of his arguments on anyone who doubts the veracity of these sources. This is similar to Paula Treichler's discussion of how Gallo's group established their research results as crucial to the claim that HIV caused AIDS: "The research laboratory of the virologist Robert C. Gallo at the National Cancer Institute . . . was able to stake out fairly ambitious territory: by repeatedly citing each other's work, members of a small group of scientists quickly established a dense citation network, thus gaining early (if ultimately only partial) control over nomenclature, publication, invitation to conferences, and history."[32] Apparently the function of closed citation networks is to control what counts as a fact and to disseminate arguments as truths that have the backing of authorized individuals. In these ways denialism does not always function differently from science as usual, even if its claims are repudiated by mainstream scientists.

This is where science studies can offer those who want to repudiate denialism some much-needed analytic advice. It is the study of the cultural context and the social meaning of scientific ideas that offers the best answer to AIDS deniers, not scientific reaffirmations of the evidence for HIV as the cause of AIDS. This is in part why AIDS deniers make their case on scientific grounds. Their rhetorical strategies are not rhetrickery in Wayne Booth's sense, that is, calculated manipulations of language to fool people, but strategies to cast doubt on mainstream scientific portrayals of HIV and AIDS. It is true that they use distrust of science and governmental control of science funding to convey their arguments, but they also try to unseat AIDS science through scientific claims. Indeed, many AIDS deniers argue that culture matters too much in scientific endeavors, believing that a science cleansed of sociocultural influence (that is, politics) will demonstrate the false premises of contemporary consensus thinking about HIV/AIDS.

I offer the counterargument that "more culture makes better science." This is a typical feminist science studies argument to "situate" scientific knowledge production in the "partiality" of individual circumstance and perspective.[33] Significantly, one cannot identify a denialist just by demonstrating bad science or faulty evidence. A person can be a bad scientist without being a denialist. To understand denialism one must understand the rhetoric of the argument, its shape and purpose, which I have discussed here. These classic forms of refutation—the scattershot presentation of evidence and argument, the attack on all truth claims associated with mainstream positions, and the suggestion of a concerted and organized conspiracy—are not altogether different, in an academic sense, from the kinds of challenges routinely lobbed against the science establishment by science studies scholars, and certainly not distinguishable from some claims emerging from lay perspectives. Denialism, as I try to show in the next chapter, may be a response structured by marginalization. Certainly, it is a claim lodged against a powerful body or idea by those who represent themselves as disempowered in comparison.

Conclusion

So how do we tell the dissenters from the quacks? There may seem to be a thin line between denialists and those who engage in controversies within

AIDS science. Of course, one's perception of the line and its ability to demarcate dissenting scientists from all-out deniers depends on where one stands with respect to AIDS research and the validity of scientific data it generates. Identifying denialism—or verifiable scientific data, for that matter—always depends on one's positionality.

In my chapter on the U.S. National Breastfeeding Awareness Campaign, I argued that scientific facts depend on a cultural consensus to establish their veracity in the public sphere. In the case of the NBAC, the Ad Council tried to use science to establish a new consensus concerning the risks of formula feeding but found itself under attack for misrepresenting risks and making mothers feel guilty. This is because, in part, the existing consensus (a belief that replacement feeding confers few, if any, significant health risks) results from entrenched social structures and systems of meaning that demand women's bodily separation from their infants and flexible activities as autonomous adults.

Infant formula manufacturers and those who support infant formula use in the United States are not labeled breastfeeding denialists. The cultural consensus favors their practices, even if the preponderance of scientific evidence demonstrates the contributions that breastfeeding makes to the health and well-being of mothers and babies. Those who refuse to believe that HIV causes AIDS can be called denialists because the cultural consensus supports the opposite position, the "mainstream view" that is the basis of AIDS science globally. It is cultural belief—and not some absolute veracity of scientific data—that makes some positions denialist and others common sense. Because of this, the belief of some scientists that better science education and clearer communication by scientists will make the public less vulnerable to the arguments of denialists is implausible as a response to denialism of any stripe.[34] To challenge denialism, one must investigate and understand its rhetorical forms and its cultural functions, not simply its reliance on faulty logic or misinformation. Those are only the mechanisms of its persistence and dissemination.

This issue is made very clear in academic and public conversations about official state denialism in South Africa. The next chapter reviews current academic treatments of AIDS denialism in South Africa, in order to demonstrate how, based on context, denialism can itself serve a variety of political functions. AIDS denialism, it turns out, is not one thing, but a shape-shifting set of beliefs. Understanding AIDS denialism in South Africa, from multiple positions, helps us to understand why some breastfeeding advocates established alliances with AIDS denialists in their response to global health policy decisions about MTCT. AIDS denialism seems to offer breastfeeding advocates a discourse that allows them to challenge mainstream public health guidelines on infant feeding practices in the context of maternal HIV infection. There are rhetorical and substantive benefits from this alliance, although the political ramifications are, in my view, disastrous.

Perhaps it matters less who the quacks are, in comparison to the dissenters, than what cultural purposes those in both categories fulfill. Denialists do not spur scientists to create better science, because they are jettisoned from the establishment and forced into increasingly marginal positions, from which their voices seem ever more shrill. Clearly, denialists serve a variety of cultural functions, one of which is to comment on (and challenge) how hegemonic ideas are established and maintained by privileged groups. One could say that denialists identify ideological structures and the ideologies these produce—except that then denialists seem like privileged seers, the marginalized downtrodden who are able to discern the truth amid oppressive situations. This is clearly an image denialists would like to cultivate. It is more accurate to say that studying denialism demonstrates the workings of ideology on all sides.

Responding to denialism, many scientists take on the mantle of exceptional truth-seekers, denying their role in the maintenance of hegemonic forms of knowledge and privilege. Denialism takes root in the general population in part because the magnitude of the scientific problems seems unbelievable or because denial is a more plausible position than the doomsday scenarios spun by the scientists.[35] Or denial resonates because science promises more than it can deliver, especially in the area of biomedicine, and people learn to distrust its claims. Whatever the case, denialism is a response embedded in particular social contexts in which its meanings are politically situated and culturally resonant—whether it is promoted by scientists or laypeople, its function is a cultural challenge to authority and what is perceived to be hegemonic belief. It is to this issue that I turn in the next chapter.

CHAPTER 12

Situating Denialism

DENIALISM MAKES for strange bedfellows.

In 2001 I was introduced to AIDS denialism at the biannual La Leche League International convention in Chicago. Former La Leche League (LLL) founder and board member Marian Tompson, along with other breastfeeding advocates, had organized a nonprofit organization called AnotherLook, which focuses attention on scientific debates and public health directives concerning breastfeeding and HIV/AIDS. AnotherLook sponsored a session at the LLL convention called "Perspectives on HIV, AIDS, and Breastfeeding Research," which included David Crowe's presentation, "Infectious HIV in Breastmilk: Fact or Fantasy?"[1] At the time of the conference, I knew little about HIV transmission through breastfeeding, and I was struck by the questions about HIV and AIDS that Crowe raised in his presentation. I had my own questions—was it true that there were legitimate reservations about HIV as the cause of AIDS, or, more specifically, the infectiousness of HIV in breast milk? In the margins of the presentation handout, I have numerous scribbled notes and stars. Two stars accompany this statement made by Crowe: "Unquestioning acceptance of current dogmas about HIV and AIDS is one of the biggest threats to breastfeeding."[2]

Curious after the LLL convention in July 2001, I explored the AnotherLook Web site. In its approach to breastfeeding and HIV, AnotherLook tries to cast doubt on the science of AIDS with respect to mother-to-child transmission (MTCT) through breastfeeding. On its Web site, the organization states that it looks for "scientific proof that infectious HIV virus is present in breast milk and is transmitted from mother to baby through breastfeeding." On its home page, the mission statement reads, "The issue of HIV and human milk has been clouded by possibly questionable science, lack of precision concerning the definition of breastfeeding, and premature public policy statements."[3] While "lack of precision concerning the definition of breastfeeding" is a noted and recognized problem in all research on lactation, these questions and statements all demonstrate the scattershot strategy of denialist rhetorics.

In this chapter I explore what appears to be AIDS denialism in breastfeeding advocacy. Of particular interest are distinctions between outright denialism and the way that questioning biomedical studies and recommendations can seem like denialism. Such questioning demonstrates the thin line that separates controversies within scientific communities from controversies that deny the considerable scientific consensus surrounding a particular disease phenomenon. Some breastfeeding advocacy participates in AIDS denialism, using existing controversies within biomedical approaches to infant feeding in the context of maternal HIV infection to promote a broader denial of mother-to-infant transmission. The point here is to understand why denialist rhetorics are attractive to these breastfeeding advocates.

I explore this issue initially by examining AIDS denialism in South Africa. There is a vibrant, and somewhat sympathetic, academic discussion of South African AIDS denialism, an official government position questioning HIV as the cause of AIDS, which created barriers to the general availability of ARVs for years. While public sentiments about the South African situation seem uniformly incredulous that the poorest continent's most wealthy country would take a stand against biomedical approaches to HIV disease, some of the academic literature on this question is more forgiving. Indeed, a varied group of scholars tries to understand South African state denialism in its cultural and political contexts, producing "situated knowledge" about what is generally thought of as an abhorrent and neglectful policy of evasion, studied ignorance, and refusal to acknowledge scientific facts.[4]

If we can understand AIDS denialism in South Africa as situated and meaningful (while also abhorrent and misguided), then we can also understand breastfeeding advocates who gesture toward denialism, as well as the general circumstances that stimulate denialist thinking. Such understanding can inform responses to individuals and groups that repudiate public health efforts on their behalf. More significant, understanding the cultural functions of denialism forces analysts of HIV/AIDS to acknowledge how contestations within and about modern biomedicine affect people's responses to medical treatment. Denialism, which often seems like a head-in-the-sand response to objectively determined facts, is also about beliefs and values, and serves as a discursive option in circumstances of intense cultural and biological controversy.

South Africa's State of Denial

AIDS in South Africa initially emerged similarly to the United States, among urban gay white men in the early 1980s.[5] However, in the late 1980s, the first documented case of AIDS in a black South African heralded a shift in the country's situation. In the 1990s, the AIDS epidemic in South Africa developed into one of the worst in all of sub-Saharan Africa.[6] South Africa, with over five million HIV-positive adults in 2006, has "one of the highest numbers of HIV-positive persons in the world."[7] The rapid increase in HIV prevalence and AIDS deaths coincided with the end of white-minority rule and the democratic elections that put the African National Congress in charge of government.

Those elections, held in 1994, brought Nelson Mandela to power. Already AIDS was a significant and growing problem in the country, even though the previous white-minority government had set up an AIDS advisory group in the 1980s. Mandela's administration acknowledged the problem of high HIV infection rates but there is evidence that the government's response to the epidemic lacked leadership. Under the presidency of Thabo Mbeki, which began in summer 1999, the government began to promote dissident positions with respect to the causes of AIDS, as well as to resist efforts to provide antiretroviral treatments for HIV-positive individuals attending public hospitals and health clinics. At the 2000 International AIDS Conference in Durban, South Africa, Mbeki avoided reference to HIV and spoke about poverty as an incipient cause of AIDS. He also brought AIDS denialist scientists like Peter Duesberg to South Africa to consult on the epidemic there. While activists working through the Treatment Action Campaign (TAC) took the government to court, leading to the 2002 High Court ruling that the government had to make ARVs available to HIV-positive pregnant women, South Africa's health ministry officials "remained hesitant about providing treatment for people living with HIV."[8] Even in 2006 the government was criticized for having "small baskets of garlic, lemons, and beets" at the country's exhibit at the International AIDS Conference in Toronto.[9] Shortly after the August 2006 conference, the Mbeki administration officially ended its public AIDS denialism, moving the responsibility for action on HIV/AIDS from the health minister hostile to antiretroviral treatments to a deputy minister who "publicly acknowledged the weakness of government leaders on HIV/AIDS in the country."[10] However, as late as fall 2008, newspapers were reporting that only then did the health ministry break "dramatically . . . from a decade of discredited government policies on AIDS, declaring that the disease was unquestionably caused by HIV and must be treated with conventional medicine."[11]

There are numerous academic treatments of the South African government's denialism. Much of this literature tries to detect a logic behind such an irresponsible public position. This trend in the scholarship analyzes why Mbeki and his administration blocked public provision of antiretroviral medicines after their efficacy was accepted in the scientific community and why they questioned HIV as the cause of AIDS. In general, scholars who pursue this line of thinking recognize the value of biomedical approaches to HIV/AIDS and deplore the lives lost to postponed treatment opportunities, but do not want the Mbeki administration's response to the South African epidemic to be defined as wholly irrational. To accomplish this task, these scholars explain South African denialism in the context of national and global conditions, particularly colonialism and the legacies of scientific racism.[12]

Five main factors driving the postapartheid government's AIDS denialism are outlined by Mandisa Mbali: (1) "the medical findings of certain dissident scientists," (2) "the extent of the crisis brought about by the epidemic, which has prompted denialism because the government cannot deal with it," (3) a mechanism "to avoid conflict over intellectual property rights of essential medicines," (4) "the impact of poverty on the course of the epidemic, which has led to government denialists positing poverty as a counter explanation to the virological cause of AIDS" or as a "smokescreen for the government's adoption of poverty sustaining neoliberal economic policies, which may be blocking further public spending on AIDS," and (5) "the history of constructions of 'the African' as the inherently diseased racial and sexual other in both colonial and post-colonial times." Mbali charges that the main motivation for the denialist stance was "a wider belief that several key tenets of science around AIDS are racist, with denialism being a defence of Africans against racism and neoimperialism, a belief well-established within certain circles in the African National Congress (ANC). . . . [The] government's denialism appears to have attempted to throw out altogether the Western biomedical/scientific paradigm relating to AIDS," or, as she asserts later, "government AIDS denialism [was] heavily affected by the legacy of racist public health discourses."[13] These general arguments surface in the work other scholars and constitute the core sympathetic interpretation of denialism in South Africa.

For example, Joy Wang, in her analysis of the ANC's 2002 anonymous AIDS denialist document entitled "Castro Holongwane, Caravans, Cats, Geese, Foot & Mouth and Statistics: HIV/AIDS and the Struggle for the Humanisation of the African," argues that "it is the legacy of racism and dehumanisation, compounded by the 'global apartheid' of the neocolonial economic order, through which AIDS denialism and its consequences must be read." Using Franz Fanon's article "Medicine and Colonialism" as a reference, Wang suggests that while "western medicine" has "made important advances" in Africa, the situation of colonization and its aftermath makes these contributions ambivalent.[14]

Anthony Butler argues that a biomedical paradigm concerning AIDS existed in conflict with an "ameliorative and palliative" alternative that favored traditional medicine and nutritional approaches to the disease, an alternative supported by ANC leaders. In the ANC analysis, three factors, "inequality, violence, and particularly mobility," are key circumstances contributing to the virulence of the HIV/AIDS epidemic in South Africa, and these were "products of the continent's colonial and segregationist history, and apartheid bequeathed a legacy of racialized HIV prevalence." Noting also the lack of public health infrastructure to provide direct medical support for ARVs (he suggests that South African public health institutions lacked proper staffing due to emigration in the early to middle 1990s), Butler concludes that numerous factors came together to stymie efforts to rally behind the biomedical response to HIV.

South Africa's public and political institutions predisposed many policy-makers to support an ameliorative/nationalist paradigm and to reject a mobilizing/biomedical alternative. The intellectual discourses of the liberation movement created an inhospitable environment for a biomedical science that lacked an appealing social epidemiology of the virus. A history of apartheid division, exile, and racist science predisposed numerous powerful and rational decision-makers to doubt the benevolence and coherence of the biomedical/mobilization paradigm. Political and economic calculation, in the face of the government's cruel inability to muster human re-

sources for a universal ARV programme, may have further predisposed the government towards delay and obfuscation, and encouraged it to disperse responsibility for the epidemic across society as a
whole.[15]

Steven Robins also argues that "the questions of race and identity . . . lie
at the heart of responses to the AIDS pandemic." Robins agrees with Wang,
in that "Castro Holongwane" can be read as "an African nationalist defence
of the AIDS dissident position in the face of what its authors claimed was a
racist representation of AIDS as a 'black disease' associated with sexual
promiscuity and the inability of Africans to control their sexual appetites."
He also suggests that support of actual dissident science "may have been
limited to a relatively small circle of intellectuals, journalists and politicians," but "this position resonated with, and possibly gave credibility to,
'popular' forms of AIDS denial and alternative and 'traditional' explanations for AIDS and illness." In this analysis, state denialism was partly successful because it was able to call upon a cultural consensus of popular
views of AIDS. In addition, Robins argues that the dissident science position on HIV was attractive because "the stigma of its early associations with
homosexuals, bisexuals, blacks, sex workers and drug users has continued
to stick . . . [which] explains the intense sense of shame associated with
AIDS as well as the attraction of dissident AIDS science and nationalist
views, especially amongst young, educated black South Africans." However,
in opposition to the government, the Treatment Action Campaign (TAC)
was able to capitalize on the experience of young, often less well-off, heterosexual women who were HIV-positive and desperate to avoid transmission to their children: "the abstract and ideological language of the cultural
nationalist response to AIDS and AIDS science did not resonate" with
them.[16] It is no wonder that the TAC's first successful court battle against
the government was about the provision of ARVs to pregnant women in
prenatal clinics and public hospitals.

Adam Sitze's wide-ranging article, simply titled "Denialism," situates
South Africa's position in a global network of denialisms. Noting that Susan
Sontag identified "a denialist kernel lodged in the very discourse of emergence that has framed the northern approach to the pandemic from the
very beginning," he goes on to suggest that denialism has also "informed the
decisions of the dominant institutions of globalizing capital, which have
acted precisely to refuse the biopower called into being by the new biomed-

ical technologies on the basis of a fundamentally racist approach to global populations." By this Sitze means that international law and custom, through the General Agreement on Tariffs and Trade (GATT), the World Trade Organization's (WTO's) Trade-Related Aspects of Intellectual Property Rights (TRIPs), and the International Monetary Fund's (IMF's) Structural Adjustment Policies (SAPs), made it seem reasonable to believe that it was impossible—both too expensive and a violation of international law—to treat everyone who needed ARVs to fight AIDS. In addition, international pharmaceutical companies, bolstered by the U.S. government, fought to maintain their patents on AIDS drugs in an effort to safeguard profits, even though the majority of HIV-positive people live in countries with limited means to purchase them. Sitze identifies these behaviors and beliefs as a disavowal at the heart of capitalistic approaches to HIV, a situation that predisposed South Africa to a "general economy of denialism."[17]

He goes on to identify the denialist irony at the heart of anti-AIDS efforts in the global north.

> Denialism's crowning achievement is an absurd but not unfamiliar geopolitical condition in which the leading institutions of globalizing capital daily reiterate their commitment to the fight against HIV/AIDS—a geopolitical condition, then, where people with HIV/AIDS have never attracted more compassionate spokespeople, charitable organizations, concerned onlookers, professional mourners, pitying philanthropists, and rock-star advocates—and yet where, fifteen years after ARVs emerged as a distinct biomedical possibility, they are available to only 50,000 to 75,000 of the 4.1 million in sub-Saharan Africa who will die without immediate access to them.[18]

Noting that "a certain denialism defined the apartheid state's relation to HIV/AIDS from the very beginning," Sitze wonders less at Mbeki's denialist actions than at the idea that his administration could have escaped some form of them.[19]

Less radical discussions of South Africa's denialism attempt to demonstrate how the value of portions of Mbeki's critique were lost in the general outcry that he was abandoning the principles of scientific medicine in favor of quack approaches to health. In her introduction to *HIV and AIDS in Africa: Beyond Epistemology,* Susan Craddock writes that "the incontrovertible dominance of biomedical models placing HIV front and center have silenced Mbeki's more insightful statements on poverty's role in creating AIDS in the South African context."[20] In addition, a number of the authors discussed here point out that accepting HIV as the cause of AIDS meant accepting a pharmaceutical answer to the epidemic. Indeed, the focus on technological responses within a traditional biomedical paradigm has been criticized even at the biannual international AIDS conferences, where ethnographic and behavioral approaches are subordinated to technoscientific solutions. Denialism in this analysis may be linked to a desire to foreground the social contexts of disease and its communicability, which in public health terms are not less significant than its microbial status and the medicines that treat it.

Nicoli Nattrass reviews most of the above arguments in her article "AIDS and the Scientific Governance of Medicine in Post-Apartheid South Africa" and book *Mortal Combat,* but repudiates each as insufficiently explanatory of Mbeki's denialism, concluding, "We will probably never know the balance of factors which underpinned his championing of the AIDS denialists—and, to a large extent, it does not matter what they were. What is clear is that Mbeki has never repudiated his earlier defence of them and he continues to question rather than endorse the science of AIDS."[21] In *Mortal Combat,* she specifically refutes the argument that "AIDS denialism was actually about economics" because "it requires us to believe that Mbeki was the public face of a deeply cynical government agenda to mislead the public on AIDS in order to balance the budget. This story is inconsistent" with various struggles between Mbeki and his own minister of finance over the HAART rollout, and "it ignores the fact that politicians are human beings who do not easily sacrifice the lives of children for a few cents." In reviewing all of the arguments about why Mbeki maintained a stance of AIDS denialism, she repeatedly suggests that the situation is a "puzzle" but implies that he may have become caught up in "the self-referencing and self-reinforcing AIDS denialist community."[22]

In the end, Nattrass indicts Mbeki's administration by identifying its most "pernicious legacy": "the erosion of scientific regulation of medicine in South Africa."[23] Like Mandisa Mbali, Nattrass grounds her arguments in a belief that contemporary biomedicine is a neutral and technical field of endeavor. Mbali writes that AIDS science and activism had, by the time of South Africa's denialist episode, shifted into a "rights-based, anti-discrimination discourse and . . . a medical, technical, non-'moralistic'/stigmatising approach." South Africa, she argues, must end the "policy gridlock partially created by AIDS denialism" by using "both human rights discourse around access to treatment and the human dignity of South Africans infected with HIV, and the *predictive and interpretative power of biomedicine.*" While Mbali acknowledges a historical racism in Western biomedicine, she is eager to argue for what it offers in a "rational" fight against AIDS: "At a microbiological level, Western biomedicine provides a powerful model for understanding the direct physical causes of disease and developing effective treatments, preventative methods and cures for them." Especially when it comes to HIV/AIDS, Mbali suggests, global public health had moved away from its biased history "to more human rights based discourses around policy responses to AIDS."[24]

Mbali and Nattrass, within this admittedly select group of scholars, are the most unforgiving of Mbeki's denialism, precisely because of the value they place on biomedicine as a scientific project that has surpassed the politics and cultural conflicts that the other scholars focus on. Those, like Sitze, who identify myriad other forms of denialism structuring the South African government's responses, embed medicine in a broader cultural context, refusing its special claims to truth. In his analysis, the medicinal value of ARVs is not denied, but their inextricability from culture and, especially, politics is emphasized over, or in conjunction with, their biological impacts.

Explanations of denialism must confront why scientific evidence becomes suspect or questioned in particular circumstances. As I argued with respect to the National Breastfeeding Awareness Campaign, the health risks of formula feeding are neglected or not recognized in the United States largely because important social and economic structures and beliefs depend on the separability of mothers from babies. The cultural consensus that acknowledges maternal guilt as a risk of infant feeding practices (but not juvenile diabetes and childhood leukemia, for example) is based on historical foundations and social institutions that continue to inform current practices. Scientific evidence for the risks of replacement feeding confronts a strong cultural resistance based in established institutions and economic structures.

In South Africa, and with respect to HIV/AIDS, distrust of traditional biomedicine was fueled by the racist history of public health under white minority rule. Jeremy Yoube's analysis of South African denialism in *AIDS, South Africa, and the Politics of Knowledge* offers a detailed discussion of this history, which provided the foundation for a pronounced cultural disinclination to trust "Western science" in the new government focused on "African solutions to African problems."[25] The fact that AIDS dissident scientists tended to separate the epidemics in Africa and elsewhere—arguing that these were not the same disease because of the divergent epidemiology and patterns of population risk—helped make what Yoube calls the "counter-epistemic community" appealing to Mkebi and his administration.

> It is true that most AIDS dissidents come from Western countries. Despite that, their suggested policy responses largely echo many of Mbeki's ideas. They want to encourage locally-produced and locally-developed responses. They see the distinctness of Africa's AIDS epidemic and believe in responding to the unique conditions that gave rise to it. They challenge the major (Western) pharmaceutical companies' intentions and argue that African states must break free. These dissidents may not be Africans themselves, but their policy ideas . . . strongly resonate with finding locally-appropriate solutions to the local manifestations of the problem.[26]

The critique of the AIDS dissident scientists also fit with Mbeki's perspective as a result of a preexisting suspicion of Western science, based on the history of its racist utilization during the apartheid era: "The colonial experience is rife with examples of justifying repression [of blacks] in the name of protecting the [white] public's health." Furthermore, "defenders of a denialist stance have often positioned their views as a response to the perceived (and, in some cases, overt) racism they see within the orthodox position on HIV and AIDS."[27] In Yoube's analysis, the AIDS dissident scientists produced a theory that resonated with the Mbeki administration's goals for an African-oriented South Africa, its wariness of public health solutions that targeted Africans as diseased or sexually depraved, and its concerns about a biomedical theory that pointed toward expensive solutions benefiting international corporations from the global north. Because of the availability of this "counter-epistemic community" and its desire for legitimacy, South African state denialism was able to use it to promote its own agendas just as the denialists gained currency (in some circles) from their public role as advisers to the Mbeki administration.

A crass reading of *AIDS, South Africa, and the Politics of Knowledge* suggests that Mbeki essentially appropriated the discourses of denialism to fit his agenda. As I have already discussed, the extent of Mbeki's personal belief in denialism is unclear and undecidable, and some scholars question whether he would knowingly manipulate AIDS policy for other reasons. Yoube does report, as do others, that Mbeki seems to have gotten much of his information about AIDS dissident discourses from surfing the Internet. If this is true, he represents the promise and peril of the information age, in which knowledge circulates without many of the authenticating frameworks of previous eras.[28] In any event, the fact that denialism exists as a discourse that can be appropriated is what is important here. Whether we think of it as a counterepistemology, or a dissident position within a scientific controversy, or an outright denial of reality, denialism operates as a discourse—that is, as a particular set of ideas articulated through predictable rhetorical strategies, including claims, arguments, and word use. Discourses are not locked into the circumstances of their original articulation; they can be appropriated for other purposes.[29] If the South African leaders utilized denialism in an attempt to create an African response to AIDS, it was because the denialists' ideas and strategies were available and worked for their purposes.

Denialism operates as a discourse articulated from the margins toward the hegemonic positions of the center. Yoube argues that many AIDS dissidents were credentialed scientists, which made it difficult to simply repudiate their claims. Since the causation controversy was black-boxed by the proven efficacy of HAART, the dissidents have been marginalized from mainstream publications and conferences.[30] Their denialism has crystallized in the context of this marginalization. Breastfeeding advocates often perceive that they share that position of marginalization in global public health debates about infant feeding and maternal HIV infection.

Denialism and Breastfeeding Advocacy

Some breastfeeding advocacy arguments challenge certain mainstream views about how to address pediatric HIV infection via breastfeeding. Some advocates seem to be so committed to breastfeeding as a public health strategy that they appear to hedge on the impact of breastfeeding on pediatric AIDS. For example, in a 1997 *New York Times* article reporter Barry Meier wrote,

> A growing number of critics contend that the United Nations has failed . . . to offer adequate guidance in sorting out the issues of breast-feeding and H.I.V. Much of the anger has been directed at

Unicef. While even the agency's harshest critics praise its efforts to raise breast-feeding rates, they add that Unicef officials have become so wedded to breast-feeding that they have lost the flexibility to deal with crises such as AIDS. "They are in denial," said Mr. Leonard of the Community Nutrition Institute.[31]

Most breastfeeding advocates are not AIDS denialists: they do not question any and all foundations of biomedical approaches to HIV and AIDS, as the denialists are wont to do. Some, however, have joined forces with denialists—or used their discourses—in their pursuit of breastfeeding-friendly policies concerning MTCT. Both groups—the breastfeeding advocates who accept the existence of HIV and believe that it causes AIDS and those who do not—share a belief that the primary problem in global approaches to infant feeding is a general lack of understanding of the enormous contribution that breastfeeding makes to human health.

An exploration of the AnotherLook Web site offers an interesting evaluation of AIDS denialism within breastfeeding advocacy. What I discuss in this section of the chapter are ways the presentation of breastfeeding and HIV on this Web site—the Web site of an organization "dedicated to gathering information, raising critical questions, and stimulating needed research about breastfeeding in the context of HIV/AIDS"[32]—utilizes, flirts with, or repudiates denialist discourses. In my analysis I will not be assessing the veracity of the information presented on the pages, but looking instead at the rhetorical strategies enacted on the site. What becomes clear is that breastfeeding advocates' challenges to global public health guidelines concerning infant feeding in the context of maternal HIV infection can be similar to the discourses of AIDS denialism. At times they even use denialist rhetorics, explicitly articulating AIDS denialist arguments. This is not, however, the predominant tendency on the Web site or in the breastfeeding advocate community. More common is a similarity of style and strategy. Nevertheless, the appropriation of AIDS denialist rhetorics for breastfeeding advocacy should give us pause, as it represents a political alliance forged on troublesome, and damaging, terms.

The opening page for the AnotherLook Web site states, in bold letters, "The issue of HIV and human milk has been clouded by possibly questionable science, lack of precision concerning the definition of breastfeeding, and premature public policy statements."[33] This statement sets the tone for the entire Web site and links the organization's focus to AIDS denialism through the idea that there has been questionable science with respect to HIV transmission through breastfeeding. The "About Us" page and the "Call to Action" both mute this idea by focusing on specific concerns within the scientific controversies concerning breastfeeding and HIV—asking questions such as "how protective is breastfeeding in resource-poor contexts?" "does breastfeeding provide immune protections for infants even when the mothers are HIV-positive?" "what are the relative rates of morbidity and mortality in relation to infant feeding method?" and so on—yet reiterate the claim that strong or verifiable scientific evidence for current policy and practice encouraging replacement feeding does not exist.

For example, the Call to Action begins with the following statement.

> AnotherLook is issuing a Call to Action to assure the best maternal/infant health outcomes in relation to infant feeding in the context of HIV/AIDS. This call is needed because current research, policy, and practice, often based on fear, are focused on the reduction of transmission while neglecting the impact on morbidity and mortality. This not only may be misleading but may inadvertently set back critical gains already achieved in public health as a result of the protection and promotion of breastfeeding.

The following paragraph reads, "We acknowledge the possibility that HIV may be transmitted through breastfeeding and that there is an urgent need for feeding guidelines. However, there is currently no published scientific evidence showing that infants born to mothers who are HIV-positive would be healthier and/or less likely to die if they were not breastfed." The recurrent insistence that scientific evidence concerning the effects of HIV in breast milk does not exist connects this statement to AIDS denialism. The rest of the Call to Action frames the discussion within the terms of a scientific controversy, pointing out that guidelines concerning infant feeding must take into account overall morbidity and mortality associated with each method, that infant feeding practices are embedded in "social, cultural, and economic environments," and that there are significant "impact[s] of spillover mortality/morbidity associated with infant formulas," as examples.[34]

Another section of the call demands "concise, consistent definitions of feeding methods, testing methods, HIV infection and AIDS."[35] This is another sign of the linkages to denialist discourses. As was evident in the work of Celia Farber, denialists argue that testing methods are not consistent or accurate and that the changing definition of AIDS suggests scientific imprecision. Here, an analogy is made between known problems in breast-feeding research concerning definitions of breastfeeding, and the denialists' claims that changing definitions of AIDS have made comparisons about AIDS statistics unscientific.[36] Overall, the mix of kinds of arguments on the AnotherLook "About Us" and "Call to Action" Web pages largely keep the discussion within the parameters of a controversy within science. Two other Web pages, "Position Papers" and "Presentations," are variable as well, but the linked papers and presentations demonstrate more clearly the specific ties to AIDS denialism and its rhetorical strategies.

For example, in a paper entitled "Infant Feeding and HIV: The Importance of Language in Shaping Policy," George Kent and David Crowe take issue with the following sentence from a 2002 UNICEF Fact Sheet: "The risks of HIV infection have to be compared with the risks of illness and death faced by infants who are not breastfed." Through a lengthy discussion, they make specific suggestions concerning how the sentence could be revised to offer more accurate information to mothers concerning relative risks of mortality and morbidity with respect to various infant feeding methods. Their purpose is to suggest that HIV infection does not necessarily lead to debility or death. Indeed, they consistently argue that it is only illness or death that should be mentioned, not HIV infection itself. One of their suggested revisions is based on the following rationale: "For the mother who needs to choose among different feeding methods, there is no reason to give more attention to deaths caused by HIV infection through breastfeeding than to deaths from other direct causes." The implication here is that HIV as a signifier evokes fear and irrational responses and leads to (illogical) abandonment of breastfeeding. They also insinuate that the entire health industry is focused on ending HIV transmission regardless of the other impacts on morbidity and mortality that might result from lack of breastfeeding.[37]

This latter issue is one of the most consistent points in breastfeeding advocates' challenges to global public health guidelines concerning infant feeding, and it is not an insignificant challenge to make, given that infant deaths due to respiratory diseases, gastrointestinal illnesses, and malaria each outnumber deaths due to HIV. Breastfeeding provides some protection against all of these illnesses. However, in Kent and Crowe's position paper, the underlying purpose is to cast doubt on the idea that HIV infection itself is to be avoided in infants. They suggest that only overall morbidity and mortality should be addressed in infant feeding advice. Their final suggested sentence revision reads, "To help HIV-positive mothers choose a feeding method, it is important to compare the likely impacts on the infant's health status of different methods of feeding in different kinds of circumstances." In offering this sentence as the right way to articulate the issues at stake in infant feeding choice, they implicitly deny any specific significance to HIV infection. HIV infection, in this scenario, is only important if "it can be used as a surrogate marker for health outcomes," which depends on whether "(a) actual health outcomes cannot be determined readily, and (b) the association between HIV infection status and health outcomes is well known." Of course, mainstream health workers believe that HIV infection is a "surrogate marker" for negative health outcomes that are well known.

Crowe's presentation at the 2001 La Leche League convention, which is also on the AnotherLook "Presentations" Web page, repeats this strategy of casting doubt in much stronger terms. The stated object of the talk (which has the title "Infectious HIV in Breastmilk: Fact or Fantasy?") is "to weigh the evidence for HIV existing as infectious particles in breastmilk."[38] Divided into sections that question scientists' ability to detect HIV, the presentation aims to cast doubt on anyone's ability to demonstrate that there is HIV in human milk. Further, in the presentation Crowe asserts that "no HIV tests have been properly validated" at all, a clear attempt to question the general existence of HIV, which is reiterated in the summary ("There is no test that can directly detect HIV in breastmilk. All indirect tests are subject to false results, particularly in third world countries."). Significantly, while the presentation provides an extensive list of seemingly standard biomedical references at the end, its "Resources" section (shown as part of the live presentation) comprises the following.

- http://www.virusmyth.com—many links
- http://aras.ab.ca—referenced quotes on testing, surrogate markers and negative effects of AIDS drugs. Plus links.
- Duesburg PH. *Inventing the AIDS Virus.* Regnery. 1996.
- Maggiore C. *What if everything you thought you knew about AIDS was wrong?* American Foundation for AIDS Alternatives. 2000. [Available from our society or from aliveandwell.org]

- Package of papers by the "Perth Group," available at no charge from Dr. Valendar Turner (E-mail: vturner@cyllene.uwa.edu.au)

Thus, after suggesting that audience members can "accept the current dogmas about HIV, breastfeeding, and AIDS, and watch breastfeeding retreat in the Third World" or "ignore majority opinions. Weigh the Evidence. Be prepared to Paddle up the Creek, Build a Summer Igloo, Sail into the Wind!" Crowe sends them to exclusively AIDS denialist sources.[39]

Crowe's presentation does include the suggestion that, with regard to infant feeding, it is a "balance of risks" that must be assessed in both policy determinations and individual decision making. His question with regard to this issue—"Is a breastfed, HIV+ baby necessarily worse off than a formula fed, HIV-negative baby?"—indicates his clear position that HIV infection in and of itself is not a threat to infant survival, although not breastfeeding is. Other position papers and presentations on the AnotherLook Web site take up the question of the "balance of risks" in various ways, although none of these suggests that HIV infection is not dangerous. Instead, they point to problems in the research concerning HIV transmission through breastfeeding, specifically identifying research on exclusive breastfeeding. A good example is Pamela Morrison's position paper, "Mothers and Babies and HIV: What Is the Risk of Breastfeeding?" which addresses the balance of risks within its own recommendations, emphasizing overall infant morbidity and mortality as well as the point that the abandonment of breastfeeding itself has significant negative consequences.[40] David Crowe points toward this idea in the summary to his presentation, by stating, "Discouraging breastfeeding by HIV+ mothers will have known major negative health effects," but only does so after making significant challenges to the mainstream science of AIDS itself.

The issue of the "balance of risks" with respect to HIV and breastfeeding is crucial to breastfeeding advocates' approaches to preventing mother-to-child transmission of HIV. The overall calculus of risk in most scenarios is difficult and bleak, and yet breastfeeding advocates indicate hope that breastfeeding can be sustained and protected for the majority of the world's infants. Breastfeeding advocates believe that the contributions of breastfeeding to global health, especially in resource-poor contexts, are consistently overlooked in public health policy decisions, and that the risks of formula feeding are equally consistently underestimated. This critique of global public health guidelines is connected to their perception that few medical practitioners in the global north, and even fewer biomedical researchers, understand basic issues in breastfeeding management or the significance of human milk's immunological advantage. Many breastfeeding advocates also suspect the influence of infant formula manufacturers on prominent national and international medical and public health organizations.[41] Breastfeeding advocates are very concerned about infant formula manufacturers' attempts to develop markets in global contexts where they have previously been prevented from hawking their wares by agreements like the International Code of Marketing of Breastmilk Substitutes. Thus, breastfeeding advocates all point toward what might be called breastfeeding denialism as a core aspect of basic biomedical approaches to MTCT that must be addressed in order to get the guidelines for infant feeding in the context of HIV right.

Breastfeeding advocates have felt marginalized by international policy-making organizations dealing with issues of peri- and postnatal HIV transmission, perceiving that HIV experts have been more influential in determining infant feeding guidelines. The advocates have questioned policies by bringing up empirical deficits in research on MTCT; they have questioned the definition of breastfeeding used in key studies; and they have charged global health policy decision makers with lack of attention to breastfeeding as an overall contributor to infant and child health. The significant similarities between breastfeeding supporters (who question mainstream advice about infant feeding in the context of maternal HIV infection) and the AIDS denialists (who refuse to accept the scientific and cultural consensus about HIV as the cause of AIDS and the efficacy of antiretroviral treatments) all concern challenges posed to mainstream AIDS science and public policy.

But breastfeeding advocates who are not AIDS denialists do not use a scattershot approach, they do not question the seriousness of the AIDS epidemic or the role of HIV in causing AIDS, and they target very specific problems in research on postnatal MTCT. Foremost among these problems is the idea that feeding the babies of HIV-positive mothers with infant formula presents a realistic option in combating pediatric AIDS in most African countries and other nations in the global south. For breastfeeding supporters, Africa as a continent is important both symbolically and practically, as there has never been an appreciable population of poor mothers there who have not breastfed their infants. As advocate and researcher Ted Greiner notes in an unpublished paper based on a lecture he gave in 2002, "we still have no data on the relative risk of not breastfeeding in any African context. The reason for this in the past was understandable: few if any poor African women do not breastfeed their babies. Researchers could not locate any substantial numbers of living babies who had not been breast fed in low-income African settings."[42]

Understanding the South African situation—its history of racist public health policies, the government's attempts to bring attention to poverty and inequality as contributors to the HIV epidemic, and the way in which acceptance of HIV as the cause of AIDS mandated the purchase of expensive drugs benefiting pharmaceutical companies of the global north—helps to situate its official denialism. In the same way, understanding the arguments of breastfeeding advocates and their struggle to have the health risks of not breastfeeding recognized explains their appropriation of denialist discourses. What appears to be straightforward denial of the truth is a situated response to both scientific evidence and cultural context.

Nonetheless, the alliance between breastfeeding advocates and AIDS denialists evident on the AnotherLook Web site and in the writing of its contributors is troubling. AIDS denialism on the part of breastfeeding supporters damages efforts to protect breastfeeding in areas of high seroprevalence by aligning advocates with extremists who refuse the overwhelming scientific consensus concerning HIV infection and maternity. Situating the reasons for this alliance—a seeming lack of understanding of the contributions that breastfeeding makes to health by public health workers intent on stopping all HIV transmission, for example, as well as the steady erosion of breastfeeding support worldwide through processes of globalization and modernization—does not excuse its adherents for participating in denialist politics. Breastfeeding advocates' involvement in AIDS denialism obstructs solidarity within the global breastfeeding movement and restricts alliances with AIDS researchers and activists in combating pediatric HIV infection.

Conclusion

It is impossible to discuss questions of denial and denialism without an analysis of risk discourse, which I examined at length in previous chapters. The difference between being in denial of a specific risk to health and rationally weighing various risks and benefits of particular medical practices depends upon one's relationship to the idea of risk, one's understanding of disease causality, one's perception of the social and cultural consequences of action or inaction, and one's social position in relation to those consequences. Identifying a given individual's decision making as rational or not (in other words, as rational or being in denial) depends as well on one's perception of that individual's conformity to one's own set of risk perceptions. Those who are perceived to make decisions irrationally usually do not conform to mainstream risk beliefs or the accepted actions expected of those who hold those beliefs.

Denialism is a highly complex response to disease in the contemporary world. In this chapter I have argued that denialism is a situated response that involves history, cultural influence, and a relationship to scientific evidence. Depending on the social, political, and economic power of specific denialists, the position can, as evidenced by the situation in South Africa, lead to widespread problems in the scale-up of medically accepted treatment programs for a deadly disease like HIV/AIDS. Or, for an individual whose power extends only to what happens to her own body, it may result in a refusal to take a certain medicine, even if the stated value of the medication is for her unborn child. Denialism as a rhetoric offers a discourse to those whose personal practices may contravene widely accepted medical standards.

This is the case with those mothers in the global north who breastfeed even though they are HIV-positive. The resort to a denialist rhetoric in these cases occurs because there is not an available public discourse supporting maternal informed choice with respect to breastfeeding and HIV. In the United States, like many countries in the global north, there is simply not a strong cultural consensus about risks to replacement feeding—there is a public health rhetoric, one which is subscribed to by many women, but the shift to formula feeding for any number of reasons is not perceived (except by those thought of as the zealous few) as involving much risk to health or well-being. As a result, replacement feeding is normative, and the advice to HIV-positive women not to breastfeed seems normal. Breastfeeding in the context of HIV can only occur, in the United States and most other highly industrialized countries, as an anomalous practice bolstered by a denialist discourse.[43]

AIDS denialism should serve as a reminder that solely technocratic and biomedical approaches to epidemic diseases like HIV/AIDS are not realistic, even if denialist arguments themselves rely on scientistic approaches. As I argued in the previous chapter, denialist rhetorics take advantage of widespread cultural skepticism in challenging scientific orthodoxies. Because of this dependence on cultural belief (or lack of it), denialisms suggest the cultural aspects of practices targeted for public health interventions. As Brooke Grundfest Schoepf writes, HIV "prevention was essentially viewed as a technocratic problem of behavior change based on access to information and condoms."[44] The same might be said about postnatal MTCT, that it can be prevented through "behavior change based on information" as well as (limited) antiretroviral treatments and infant formula. Yet behaviors around sex and infant feeding are embedded in cultural traditions and, consequently, are meaningful activities linked to other social significations. They are both deeply symbolic and absolutely material in their typical expression as routine biosocial activities. Meanings around infant feeding—including expectations for infant behaviors and ideas about child development—changed precipitously in the global north as rates of breastfeeding fell initially throughout most of the twentieth century and then began to rise in the final quarter. Those changed meanings continue to constrain increases in rates of breastfeeding to the first few months of babies' lives. Denying the significance of those changes and their connection to other enormous transformations in family life is a kind of denialism that pervades modern perspectives on the biological and social meanings of breastfeeding globally.

The problem of HIV transmission through breastfeeding is a global public health problem—indeed, a global public health nightmare—but the solutions to this problem are circumscribed, given that (as with sex) all breastfeeding cultures are local. The only way to fully understand why mothers do what they do—especially when such behavior seems to contravene proven practices to combat disease transmission—is to comprehensively address their worldview, their specific experiences, and their reasons for acting as they do. It seems to me that such an understanding is largely beyond the comprehension of those committed to biomedicine as the arbiter of proper maternal behavior, as well as of those unable to appreciate the significant contribution that affluence makes to perceptions of rational behavior. But the problem is even deeper, insofar as most Americans, and perhaps most inhabitants of the global north, do not have a working knowledge of fundamental social relations obtaining in African societies, as well as how living in cultures where breastfeeding is normative affects public health efforts concerning HIV and infant feeding. The next chapters explore this issue through an analysis of the concept of choice as a guide to decision making for HIV-positive mothers in the global south.

CHAPTER 13

Representing African Women

THE *NEW YORK TIMES* reported on January 30, 2005, that the "U.S. is close to eliminating AIDS in Infants." The accomplishment is impressive: in 1990, 321 New York City newborns were infected with HIV; in 2003, "five babies were born with the virus." According to the article, the dramatic decrease in pediatric HIV infection is due to the success of antiretroviral treatments during pregnancy and the passage of laws allowing HIV-positive infants to be identified through immediate testing of newborns. In New York, mothers could only be identified and treated when newborn testing was not "conducted blind, meaning that no names were attached to the data," which occurred after a change of test reporting practices in 1997. In 1998, a law required the immediate testing of newborns. The author writes, "As the struggle with pediatric AIDS shows, much can be accomplished when there are a clear focus and a concerted effort."[1]

One aspect of that effort that remains neglected in the article is the infant feeding protocol for HIV-positive mothers. Rates of pediatric AIDS cannot fall to zero without specific interventions into the mode of infant feeding conducted by mothers who are HIV-positive. That the article fails to mention this fact is perhaps startling only to breastfeeding advocates, but as global public health debates concerning mother-to-child transmission are focused on both drug treatment for pregnant women and infant feeding advice and practices, the absence of a discussion of infant feeding in relation to the victory over pediatric AIDS in the United States is notable.

In its lack of interest in infant feeding protocols in the context of maternal HIV infection, the article articulates a perspective on HIV/AIDS typical of highly industrialized countries. This perspective is exemplified by its narrative iteration of the cause of HIV infection in children: "As AIDS spread from the gay community to drug users, women, and finally their children,

. . . frustration and hopelessness grew."[2] Such a view is not insignificant, as the so-called Pattern I countries offer a specific epidemiology for disease spread that affects public health measures.[3] However, the American experience with regard to HIV/AIDS is best placed in a global context of comparison and contrast, especially when it comes to mother-to-child transmission. Most HIV-positive mothers worldwide do not live in contexts in which replacement feeding is normative culturally. By not commenting at all on infant feeding as a factor in stopping MTCT, the article about the situation in the United States makes it seem that drugs and reporting are the only issues of consequence, neglecting some of the most important aspects of the problem for women in other parts of the world.

By not placing the American situation in a global context, it comes to be seen as a model for all relations of mother to baby, which can lead to misunderstanding of the intense global controversies about infant feeding and HIV infection, especially concerning the question of whether provision of artificial baby milks is called for. For example, in a 2000 letter to the *Wall Street Journal,* sociologist Amitai Etzioni wrote the following.

> It is great news that Americans are telling African mothers who are HIV-positive not to breast-feed their infants ("Sparks Fly at AIDS Meeting Over Breast-feeding," July 12). Studies show that if such a mother provides her infant with medication for a very short period and uses formula instead of breast milk, the infant has a high probability of throwing off the horrible illness.
>
> In 48 of America's states, testing of newborns for HIV is not required despite the fact that their blood is already being tested for other illnesses (especially PKU) in all states. And if an infant is somehow found to be HIV infected, the mothers are not told because of civil libertarian opposition. They argue that such disclosure would cause discrimination against the mothers, violate their privacy, and that prenatal care is superior. As a direct result, many babies who do not get the necessary drugs and are breast fed, die. It seems that only in Africa can our representatives effectively campaign for what must be done.[4]

While the author tries to show how the United States is bungling public health measures with respect to pediatric HIV, what is interesting here is how the American context is assumed as normal, even though Africa is heralded as a place where "what must be done" is actively fought for. Replacement feeding is only safe in contexts where clean water is readily available and formula is made available to and affordable for poor mothers. In reality, what "must be done" in Africa is debated because breastfeeding is understood to be crucial to the life of most babies on that continent. The author's mistaken belief that there is a clear-cut answer to mother-to-child transmission of HIV in Africa fuels his conviction that the same clear-cut answer is being purposefully avoided in the United States.

Etzioni is addressing what he clearly feels to be denial in the American context, and the *New York Times* article cited at the start of this chapter demonstrates that since he wrote the letter to the *Wall Street Journal,* unblinded HIV testing of infants has indeed contributed to lowering the incidence of pediatric AIDS in the United States. But Etzioni does not consider the cultural importance and meaning of infant feeding—let alone its biological contributions to health—for women and babies in varied circumstances. Because formula feeding is an accepted and ordinary practice in the United States and other industrialized countries, women are not ostracized (or stigmatized as HIV-positive) as a result of feeding their babies with bottles. Infant formula is understood as a reasonable and healthful substitute for human milk. Infant feeding has a variety of cultural meanings attached to it in the United States, but as we have seen there is a strong social consensus that women must not be criticized for their choice of method. Even as many bottle-feeding mothers complain about cultural and medical pressure to breastfeed, the actual numbers of women who never breastfeed (between 25 and 30 percent) or who are not breastfeeding when their babies are six months old (between 55 and 60 percent of all mothers) suggest that the cultural norm is limited breastfeeding in the months following birth followed by predominant bottle feeding. In the United States, most women do not follow medical advice concerning infant feeding (six months of exclusive breastfeeding, followed by at least another six months of nursing along with complementary feeding). This cultural context, biased as it is toward normative replacement feeding, has skewed U.S. perceptions about women's struggles globally.

In this chapter I look at how articles in U.S. news media portray HIV-positive African mothers and their infant feeding choices. I am particularly interested in the use of African women to consolidate and affirm decisions routinely made by American women. The articles I analyze here demonstrate the difficulty of imagining, from the affluent contexts of the global north, decision making by poor mothers in the global south. Furthermore, in these articles infant formula and bottle feeding are resymbolized in images that clearly counter the previous, prevailing tendency to equate replacement feeding in the global south with infant death, established during the Nestlé campaign in the 1970s and 1980s. As we saw in the letter by Etzioni, solutions to infant feeding in cases of maternal HIV infection are simplified, here through pictures that provide rhetorical support for replacement feeding as an answer to MTCT. These articles and their illustrations, then, work as arguments to impose a particular consensus about infant feeding on situations that resist clear-cut solutions.

African Women Are Black Women

Stories in U.S. media about postnatal transmission of HIV from mother to child neglect a multidimensional portrayal of breastfeeding or ignore breastfeeding altogether. Another blind spot that occurs is the implicit racialization in discourses about African women. Most HIV-positive women in the world are not white. The images of dead babies that bolstered the Nestlé boycott and campaigns against infant formula marketing in developing countries were of black and brown infants exploited by the products of industrial food manufacturers whose headquarters were situated in the white global north. The new dead baby images are AIDS babies; they are black and brown infants whose exploitation still has to do with the provision of infant formula, although as we shall see the causal relation is reversed.

In December 2000, the *Wall Street Journal* published an article about formula companies and the AIDS crisis that speaks to all these issues. The title, "Bottled Up: As UNICEF Battles Baby-Formula Makers, African Infants Sicken," is quite accurate to the article content. A response to this article published in the *British Medical Journal* highlighted the general complaint that the *Wall Street Journal* took the side of the formula companies in representing them as "white knights" who would save potentially sick children in Africa who are not well served by UNICEF or other global agencies meant to look after their interests.[5] In my reading, the *Wall Street Journal* does provide some criticism of the companies' practices, identifying, for example, complaints that they continually break the International Code of Marketing of Breastmilk Substitutes. Yet the newspaper is clearly on the side of the corporations, which show up as the champions of African children, foiled again and again by the bureaucracies of aid organizations and their unfounded prejudice against the business of infant food manufacturing.

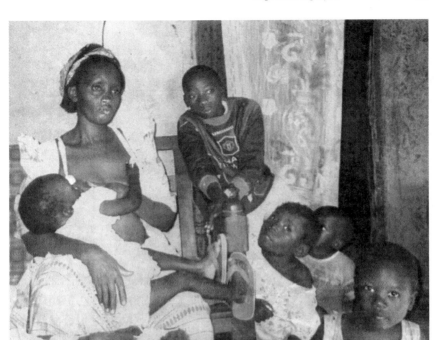

Fig. 2. Photo accompanying "Bottled Up: As Unicef Battles Baby-Formula Makers, African Infants Sicken," by Alix M. Freedman and Steve Stecklow, *Wall Street Journal*, December 5, 2000, A18. (Reprinted courtesy of UNAIDS.)

One imputation of this article is the notion that any HIV-positive mother who breastfeeds is necessarily making the choice for her child's eventual death. This point is of course reiterated in the question discussed in chapter 10, Tina Rosenberg's query "Why would a mother choose to condemn her baby to death?" But, as I have suggested, there are significant controversies within AIDS science concerning the transmission of HIV through breast milk, especially in terms of the effect of poverty environments on feeding method. The mother's body is not so absolutely identifiable as a cause of death for the child. To disentangle this particular knotty set of meanings, I'd like to discuss the main visual image of the *Wall Street Journal* article "Bottled Up," comparing the picture and the mother's story with another mother referred to in the text but not pictured.

Joyce Ganyana, shown in figure 2, is described this way: "Joyce Ganyana, an HIV-positive mother who lives in a Kampala slum, says she can't afford to buy a liter of cow's milk for 43 cents, let alone a one-pound tin of formula, which generally costs $6. 'If I stop breast-feeding, the baby will fall sick and die because she'll starve,' says Ms. Ganyana, 40, who ekes out a living selling vegetables. 'Formula is for the rich ones who can afford it.'" Another HIV-positive woman featured in the article but not pictured made a different choice about infant feeding.

> For example, after being counseled about the pros and cons of breast-feeding and formula at Nsambya Hospital in Kampala, 23-year-old Betty Nanfuka chose formula and was taught how to prepare it. Now she recites how she boils water twice a day on charcoal left over from meals and mixes two scoops of water for every two "level" scoops of formula she puts in a clean flask. The HIV-infected mother says that to preserve her secret, she always feeds her baby inside the house. Says Ms. Nanfuka: "If women are given a chance and told what to do, they can carry it out." So far, her baby, Maureen, has tested negative for the AIDS virus.[6]

Readers are not told if Glydesi, the two-year-old daughter of Joyce Ganyana pictured nursing, is HIV-positive, although we have already been informed that eleven-month-old Latshia Scovia, also nursing from an HIV-positive mother, is HIV-positive and thus subject to a "death sentence."[7] The photograph of Glydesi, however, suggests a robust child, like her numerous siblings. There is no dying baby here, yet. Instead, there is potential risk, invisible risk, represented by the mother's body. This picture may indeed show how breastfeeding keeps the children of HIV-positive mothers alive. Yet we are asked to see that this mother is feeding her child to death.

Three other aspects of this photo deserve comment. The mother's body is disarmingly disrobed, at least for an American audience not used to seeing uncovered breastfeeding bodies. The "baby" is two years old, far beyond the age considered acceptable in the United States for a child to nurse. Indeed, the notion that a two-year-old needs to nurse for nutritional reasons (otherwise she'd starve, her mother stated) seems ludicrous from an American perspective, yet breastfeeding advocates know that many children around the world depend on breast milk as a staple of their diets for two years or longer. From the American perspective, nursing a two-year-old is often considered repugnant, a self-centered behavior on the part of a mother. There is a sense, then, that this mother is willfully risking her child's health for an unnecessary practice that may be mere self-indulgence.

Finally, the four other children, all seemingly close in age, make this representation of a black mother reminiscent of the public U.S. conversations about poor women who give birth to children indiscriminately and rely on the state for financial assistance in bringing them up. "Why is this mother a mother at all?" is a hidden question suggested by the photo in its publication context of the *Wall Street Journal*. It is interesting, then, that a photograph of an HIV-positive woman and her child, in an article that strongly suggests that formula manufacturers are being inhibited by international aid organizations and their bureaucratic regulations in the companies' attempted rescue of dying babies, is presented in such a way as to suggest the mother's own culpability in the possible transmission of HIV to her child.

The good mother, Betty Nanfuka, is not pictured, perhaps because her bottle feeding must be hidden in the confines of her home due to stigma, or perhaps because in December 2000 it would have been difficult to portray an African mother feeding her baby with a bottle without conjuring up the dead bottle-baby pictures from the Nestlé campaign. Fast-forward a few years, and a reconceptualization and resignification of baby bottles is in full swing.

Fighting Stigma with Infant Formula

A 2006 article in the *San Antonio Express-News* describing a comprehensive prevention of mother-to-child transmission of HIV (PMTCT) program in Zambia reveals some of the pitfalls that occur when the American experience of HIV/AIDS is understood as paradigmatic. "In Zambia, A Formula to Fight AIDS" describes a program sponsored by San Antonio's Sisters of Charity of the Incarnate Word. The nuns conduct the program at their mission in Mongo, Zambia, where they "teach at Catholic schools, run an AIDS hospice, and give food and financial help to orphans." The author describes the "growing milk program" as

> contradict[ing] decades of the "breast is best" philosophy that a mother's milk is far safer and provides better nutrition than any other type of food—an ideology that prevails in much of Africa even in the face of HIV.
>
> Because infected women face only a 10 percent to 20 percent chance of passing along the virus in their breast milk, proponents say the benefits of breastfeeding outweigh the risk of HIV.
>
> The U.S. has all but eliminated the spread of HIV from mother to child by cutting out breast milk and using sophisticated medicines that keep the virus at bay.
>
> In African countries like Zambia, the recent arrival of a cheap and

easy drug treatment has underscored the breastfeeding dilemma. Women take a single pill of a drug called nevirapine during labor, and babies are given a few drops of it after birth. The treatment reduces the chance of infection [during labor and delivery] by nearly half, but the very same babies who are saved from HIV may become infected months later from breastfeeding.

The insertion of information about the United States and its methods of preventing pediatric HIV infection through avoidance of breastfeeding and the use of "sophisticated medicines" are cues that the article represents a northern perspective on preventing MTCT. Claiming that the "breast is best" philosophy is "an ideology that prevails in much of Africa even in the face of HIV" is disingenuous. It is not an ideological commitment to breast milk that promotes breastfeeding among public health systems in Africa and elsewhere, but lack of suitable alternatives, given poverty environments, lack of clean water, and low availability of medical care necessary to treat babies for illnesses against which breastfeeding is protective. Breastfeeding has been promoted because of the clear consensus that replacement feeding is risky in the poverty environments of Africa and the global south. Later in the article, the reader finds out that the Zambian babies in this program are offered "a year's supply of medicine to guard their babies against pneumonia, the No. 1 killer of children under age 5." Breastfeeding protects against pneumonia.

The author does point out that in resource-poor contexts the issue of clean water for formula preparation is paramount, because "water tainted with intestinal bugs can cause diarrhea, and infants who don't exclusively breastfeed are 25 times more likely to die from it, according to UNICEF." Women in the nuns' program receive instruction on treating water, as well as chlorine, soap, plastic containers, and feeding devices like bottles and cups. In addition, "nurses examine the babies each week and teach the mothers how to safely prepare the milk." Nevertheless, one of the children focused on in the article had been to the hospital four times in her first year of life, for her "frequent bouts with malaria, diarrhea, and skin rashes." In addition, she was smaller than her mother's older children. The worried mother "scrutinized the baby's every cough."[8] The free provision of infant formula clearly entails a significant commitment of resources to the health care of the babies who are not protected from routine illnesses by the immunological properties of breast milk.

The mothers taking part in the replacement feeding program are represented in the article as heroic in their decision to fight the negative social consequences of being identified as HIV-positive. The article details the harsh social stigma faced by the mothers who choose to feed their babies with formula, as bottle feeding often signifies HIV-positive status in contexts where breastfeeding is the norm. This representation allows the production of a heroic narrative concerning the mothers' sacrifice of social position, conjugal and familial relationships—even contact with older children taken by spouses who leave after disclosure of the women's positive HIV status—in order to decrease the reported 10 to 20 percent risk of postnatal HIV infection through breastfeeding.

I do not underestimate the actual sacrifice that the women in the program undergo in their attempts to keep their babies HIV-free. But the heroic narrative allows the U.S. author to focus on the mothers' challenge to the prevailing cultural norms rather than the significant resources necessary to keep their babies well once the mothers decide not to breastfeed. It is a matter of emphasis, to be sure. After all, if the United States "has all but eliminated the spread of HIV from mother to child," shouldn't other countries have a crack at it as well? By suggesting that the mothers are fighting stigma by bottle feeding, the bottle itself comes to signify their heroic, sacrificial gesture, changing rather dramatically the meaning of baby bottles produced through the Nestlé boycotts in the 1970s and 1980s.

Conclusion

Readers in the United States do not see, as a general rule, any negative risk to formula feeding, as I have discussed previously. Thus the idea that mothers might have a difficult decision to make with regard to infant feeding choice in the context of HIV infection is not an intuitive one for Americans. Even when told that a child needs to take medicine to ward off pneumonia, or that a child has been hospitalized four times as an infant with malaria and diarrhea, middle-class American readers are unlikely to consider the economic or medical impacts that this might make on the child's eventual survival or the family's well-being. These are simply represented as trade-offs for an HIV-free future, even if these other illnesses eventually prove fatal to vulnerable infants in poverty environments. After all, most American mothers practice their mothering under the authority and supervision of medical professionals. It is much easier to focus on stigma as the limiting factor for mothers' options than to consider an algorithm of risk in which no option is necessarily a good one.

Furthermore, another prevalent narrative about infant feeding in the United States concerns an alleged pressure to breastfeed, exemplified by the *New York Times* article entitled "Breast-Feed Or Else," discussed in chapter 7.[9] In keeping with this theme, narratives about fighting cultural norms and stigma that challenge breastfeeding as the proper method of infant feeding resonate with a public who thinks that breastfeeding is difficult or impossible for many women and that cultural pressures to breastfeed are themselves improper intrusions into women's private choices.

Representations of African mothers in U.S. media demonstrate the difficulty of portraying and appreciating the material circumstances of life in the global south. This was clear in the *Washington Post* articles about maternal mortality in Sierra Leone discussed in chapter 8, as well as those analyzed here.[10] Situatedness, Donna Haraway might suggest, always leads to partial perspective, which is seldom recognized or acknowledged.

Of course, it is no surprise to many that U.S. reporting on African women, infant feeding, and HIV/AIDS would be rife with ideologically inflected perspectives that mystify the women's practices or accommodate them to American norms and stereotypes. Global public health debates about infant feeding in the context of maternal HIV infection are more attentive to the material conditions of women's lives in the global south, as these are the specific scenarios that public health workers address in their work. Yet conflicts abound in these discussions as well. The circumstances of poverty, lack of infrastructure development, and the meaning of HIV/AIDS in women's lives all contribute to the difficulty of maternal decision making about infant feeding. "Informed choice" became a way for public health policymakers to accommodate the myriad uncertainties influencing mothers' decisions. But informed choice has always been and remains a contested global public health guideline. Debates about the appropriate approach to ending MTCT continue in the medical and public health literature, and it is to these, and the meaning of "choice" in infant feeding decisions in both global north and south, that I now turn.

CHAPTER 14

Informed Choice

FOR MOST WOMEN around the world, partial, prolonged breast-feeding is the cultural norm, especially in areas of high HIV prevalence among childbearing women. This group includes most women who are targets of global efforts to prevent mother-to-child transmission of HIV. Since 1997, these efforts have focused on informing women of the choices they might make concerning how to feed their babies and on supporting their chosen practices. While the international agencies have backed off from the 1997 "informed choice" doctrine to emphasize the balance of risks for women and their babies in these circumstances, many breastfeeding advocates continue to object to the principles underlying the infant feeding guidelines. They argue that many poor mothers are not able to make good choices because of pervasive structural, cultural, and personal constraints on their behavior. In other words, many breastfeeding advocates see informed choice—bolstered or not by AFASS criteria—as a sham.[1]

Cultural patterns of infant feeding in areas of the world with high seroprevalence mitigate against the fully empowered sense of choice that has supported global infant feeding guidelines since 1997. Even in fully industrialized settings there are problems with choice as a way of construing decisions about infant feeding. The ideological strength of choice as a hallmark of individuality and personal freedom obscures the extent to which even intimate choices are constrained by social circumstance and cultural forces. Infant formula companies have appropriated choice as a way to promote their products, further supporting the notion that health promotion campaigns about breastfeeding pressure women and make them feel guilty about choices freely made. And even the use of the word *choice* with respect to reproductive rights, some U.S. feminist scholars have argued, has obscured the extent to which the right to abortion has really been a privilege available to select few. If we shift this critique of choice to infant feeding debates, it seems clear that decisions about breastfeeding, in the global north, or formula feeding, in the global south, are the result of privilege rather than choice.

Analyzing discourses about choice and infant feeding, it is clear that choice and denial operate symbiotically in public discourses about maternal behavior. If informed choice is a way of pretending that mothers have agency in decisions about infant feeding, denial is a way of identifying when they have made the wrong choice. For many women in the world, choice and denial characterize interpretations of the no-win situations that define their lives. This chapter explores medical debates about replacement feeding in the global south, seeking to foreground thoughtful consideration of the material conditions that tend to be obscured by ideologies of modern individuality. I begin with an image of a baby with a bottle in the global south.

Public Health Debates in Images and in Print

Resignifying poor black women feeding babies with bottles is an element of the representational politics concerning the prevention of pediatric AIDS. The cover of the 2004 Annual Report of the international nonprofit Partners In Health (PIH) demonstrates this fact rather overtly (fig. 3). Yet symbolic changes, especially in media whose primary audience is made up of educated whites from the global north, do not address the circumstances within which HIV-positive black and brown women in the global south make decisions and engage particular infant-feeding practices. The bottle, seen as a weapon against stigma, the conveyor of love, or a vessel for a pure substance that will protect an infant against HIV infection, is wielded without reference to the material contexts and cultural constraints that make MTCT so difficult to address in the global south.

Disagreements about precisely what makes up those contexts and constraints preoccupy global public health debates about infant feeding and maternal HIV infection. Paul Farmer and Partners In Health have promoted a model "to prevent the embodiment of poverty and social inequalities as excess mortality due to AIDS, TB, malaria, and other diseases of poverty." Their strategy is to remove "clinical and community barriers to care" because "diagnosis and treatment are declared a public good and made available free of charge to patients living in poverty." This strategy in-

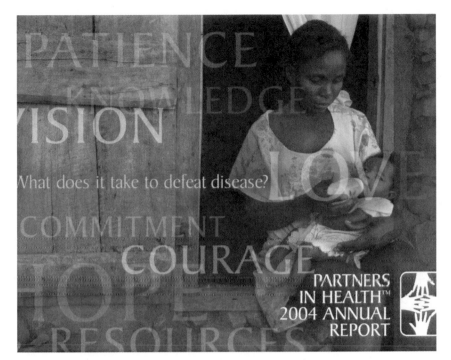

Fig. 3. Cover photo of Partners In Health, *2004 Annual Report*, Boston: Partners In Health, 2005. (Reprinted with permission.)

volves a model of care in which the removal of economic barriers is a basic aspect of the treatment program, and the standard of care is itself modeled on the standard of industrialized countries. In *Infections and Inequalities: The Modern Plagues,* Farmer argues that it is not only immoral, but also medically inadvisable, to use a different measure for standards of care in resource-poor contexts, especially when it comes to infectious disease. Because industrialized countries have diminished pediatric AIDS with treatment programs that provide antiretroviral drugs to mothers during pregnancy and at delivery, as well as full replacement feeding for infants, PIH's approach to MTCT in resource-poor settings in the global south engages the same strategies.[2]

Critics of PIH's model call it "formula plus" to indicate the increased resources necessary to ensure safe replacement feeding (similar to the resources offered to the Zambian women in the project described in the previous chapter). It is telling that Farmer et al. state in a discussion of a PIH project in Rwanda, "Unsurprisingly, opposition to the PIH model did not come from rural Rwandan women living with HIV. Rather, we faced the most resistance to this approach from local and global health policy makers who continued to promote universal breast-feeding, a policy which made eminent sense prior to the advent of HIV. Instead of trying to overcome programmatic barriers, the experts argued that formula-feeding was simply not feasible in rural Rwanda and that HIV-related stigma would prevent women from enrolling in such projects."[3]

In the *PIH Guide to Community-Based Treatment of HIV in Resource-Poor Settings,* there is no stated fear of spillover effect and there is no attention paid to the possibility of stigma involved with bottle feeding. Indeed, the *PIH Guide* suggests that counseling formula feeding (in the context of "aggressive diarrheal prevention") is both "practical and ethical." The critical view, exemplified in an article by Anna Coutsoudis and colleagues, is that breastfeeding is embedded in "biological, social, cultural, economic and political contexts" and is not easily extricated from these. Coutsoudis et al. are suspicious of attempts to ameliorate the effects of poverty on health that do not actually "improve the poverty status of mothers." In this criticism they are responding directly to PIH projects. They argue that global divides in wealth must be taken into account in public health guidelines and programs. Exclusive breastfeeding is, for them, a strategy for existing poverty contexts, in which "the child population as a whole" is put at risk by "the unrestrained promotion of infant formula." They also identify specific negative consequences of the "formula plus" model—its potential "side effects," as it were. Not only are the formula and other goods necessary to make formula feeding safe in these contexts always subject to resale, but "resources provided only to some households and not to others can increase inequities." Thus for Coutsoudis et al. breastfeeding itself is a fundamental value and preserving it—even in the context of HIV infection—is important. Breastfeeding is identified as "an unfailing anchor of child survival." Finally, they point out that infant mortality increased under the "formula plus" program and criticize the idea that rates of HIV infection should be the only markers of program success, suggesting that overall morbidity and mortality rates must be taken into account.[4]

Reading Farmer's *Infections and Inequalities,* I was struck by the philosophy undergirding his argument—that it is not culture that forms a barrier to treatment in poor communities (that is, it is not culturally specific beliefs about illness that lead the poor to be noncompliant with biomedical treatment protocols) but economic barriers and a lack of material commitment, on the part of government officials and public health authorities, to treating the poor. The larger analysis proffered is convincing, in that Farmer demonstrates how inequality spurs epidemic infections in poor communities. In other words, he shows that it is not simply poverty but the gap between the wealthy and the poor that causes the concentration of epidemic disease in poor populations. Farmer also argues convincingly that biotechnically sophisticated treatments should be made available to treat disease in the poorest communities on earth. With respect to breastfeeding and HIV transmission, the assumption is that emulating the practices of successful medical interventions—those considered routine and standard in the global north—is what needs to be done to stop pediatric HIV infection in the global south. If breastfeeding is contraindicated in the global north, it should be in the global south, and economic and practical barriers to the implementation of full replacement feeding for all affected infants should be overcome as a basic part of the treatment package. In "Structural Violence and Clinical Medicine" he and his coauthors state simply, "we show it is possible to address structural violence through structural interventions."[5]

Yet for Farmer and PIH, the fundamental value of breastfeeding as an aspect of global public health is never stated. It is not completely clear why this is so. After all, breastfeeding is considered by so many in public health as a crucial element of disease prevention in poor populations around the world. But Farmer's position may be precisely that breastfeeding is perceived to be necessary only for poor populations (and merely an added benefit for the wealthy). Farmer is adamantly against dividing the world in this way. Such division is an aspect of the "structural violence" that already condemns so many of the world's poor to vulnerability and disease.

If I can extrapolate based on my reading of *Infections and Inequalities,* Farmer's position would be that the only medically and ethically defensible act would be to provide all HIV-positive mothers with appropriate medicines and replacement foods for their infants, as well as the materials necessary to make such feeding safe, affordable, and sustainable.[6] As Farmer et al. point out, breastfeeding makes sense as a public health measure in the absence of maternal HIV infection. One gets the feeling that he would scoff at the idea that most mothers' lack of knowledge concerning their HIV status should affect policy on this issue. If knowing their status is essential to providing them equitable medical care, then mothers should be tested and those who are HIV-positive should receive the kind of care and treatment protocols available to women in highly industrialized settings. The PIH model is fundamentally a biomedical model, enhanced by anthropological understanding of how to make such capital-intensive treatments available to the world's poor.[7]

All of this begs the question of why Partners In Health would superimpose the word *love* over the picture of a black Haitian woman bottle-feeding her baby on the cover of its 2004 annual report. The strength of the PIH model is in its ethical and medical components, but the cover suggests that even these need rhetorical support, at least for the readers of an NGO annual report. Readers of such literature, educated inhabitants of the global north for the most part, may need the resignification of baby bottles (and maternal love) in order to feel comfortable with a shift in global public health policy concerning infant feeding. Even though most of these readers live in contexts where bottle-feeding is normative, they are not used to thinking the same for the women targeted by PIH efforts. After all, these readers are likely to be knowledgeable about ongoing public health efforts to support, promote, and protect breastfeeding around the world, and to be familiar with the dead baby images of the Nestlé campaign. These readers, I am suggesting, need bottles resignified for them as one part of a larger strategy to scale up their vision of appropriate medical care for HIV-positive mothers and their babies.

Another perspective on appeals to "mother's love" in programs to prevent pediatric AIDS is more pointed. Anthropologists Karen Marie Moland and Astrid Blystad argue that "emotional and moral appeals to 'mother's love' [in prevention of MTCT programs] articulates well with local values. But . . . counting on mothers' [*sic*] love without enhancing her survival chances is not an adequate public health response to the problem of MTCT. Neither is it an ethical response to one of the most disturbing public health problems of our time." The cover of PIH's 2004 annual report underscores the extent to which maternal love circulates as a universal given within public health programs to combat pediatric HIV infection. Yet the success of such programs does not depend on the intensity or depth of a mother's love. Moland and Blystad report that even though "HIV-positive mothers across the 5 study sites suffer and make sacrifices both in terms of their own health and social life and in terms of the family economy to secure an HIV-negative child . . . many women, despite their dedication to the course and despite their maternal love, do not manage to adhere to the demanding infant feeding prescriptions." Other circumstances, including family pressures, perceptions of infant hunger or well-being, poverty, and conflicting advice from nurses and feeding counselors affect mothers' ability to translate their love into practices that follow one or the other feeding protocols recommended for the infants of HIV-positive women. Moland and Blystad suggest that concerns about maternal mortality continue to lag in global efforts for "mother and child" health, implying that "mother's love" stands in for financial and political commitments to HIV-positive mothers themselves, as their importance to PMTCT programs continues to be understood only insofar as they themselves are "a threat to infant survival."[8]

Mothers' love cannot overcome the effects of poverty on maternal practices. The conflict between Partners In Health and Coutsoudis et al. has at its base a difference of view about the meaning of the material conditions of poverty in decisions about infant feeding. It is also a conflict about the value of breastfeeding to global public health and how interventions into infant feeding practices affect the sustainability of breastfeeding worldwide. Both sides feel that their evidence suggests a clear path forward—"formula plus" for PIH and exclusive breastfeeding for Coutsoudis and her group. Neither, it would seem, supports the existing framework of choice that continues to characterize global guidelines for infant feeding in the context of maternal HIV infection.[9] It is to this topic, and its ramifications in the global north and south, that I now turn.

"Informed Choice" or HIV-Positive Motherhood in the Global South

Informed choice has been the main public health strategy concerning global infant feeding guidance since the 1997 WHO statement. Recent changes, in 2000–2001 and 2006, have shifted back somewhat toward the earlier 1992 reaffirmation of breastfeeding as the first choice for infant feeding for most women in the world, but they have not extricated the guidelines from an emphasis on maternal decision making. Researchers in the field have documented numerous obstacles to the implementation of truly informed choice for mothers in the global south. Marina Manuela de Paoli, in a 2004 dissertation, identifies a variety of problems, including the custom of prolonged, partial breastfeeding in many locations with high rates of maternal HIV infection; low self-efficacy among mothers, given their generally low social status; stigma associated with complete replacement feeding; the role of other family members, especially mothers-in-law, in determining feeding patterns and especially in introducing other foods and water early on; high rates of infant morbidity and mortality in resource-poor settings; lack of access to clean water; and poverty and thus a lack of cash for replacement food.[10] The evidence begs the question, what is *choice* in these contexts?

It is clear that choice entered public health guidelines concerning support and advice for HIV-positive mothers as a result of a public health dilemma. Guay and Ruff suggest that although "in resource-poor settings, withholding breastfeeding was known to significantly increase infant morbidity and mortality due to infectious diseases and malnutrition . . . the risk-benefit ratio for an HIV-infected woman was not constant throughout resource-poor settings: some women in such settings might in fact be able to provide safe breast milk alternatives to their infants. This led to the need to assess the risk-benefit ratio on an individual basis." As Pamela Morrison and Ted Greiner point out, "Mothers are faced with a dilemma of competing risks." Public health workers who had previously stressed the overwhelming contributions that breastfeeding makes to health in resource-poor settings could no longer make such recommendations with complete confidence, in the context of maternal HIV infection. Yet breastfeeding advocates point out that the acknowledgment of individuality in determining the capacity to comply with the sanitary and resource requirements for replacement feeding simply shifts the burden of decision making to mothers, many of whom are not able to adequately weigh the balance of risks in their own situations. Ineke Buskens comments, "Mothers' intent to save their infants opens up tension between public health goals and personal conceptualizations of safety and risk." She and de Paoli emphasize other people's influence on infant feeding practices, particularly male partners, mothers, and mothers-in-law, and the difficulty of mothers to adhere to specific feeding regimes that counter the social norms of their communities.[11]

The language of research articles on this topic is telling: some examples include "HIV and Infant Feeding—An Ongoing Challenge," "Preventing Mother-to-Child HIV Transmission in the New Millennium: The Challenge of Breastfeeding," "How to Counsel Infant Feeding Practices in Southern Africa in a Time of HIV/AIDS?" "Child Mortality Associated with Reasons for Non-Breastfeeding and Weaning: Is Breastfeeding Best for HIV-Positive Mothers?" "Free Formula Milk for Infants of HIV-Infected Women: Blessing or Curse?" "Infant Feeding Dilemmas Created by HIV: South African Experiences," "The Dilemma of Postnatal Mother-to-Child Transmission of HIV: To Breastfeed or Not?"[12] While clearly not an exhaustive list, these titles demonstrate tension and conflict, indicated in the use of words like *challenge* and *dilemmas* and the frequent use of questions in the titles.

The impact of the dilemma is made clear in a short paper presented at the 8th Conference on Retroviruses and Opportunistic Infections in February 2001: "A Tale of Two Worlds: Stopping Global Mother-to-Child HIV Transmission."[13] The title alone tells us that the backdrop to the global problem is the fact that MTCT in the global north has been halted, while the situation in the global south is dire. MTCT dilemmas in the global south are the same as the dilemmas of the HIV/AIDS pandemic overall: how to get medicines and treatment protocols shown to be successful in wealthy countries scaled up in all parts of the world. Choice in infant feeding method became a way to mediate between the clear limitations of infrastructure and resources in poverty environments while acknowledging the treatment regimens successful in the global north. In addition, informed choice made it seem as if mothers and counselors would work together as rational decision makers to determine the best options in each individual mother-infant scenario. This put HIV-positive mothers in the global south in the position of good biomedical subjects, weighing risk and benefit. Informed choice as a policy made women in the global south seem more like the women in the global north who read *What to Expect When You're Expecting.*

On the other hand, it is difficult to not be for choice. To be against choice is to erase maternal agency altogether, to assume that mothers cannot make decisions in their own and their children's best interest. Choice indicates that mothers should be counseled to select the infant feeding method with whose requirements, in the face of HIV infection, they believe themselves capable of complying. The idea that mothers can and should be deliberative about their practices, and take an active role in choosing the one they believe themselves able to practice successfully, is a positive way of construing what is, realistically, a bad situation all around. At least allow women some degree of agency, the thinking goes. It is a position that coheres with global feminist ideals about women's capacities, even in the most dire circumstances.

Essentially, dilemmas concerning the informed-choice infant feeding advice guidelines reiterate tensions between (maternal) agency and (sociocultural) constraints. This is Paul Farmer's conflict with bureaucrats who decide that certain frontline infectious disease treatments are not cost-effective in the global south, or with breastfeeding advocates who believe that stigma is a significant constraint to replacement feeding among HIV-positive mothers in Rwanda (and elsewhere). Focusing on maternal agency, Farmer believes that HIV-positive women want to be cured, and they will comply with difficult treatment practices to stop transmission of HIV to their children. In his studies, these women seek frontline treatments and do not seem to be stymied by social or cultural constraints when structured inequalities are addressed in the treatment protocol.[14] Critics of Partners In Health's approaches, as I have shown, focus on the sociocultural and economic constraints of poverty environments and existing inequalities that make HIV treatments in resource-poor settings difficult to achieve along the model of those successful in the global north. Both Farmer and his critics are against informed choice, but for different reasons: Farmer because he believes in replicating frontline treatments in the global south rather than waffling with practices like breastfeeding, which would be considered substandard preventive practice in the global north, and his critics because they believe breastfeeding must be sustained as an overall strategy for global child health, even as specific interventions for HIV-positive mothers are studied and pursued.

Practically, researchers have found that informed choice is a difficult protocol to achieve in the prenatal counseling context. De Paoli provides an excellent discussion of some personal and economic constraints contributing to this difficulty.

> The guiding principle according to the most recent guidelines on HIV and infant feeding is that HIV-infected mothers should be allowed to make and to be supported in making informed decisions about how to best feed their infants. For these mothers, the decision about whether or not to breastfeed should be made by each mother based on full information of the options available. According to the counselors interviewed for this study, this issue (whether or not to breastfeed) created problems for most of the women. The informed choice of an infant feeding method seemed to be seriously compromised by the quality of the counseling, the lack of time to cope with the results, and the lack of follow-up support. However, in order to make informed choices, the mothers must be aware of, and have real access to the required resources, and have a real possibility of freely choosing from the recommended feeding alternatives. They must

also have good information about these available alternatives. Other studies have also shown that health-care workers' lack of knowledge, skills, and the time to conduct proper counseling, has proven to be a limiting factor in the efforts to convey correct information to HIV-infected mothers.

An HIV-infected woman is often the first person in the family with a positive HIV diagnosis. The counselors perceived that it was difficult for women to press all of these issues in the face of their husbands' coercive threats and their own emotional and economic dependence and compliant roles in relationship to men. For the same reasons, we found that the counselors perceived it to be difficult for HIV-infected women to make an informed choice about an infant feeding method. Follow-up of HIV-infected mothers was therefore regarded as a necessity in order to be able to give the needed support to the mothers who were trying to cope with a positive HIV test, adhere to an infant feeding method, and decide whether to risk involving a significant other. . . . At the pMTCT site where the in-depth study was undertaken, the health-care workers worked as counselors on their days off. This limited their capacity to follow up the HIV-infected mothers. Similar constrained working situations have been reported in other resource-poor settings, and few health-care providers seem to have been given the necessary time and training to provide proper infant feeding counseling.[15]

In addition, de Paoli remarks that in her study, counselors and nurses did not believe that the women they dealt with had real choices, given local social norms and expectations of mothers. The counselors' beliefs influenced the kind of advice that they gave to mothers. Counselors who may believe that HIV-positive mothers must breastfeed because of cultural constraints may nevertheless know little about exclusive breastfeeding practices "and said that they would not choose this method if they, themselves, were HIV-infected." De Paoli concludes, "The prevention of infant HIV-infection requires that women exercise influence over their own behaviour and decisions," which, she implies in previous discussions, they may not have due to embedded social mores that ensure their disempowerment, especially in relation to male partners, community elders, and mothers/mothers-in-law: "women's attempts to follow [counselors'] advice (choice of infant feeding method, disclosure of HIV status to partner, safer sex practices) often gave rise to problems because prevention of MTCT often conflicted with inter-personal pressures and sentiments."[16]

In the terms of the PIH model, it seems to me, informed choice would be perceived as a way of deflecting the responsibility of health care infra-structures to overcome barriers to proper treatment—women must them-selves determine if they have the resources, both financial and cultural, to pursue replacement feeding, and the system holds no responsibility for pro-viding these. All of the barriers indicated by de Paoli fall under the same la-bel—lack of will to offer effective frontline treatments. The PIH model of-fers another interesting insight concerning choice—and its obverse, denial. Maternal denial, we have seen, is called out when mothers seem to make de-cisions that fly in the face of common sense or routine medical knowledge. (Why not take a pill when your child's health, even survival, is at stake?) Much of Farmer's *Infections and Inequalities* is taken up with questions of patient compliance, and why the seeming noncompliance of the poor is re-ally evidence of a lack of will on the part of policymakers and medical in-stitutions to confront the barriers to access and treatment that bedevil the impoverished ill. Denial, of course, is another way of naming noncompli-ance with commonly accepted versions of appropriate health-seeking be-havior. Rather than offering an alternative logic to decision making, how-ever, denial suggests an active resistance to good evidence and proper action. For Farmer, noncompliance is an effect of structural violence. In my analysis, denial becomes a corollary of choice, a judgment that is the conse-quence of making perceived wrong choices.

Let me now turn briefly to the rhetoric of choice in infant feeding de-bates in the global north. Choice in the global north is the hallmark of fem-inist arguments for reproductive rights, although it has perhaps outlived its usefulness even in that sphere. Choice signifies competence, rights, and ra-tionality. It is a basis of neoliberal policies, both domestic and international, stressing individual's rights and beliefs over consensus or communal stan-dards. Choice is also the banner under which infant formula companies have chosen to operate. These discourses, and their problems, influence how informed choice has functioned globally in public health guidelines for infant feeding advice. Indeed, paying attention to articulations of choice in infant feeding debates in the global north calls into question conven-tional thinking about global north-south divides in this arena. Analysis of this issue serves to strengthen, as well as problematize, the PIH model and Paul Farmer's claims.

Choice and Motherhood in the Global North

On the Web sites of Ross Laboratories, Mead Johnson, and Nestlé/Carnation the choice to feed a baby with infant formula is presented as increasingly under fire, presumably by strong medical evidence about the health contributions of breastfeeding. Choice comes across defensively, with qualifiers about what is actually important in infant feeding. For example, in some articulations, love is more significant than breast milk or infant formula, which displaces the choice altogether onto the question of maternal emotions and, at some level, fitness. Implicitly, there's a sense that these Web sites are responding to an attack—if you feed with formula, you do not love your baby enough. The response, then, is to argue that it is love that counts in infant feeding and care, not what goes into the baby. Palpable in this rhetoric is the sense that mothers feel burdened by the need to demonstrate that they are good mothers by the way they feed their children.

What is important in these materials is the notion of an informed decision to breastfeed or feed with infant formula. The information on each site about advantages and disadvantages of each choice exists to help mothers make these informed decisions. However, the notion of an informed decision is undermined by the idea that decisions about infant feeding are made by the heart, not the head: in the end, information is not really the deciding factor. For example, on Mead Johnson's Enfamil Web site, after the discussion of "Choosing to Breastfeed," the page ends with the following statement: "Now that you're familiar with some of the advantages of breastfeeding, you have the added advantage of making an informed decision. In the end, of course, you'll do what your heart tells you. You can't go wrong. After all, that's the organ that's pumping out all that love for your baby."

Another Enfamil Web page discusses "It's Your Family's Decision": "Only mom and dad know what will work best for their family. So, be confident in the choice that you make. The best way to deal with people who question your choice is to simply tell them, politely but firmly, that you have discussed how to feed your baby with your baby's doctor. Feel good about your decision and be confident your baby is getting the essential nutrients he needs."[17] Decisions made through love are thus bolstered by references to medicine and its authority. Love also becomes the affective mechanism for determining correct choices and practicing good mothering; this linkage is evident in figure 3 (this chapter), the cover photo from PIH's 2004 annual report.

The representation of choice or decision concerning infant feeding in these product-oriented informational sites clearly echoes some aspects of the discourses of reproductive rights struggles in the global north. Some feminist historians have struggled with the concept of choice with respect to abortion rights, seeing it as a figuration of consumerism right from the 1970s, when *Roe v. Wade* made abortion legal in the United States. Rickie Solinger has shown that the rhetoric of choice obscures the importance of rights with respect to abortion and reproductive freedom. In an article "Poisonous Choice," and her subsequent book *Beggars and Choosers*, Solinger criticizes the use of choice to articulate abortion rights, and demonstrates how choice operates to stratify mothers into categories of good and bad choosers (i.e., good and bad mothers). First, she demonstrates how the concept of choice moved abortion rights from a rights framework to one focused on women as consumers, arguing that choice was already being used in terms of consumer privilege with respect to reproductive rights in the initial aftermath of *Roe v. Wade*. The use of choice instead of abortion rights made an alliance between the right to control one's fertility through pregnancy termination and the consumerist connotations of choice. Any decision a woman makes about reproduction thus becomes vaguely connected to her rights as a consumer (a right to choose this over that), rather than her rights as a human being.[18]

Then Solinger argues that the articulation of abortion rights as choice opened up the possibility of women being criticized for making wrong choices. The rhetorical links of choice to consumerism, and the ability to turn the discourse of choice into one of blame, led to choice becoming a very narrow political slogan that foregrounded the experience of middle-class women and made all other women vulnerable, because what are construed as rights in this scenario turn out to be privileges available to very few.

If Rickie Solinger is correct, choice has only meant the right of access to abortion for middle-class women, and thus it has never really meant choice, nor rights, in a universal sense. Choice in infant feeding method has not liberated women in the global north from the social burdens of maternity, although many women have benefited from entry into waged labor made possible under current constraints by replacement feeding. It is possible that the pressures felt by women who do not breastfeed, who feel that others look at them as if they have made a bad choice, are a legacy of the way choice rhetorically operates in relation to motherhood, functioning to distinguish mothers who choose well from those who do not. Since we know that in the United States, the constraints on breastfeeding are far harder to overcome for poor women, young women, women of color, and women with less education than for those women with education, resources, and more life experience, we can apply Solinger's analysis of abortion to infant feeding and notice that choice operates similarly to distinguish women who make good choices from those who do not, as if those choices are unconstrained.

In the introduction to their anthology, *"Bad Mothers": The Politics of Blame in Twentieth-Century America*, Molly Ladd-Taylor and Lauri Umansky write that "the 'bad' mother serves as a scapegoat, a repository for social or physical ills that resist easy explanation or solution. Scapegoating, as a process, does not engage principles of equity or evenhandedness; it seeks pockets of vulnerability."[19] In Paul Farmer's terms, scapegoating is a ritual that obscures the structural violence endemic to unequal societies, because it covers over systems of constraint that contribute to poverty. Scapegoating isolates the effects of inequality in individuals, and then blames them for causing their own inequality and impoverishment. Choice is a structure accommodating these scapegoating mechanisms and functions, as it shifts responsibility for public health risks to individuals, relieving government, the medical profession, and other institutions of their responsibility to safeguard community health.

In addition, choice means that information becomes the currency of public health endeavors, rather than structural supports or reforms, such as ending poverty, providing clean water, or making medical care accessible to all. In the PIH model, choice is a way of deflecting the responsibility to provide first-line treatments for infectious disease in poverty environments.[20] Thus, even though the contexts for infant feeding debates differ in the global north and south—in the sense that the outcomes of specific choices are understood to involve different variables of morbidity and mortality— overall choice has a similar structuring function in both rich and poor countries. It operates as a discursive mechanism to make an important public health issue (feeding babies) a private consideration of mothers.

Conclusion

The modern project of individuality is played out in infant feeding debates, just as it is played out in reproductive rights debates. We become individuals and we are modern, in part, through our choices, through having choices at all—that is, in not having to live through traditional patterns preset for us by others. In this sense, informed choice as a public health guideline for advice to HIV-positive mothers in the global south seems to draw these women into modern modes of maternity. And, as I noted previously, it is difficult not to herald choice as a step forward, as it emphasizes maternal agency and the capacity of mothers to understand their own circumstances better than others and to make decisions about their own lives based on this intimate, self-authorized, knowledge.

As breastfeeding advocates and researchers remind us, however, informed choice as a public health policy seems to ignore the constraints that poverty environments place on mothers' ability to follow through on decisions. After all, all environments place constraints on mothers' practices. We have seen in previous chapters that all sorts of pressures, ideas, and structures of social life affect women's decisions as mothers. Poverty limits the capacity of mothers to control aspects of their environment necessary for the successful enactment of various infant feeding methods. This is why poor mothers tend to choose the default cultural norm for their particular context and why education and resources are good indicators of nonnormative choices, in the United States and elsewhere.

Furthermore, as I suggested in chapter 3, the modern project of individualization makes life seem the result of deliberative choices. Choices focus on the individual and blur the impact of the constraints within which the individual operates. From a Foucauldian perspective, choice is a paradigmatic mechanism of the modern formation of the individual—an autonomous activity that nevertheless enforces subjugation and normativity. In the context of this understanding, breast or bottle is beside the point. The enactment of choice produces mothers who take instruction from health workers or Web sites, who subordinate themselves to expert knowledges and commercial practices, and who discipline themselves through expectations of good mothering that emerge in consultation with strangers and their forms of professional information. Choice thus operates as a specific mechanism of modern medicalization.

In the context of maternal HIV infection, however, medical treatment and attention are necessary and sought after. HIV-positive mothers, by all accounts, want to prevent infection in their children and receive treatment for themselves. They may refuse specific kinds of medication, but examining these situations usually demonstrates how local knowledges about disease and structural inequities contribute to outcomes that are understood medically as noncompliance or socially as denial.[21] We see here how poor mothers can so easily be identified as in denial about their illness and their potential to pass it on to their offspring. Denial is a way of marking a person at odds with (or outside of) the information economy of health, someone who refuses to take up positively the power of choice. To deny or refuse certain types of medical care is to be nonmodern with respect to one's body, one's health, and the bodies and health of one's children. Modernity demands similar compliance with respect to risk and purity, functioning as ideological requirements for acceptable behaviors in the face of contaminants, microbes, and other bodily invaders.

There are many small research studies addressing whether and how replacement feeding can be made safe for the infants of HIV-positive mothers in the global south. Other studies focus on safer breastfeeding in the context of maternal HIV infection. Both kinds of study depend on a well-developed infrastructure of public health clinics, voluntary testing centers (so that women might know their status), and nurses and counselors who can reliably advise women in the two methods of infant feeding and help determine, with the mothers, what kind of feeding method would best fit their situations. In the case of replacement feeding studies, the provision of infant formulas to impoverished women and their families is a necessary component. Looked at from the perspective of the resources necessary to support informed choices on the part of mothers, the real problem for HIV-positive mothers in the global south is their poverty and the impoverishment of the countries they live in. What Paul Farmer calls the structural violence of global inequality is clearly the dominant factor in the bleak prevention scenario that most of these women face.

When I listened to several talks on infant feeding interventions at the 2006 International AIDS meetings in Toronto, it occurred to me that each study, with its specific and small population, its cultural particularities, and its distinct economic context, would not produce results that would be transferable to more general policy guidelines about infant feeding in the context of maternal HIV infection. Replacement feeding in certain contexts would be more acceptable to mothers and others than in other contexts, and only some mothers could really safely feed with infant formula and expect their children to survive. Exclusive breastfeeding would be possible for some women but not others. Producing a set of guidelines for *all* HIV-positive mothers in poverty environments struck me as an impossible goal. I agree with Coutsoudis et al. that the PIH "formula plus" model is not workable in all situations, and it may not even be preferable given the potential for increased morbidity and mortality of nonbreastfed infants, even if they remain HIV free. At the same time, cultural patterns of prolonged partial breastfeeding are hard to break, so exclusive breastfeeding, while feasible in some contexts, would not work for all women either. For these reasons, informed choice as a policy began to make sense within the confines of what appeared to be an impossible set of conflicts.

And yet, that is precisely its problem. It is a brokered response in the context of a dilemma that appears to have no obvious, foolproof, universal solution. Such is the impact of AIDS on public health globally, and on maternal and child health in particular. Short of massive funding infusions so that first-line treatments would be available to everyone, it is unclear that one particular way forward is possible. And if such massive funding did miraculously appear, and the PIH model was adopted for all situations of maternal HIV infection, would breastfeeding disappear from the planet as a normative mode of feeding human babies? Would it only survive as a highly mediated, medicalized practice of elite mothers?

The disappearance of breastfeeding, of course, is the nightmare scenario that breastfeeding advocates fear. One way to consider this situation calmly is to think about sexual intercourse. HIV is spread through sexual intercourse, but people have not stopped having sex. The recommendation is for safer kinds of sexual encounters. Clearly, this is a manipulation of cultural norms—condoms are not natural in sexual encounters but can be made normative through a variety of educational and social means. This is the rationale for safer breastfeeding practices, such as exclusive breastfeeding and early weaning. Such practices inevitably medicalize breastfeeding but support and protect its very existence in the context of perhaps the most significant assault on its value as a human activity.

African women are critical figures in sustaining the dreams of global breastfeeding advocacy. Prolonged breastfeeding, a staple of jokes in the United States about La Leche League, is indeed a normative practice in many African cultures and countries, although it rarely occurs in reality as it does in the particular scenarios of advocacy imaginaries.[22] Prolonged breastfeeding is also usually partial, complemented by a variety of culturally approved foods or drinks meant to stretch the time a mother can be away from her baby, allow others to feed nursing children, or supplement a substance (human milk) thought to be inadequate in quenching babies' thirst or assuaging their hunger. As long as breastfeeding's value is measured in medical terms, its actual contribution through its typical practice will always be somewhat less than is upheld by those who believe in it, because exclusive breastfeeding, the current medical norm, is rare. Nevertheless, to see breastfeeding abandoned in Africa would be, for advocates, to witness the passing of a biological aspect of motherhood that, until now, has sustained human life as we have known it. It would be a tragedy beyond human proportions.

Which is why breastfeeding advocates try hard to find ways to continue to support breastfeeding, even in the context of maternal HIV infection. Breastfeeding advocates believe in breastfeeding beyond its medicalization. As I argued in chapter 6, they use medical discourses as a way to demonstrate their belief in the value of women's bodies. They are especially concerned with AIDS researchers who do not seem to value breastfeeding or to understand how easily lost are its contributions to human communities. In areas of the United States, after breastfeeding started to be abandoned in the late nineteenth century, within two generations there was barely enough lay knowledge of lactation management to sustain its resurgence. The resurgence that has occurred has done so under the auspices of an overtly medicalized understanding of the value of nursing.

In the medical paradigm, traditional suspicions of mothers' milk intensify in light of fears of toxins and viruses that may be transmitted from mothers to babies. The resignification of bottles and bottle feeding that is transforming the meaning of replacement feeding in the global south enhances these tendencies by normalizing practices that the Nestlé boycott had successfully linked to images of dead babies. The unspoken fear that resides behind advocacy discourses and inside studies promoting breastfeeding is that, in light of (1) historical circumstances, (2) the meaning of AIDS in the social sphere, and (3) long-standing cultural suspicions about women's bodies and their excretions, offering choice to mothers newly diagnosed with HIV will inevitably lead to the widespread abandonment of breastfeeding as the customary way to feed babies. Advocates' tenacious arguments in favor of breastfeeding, their desperate appropriation of denialist discourses, and their repudiation of informed choice and the AFASS criteria are meant to stave off the realization of this dystopia, the disappearance of human milk from the ordinary relation of mothers and babies.

Notes

CHAPTER 1

1. AIDS stands for Acquired Immune Deficiency Syndrome. It is the name used for the constellation of illnesses that are caused by HIV. HIV disease is the medical name for the illness caused by infection by the human immunodeficiency virus, but usually HIV/AIDS is the combined acronym used to convey the disease and its syndromic consequences.

2. Kukla, *Mass Hysteria,* 53. See the entire second chapter, "Imbibing the Love of the Fatherland," 29–63.

3. Williams, "Milk and Murder." This speech was delivered to the Singapore Rotary Club. Cicely Williams, born in Jamaica and educated in England, was one of the first female doctors to graduate from Oxford. In 1948, she became the first director of the World Health Organization's Maternal and Child Health Services.

4. See de Wagt and Clark, "UNICEF's Support to Free Infant Formula for Infants of HIV-Infected Mothers in Africa," 9–10, for a discussion of spillover and concerns about the provision of infant formulas broadly to populations of mothers with high seroprevalence.

5. See Iliffe, *The African AIDS Epidemic,* for an extended synthetic account of these points.

6. Martin, *Flexible Bodies,* xv.

7. Booth, *The Rhetoric of Rhetoric,* 8.

8. This is a point of contention within cultural studies. Some Marxist perspectives hold to the traditional view that identifying ideologies is a method of demystification that can lead to a clear grasp of true conditions. Most contemporary cultural studies approaches trade one form of ideological constraint for another. My view is closer to the latter position.

9. Brad Lewis writes about the "global convergence of health delivery" in "The New Global Health Movement," 471–73.

10. Jaggar, "Is Globalization Good for Women?" 301 n1.

11. Escobar, *Encountering Development,* 163.

12. Jaggar, "Is Globalization Good for Women?" 299.

13. Lewis, "The New Global Health Movement," 473.

14. Ivan Illich wrote, in this regard, "The destructive power of medical overexpansion does not, of course, mean that sanitation, inoculation, and vector control, well-distributed health education, healthy architecture, and safe machinery, general competence in first aid, equally distributed access to dental and primary medical care, as well as judiciously selected complex services, could not all fit into a truly modern culture that fostered self-care and autonomy.... beyond a certain level, [however,] the heteronomous management of life will inevitably first restrict, then cripple, and finally paralyze the organism's nontrivial responses, and what was meant to constitute health care will turn into a specific form of health denial" (*Medical Nemesis*, 220).

15. "Representations of the world are always partial and inaccurate, because linguistic structure forces us to make distinctions in order to create and register meaning. How distinctions get made depends in large part on the motivations and desires of the producers. In medicine, the most obvious example is the distinction between 'normal' and 'pathological' " (Lewis, "High Theory/Mass Markets," 366).

16. Ibid., 370.

CHAPTER 2

1. See "MTCT," later in this volume, for a longer, although not comprehensive, discussion of the Nestlé boycott.

2. Breastfeeding is also thought to protect mothers. Mothers who breastfeed are less likely to become pregnant with another child during the first baby's infancy. Child spacing protects infants by ensuring their nourishment (breast milk), and it protects maternal health by not overburdening mothers with many babies close together.

3. Spelling of *breast milk* differs in international documents, even in different versions of the same document. I use the following title, International Code of Marketing of Breastmilk Substitutes, because it is the spelling used in my source, *The Breastfeeding Movement: A Sourcebook,* compiled by Lakshmi Menon for World Alliance for Breastfeeding Action. In other uses of the term *breast milk,* I separate the two words following the usage of the American Academy of Pediatrics.

4. Stehlin, "Infant Formula."

5. Lawrence, "Major Difficulties." In the United States, over 70 percent of women begin nursing in the period right after birth but just over 40 percent of all mothers are still offering any breast milk at six months and around 20 percent are still nursing at one year, the medically recommended minimum length of breastfeeding duration. "In addition, rates of exclusive breastfeeding are low" (DHHS, "New Breastfeeding Rates Published"; see also Li et al., "Breastfeeding Rates," e31).

6. Scheper-Hughes, *Death without Weeping.*

7. Wolf, "Low Breastfeeding Rates," 2000–2004.

8. Coutsoudis et al., "Influence of Infant-Feeding Patterns."

9. For issues of permeability with respect to the immune system, see *Flexible Bodies* by Emily Martin. See also Martin, "The Pharmaceutical Person," for a discussion of personhood and subjectivity in relation to pharmaceuticals.

10. Prior to this discovery, physicians had subscribed to a variety of theories concerning the causes of tuberculosis, including constitutional proclivity, direct heredity, and environment (as well as a few arguing for contagion). See Feldberg, *Disease and Class*, and Dubos and Dubos, *The White Plague*. Koch determined that the tubercular lesions of consumptives all contained bacilli.

11. Rothman, *Living in the Shadow*, 180.

12. In a book originally published in 1915, Ellen N. La Motte writes, "It is not necessary to insist on milk and eggs, certainly not in the abnormal quantities which a few years ago were considered indispensable to the treatment of tuberculosis" (*The Tuberculosis Nurse*, 148). On the following page, she indicates that three to four glasses of milk per day were sufficient (149).

13. Ott, *Fevered Lives*, 112.

14. A wide range of historical forces, including the agency of mothers themselves, made replacement feeding the dominant trend in the United States in the twentieth century (see Wolf, *Don't Kill Your Baby*). Breast milk was always understood by physicians and public health workers to be best for babies. Yet once breast milk substitutes existed and were easily available, either as proprietary formulas or modifications to cow's milk that mothers themselves would put up after having learned how from visiting or clinic nurses, a nurse's job was almost always to accommodate their use and teach women how to engage them safely. As replacement feeding became more common in the first half of the twentieth century, there were new challenges concerning food supplementation and proper nutrition for visiting nurses. These took time to learn and communicate. Thus, while the benefits of breastfeeding were known all along (and consistently articulated), practical advice on breastfeeding was lost, not communicated, or just not emphasized by health professionals and social workers, who more and more needed to address the actual needs of mothers practicing replacement feeding.

15. If the baby has been exposed, then the mother and baby should be treated together.

16. Contemporary advice with respect to tuberculosis and maternity continues to warn against breastfeeding if the mother has active, untreated TB. While separation of mother and baby is based on the difficulty of keeping the baby safe from droplet infection by the mother, the representation of information about tuberculosis and breastfeeding in some contexts encourages the reader to believe that there is TB itself in the breast milk and that its presence is infectious. For example, the American Academy of Pediatrics offers the following information on its "Special Challenges to Breastfeeding" Web page: "There are a few infectious diseases that mothers have that can be transmitted through human milk to the baby, including HIV and untreated tuberculosis." They follow this with the comment that "mothers with tuberculosis should not breastfeed until appropriate treatment has been started" (American Academy of Pediatrics, "Special Challenges," pars. 4, 5). One parents' Web site, "Breastfeeding, HIV, and Disease Transmission," quotes the AAP's 1997 policy statement on breastfeeding, which includes active TB in a list of conditions in the mother that contraindicate breastfeeding (along with galactosemia, illegal drug use, and HIV infec-

tion [in the United States]) and then states, "This suggests to me that there's evidence of transmission of tuberculosis via breastmilk" (Gunderloy, "Breastfeeding, HIV, and Disease Transmission"). Indeed, the National Institute of Child Health and Human Development's Web page on breastfeeding states, "A woman with certain health conditions, such as HIV or active tuberculosis, should not breastfeed *because she risks giving the infection to her infant through her breast milk*" (National Institutes of Health, National Institute of Child Health and Human Development, *Breastfeeding*; emphasis added). Yet Lawrence and Lawrence, who provide the most comprehensive medical discussion of breastfeeding and tuberculosis, are very clear: "In the absence of tuberculous breast infection in the mother [which is rare in the United States], transmission of TB through breast milk has not been documented" (Lawrence and Lawrence, *A Guide*, 640).

Lawrence and Lawrence add, "The real risk to the infant requiring separation is from airborne transmission. Separation of the infant from a mother with active pulmonary TB is appropriate, regardless of the method of infant feeding" (ibid.). Yet most of the readily available information on breastfeeding in the context of maternal tuberculosis infection simply suggests that an active TB diagnosis contraindicates breastfeeding without discussing reasons why this is the case. Since all other contraindications to breastfeeding concern what could be in the milk to harm the baby, TB can be, and clearly is, interpreted similarly.

17. See Verghese et al., "Urbs in Rure," for a discussion of the importance of trucking routes for the spread of HIV into the rural United States. Both Iliffe, *The African AIDS Epidemic,* and Helen Epstein, *The Invisible Cure,* discuss migrant workers, migration, and trucking as routes for infection in Africa.

18. See UNAIDS, "A Global Overview of the AIDS Epidemic," for a sense of how women are figured in international reports on the epidemic. Ironically, despite feminist claims about the invisibility of women *as women* (i.e., not as mothers) in HIV/AIDS research, at the 2006 International AIDS Conference in Toronto, Canada, breastfeeding advocates and others commented upon the virtual absence of mothers and MTCT in the program. While pediatric AIDS gained some significant attention, there seemed to be little interest in breastfeeding or infant feeding issues. Some plenary addresses that specifically mentioned pediatric HIV infections did not discuss transmission through breastfeeding or the issues attendant to it at all.

19. UNAIDS, *2008 Report on the Global HIV/AIDS Epidemic: Executive Summary,* 7; UNAIDS, *2006 Report on the Global AIDS Epidemic: Executive Summary,* 6; UNAIDS, *2006 Global Facts and Figures;* U.S. Congress Committee on Oversight and Government Reform, *HIV/AIDS TODAY Factsheets.*

20. Helen Epstein, in *The Invisible Cure,* discusses reasons why developing an AIDS vaccine is so difficult. See 15–20, 27–38.

21. Duden, *Disembodying Women.*

22. See Van Esterik, "Towards Healthy Environments for Children."

23. I discuss this term in the next chapter. It is originally from Derrida, but I found it through Emily Martin, "The Pharmaceutical Person."

CHAPTER 3

1. For example, the following claim by Anthony Giddens: "The modes of life brought into being by modernity have swept us away from *all* traditional types of social order, in quite unprecedented fashion. In both their extensionality and their intensionality the transformations involved in modernity are more profound than most sorts of change characteristic of prior periods" (*The Consequences of Modernity*, 4). Authors always hedge this claim, but one of the significant and common characteristics of theories of modernity is the idea of a break with past, or traditional, patterns.

2. This is an extension of the "primordialist thesis." See Arjun Appadurai, *Modernity at Large*, 139–40.

3. See Hausman, *Mother's Milk*, 140–50.

4. At the start of *The Consequences of Modernity*, Anthony Giddens tersely characterizes modernity: "'modernity' refers to social life or organization which emerged in Europe from about the seventeenth century onwards and which subsequently became more or less worldwide in their influence" (1). Giddens is a sociologist, so his emphasis on "social life or organization" is in keeping with his discipline; political scientists tend to look at emerging political organizations and structures. Typically, philosophers identify Kant as the epistemic break between the Enlightenment and modernity. Herbert Dreyfus and Paul Rabinow write, "Modernity is not a specific historical event, but a historical conjuncture which has happened several times in our history, albeit with different form and content: for example, the breakdown of the traditional virtues in Athens at the time of Socrates and Aristophanes, the decline of the Hellenistic world, *the end of metaphysics at the time of Kant*" ("What Is Maturity?" 117; emphasis added).

Other periodizations are more common to literary and cultural analysis, although some historians also find them useful. Modernity can be identified with modernism, an artistic and cultural movement of the late nineteenth and early twentieth centuries in Europe and America. T. J. Jackson Lears identifies rationalization as a key force and conceptual register for the "second industrial revolution" of the 1880s. He writes, "The rationalization of economic life—the drive for maximum profits through the adoption of the most efficient forms of organization—was moving into high gear, especially in the United States.... In matters of organization technical 'rationality' was becoming the dominant mode" (*No Place of Grace*, 10). He continues, "The process of rationalization did more than transform the structure of economic life; it also affected the structure of thought and feeling, of culture in the broadest sense" (ibid.). Thus Lears's interpretation of modernity, and his primary focus on antimodernism in the late Victorian and Edwardian periods, identify an element understood to be central to modernity in a number of other treatments—rationality in the service of capitalism and accumulation.

Modernity often is linked to modernization, "the struggle for democracy, the development of industry, the extension of communications, and the deep social and personal changes" accompanying these phenomena (Williams, *The Long Revolution*,

12). German sociologist Ulrich Beck identifies cultural ramifications of the technological and structural changes of modernization identified with industrialization: "*Modernization* means surges of technological rationalization and changes in work and organization, but beyond that it includes much more: the change in societal characteristics and normal biographies, changes of lifestyle and forms of love, change in the structures of power and influence, in the forms of political repression and participation, in views of reality and in norms of knowledge. In social science's understanding of modernity, the plough, the steam locomotive and the microchip are visible indicators of a much deeper process, which comprises and reshapes the entire social structure. Ultimately, the *sources of certainty* on which life feeds are changed" (*Risk Society*, 50 n1; emphases in original).

The connection of modernity with modernization is not incompatible with identifying modernity with the Enlightenment, but tends to focus attention on technological developments and industrialization. In the post–World War II period, modernization was theorized in international development circles and enacted through aid to colonized and formerly colonized countries. In modernization theory, the model of development is the United States, as well as the countries of western Europe. Modernity is what follows on the project of economic modernization and is, definitively, a pattern established by the "West."

5. Williams, *The Long Revolution*, 63. Williams compares "structure of feeling" to other concepts like "social character" (from Fromm) and "pattern of culture" (from Benedict), the former of which is "both an ideal and a mode" and the latter a "way of life" that is nevertheless an abstraction; neither alternative is quite right in his view (63–64).

6. Taylor, *Modern Social Imaginaries*, 25, 2. See also pertinent passages on pages 12, 17, 23, 45–46, 75.

7. Ibid., 45.

8. Giddens, *The Consequences of Modernity*, 21, 26.

9. "The reliance placed by lay actors upon expert systems is not just a matter—as was normally the case in the pre-modern world—of generating a sense of security about an independently given universe of events. It is a matter of the calculation of benefit and risk in circumstances where expert knowledge does not just provide that calculus but actually creates (or reproduces) the universe of events, as a result of the continual reflexive implementation of that very knowledge" (Giddens, *The Consequences of Modernity*, 84).

10. Giddens does not periodize modernity but seems to locate it most forcefully in the development of the social sciences, which would place it in the nineteenth century (see *The Consequences of Modernity*, 36–45). He argues against the idea that current reflexive tendencies signal the advent of postmodernity, arguing instead that we live in conditions of radicalized modernity (51). As a result, "living in the modern world is more like being aboard a careering juggernaut . . . rather than being in a carefully controlled and well-driven motor car" (53). Beck argues similarly: "Reflexive modernization means not less but more modernity, a modernity radicalized *against* the paths and categories of the classical industrial setting. We are experiencing a transformation of the foundations of change" (*Risk Society*, 14; emphasis in original).

11. Beck, *Risk Society,* 104 (emphasis in original).

12. Giddens writes, "The chronic entry of knowledge into the circumstances of the action it analyses or describes creates a set of uncertainties to add to the circular and fallible character of post-traditional claims to knowledge" (*Modernity and Self-Identity,* 28).

13. Beck, *Risk Society,* 23, 97. Beck points out that individualization has particularly deleterious effects on women, given that the institutional structure of the family remains constant while women's roles have undergone a radical transformation (109, 111). See also Beck-Gernsheim, "Life as a Planning Project."

14. For a good, short introduction to governmentality, see Inda, "Analytics of the Modern: An Introduction." There is some disagreement among Foucault scholars concerning terminology. Ellen Feder, in *Family Bonds,* uses biopower instead of biopolitics and does not consider biopower the overarching category including discipline, instead distinguishing the two. Her discussion is very useful in understanding how gender and race might be profitably examined using the concepts of discipline and biopower as she articulates them. However, it seems very important to have a general term, like biopower, within which a focus on the subject (discipline) and one on populations (biopolitics) can be disaggregated and understood. This is why Inda's discussion is so helpful.

15. Turner, *Regulating Bodies,* 9.

16. Peter Conrad's *The Medicalization of Society* is a good example of this approach.

17. Foucault, "The Politics of Health" (176), identifies the eighteenth century as the start of a new kind of politics of the body, in which "the state of health of a population as a general objective of policy" emerged (168; see also 169–70). Partly resulting from "the great eighteenth-century demographic upswing in Western Europe," "'population,' with its numerical variables of space and chronology, longevity and health, [emerged] not only as a problem but as an object of surveillance, analysis, intervention, modification etc" (ibid., 171). The family is the initial and ongoing locus of "the medicalisation of individuals," with children and babies receiving significant attention (ibid., 175, 174). Hygiene becomes a focus within what Foucault calls "the regime of health" and allows for "a certain number of authoritarian medical interventions and controls" (ibid., 175). Ian Hacking points out that the focus on population norms was made possible by the development of statistics in the nineteenth century, which involved a transformation of descriptive statistical regularities into probabilistic renderings of normative laws (*The Taming of Chance*).

18. See also the entire introduction, 1–25. Hoy, *Foucault: A Critical Reader.*

19. See Kelly, *Critique and Power,* for a discussion of this issue with respect to Foucault and Habermas.

20. That is, they are perceived to be unable to become modern as a result of their clinging to local traditions or their inability to commit to the cultural changes necessary to achieve modernity's goals. Charles Briggs writes, with regard to cholera epidemics in Venezuela in the 1990s, "Premodern subjects are deemed incapable of taking advantage of modern initiatives or even actively resisting them; by failing to embrace modernity when the stakes are so high, they purportedly prove that they will

never become part of the modern world, at least not anytime soon" ("Modernity, Cultural Reasoning, and the Institutionalization of Social Inequality," 684).

21. See Gikandi, "Reason, Modernity, and the African Crisis," 162.

22. Knöbl, "Modernization Theory," 162.

23. And, indeed, it is within modern social systems that science (including biomedicine) gains authority as a value-neutral, objective endeavor, which allows it to be seen as a universal good across cultural systems. (Thanks to Heather Switzer for this thought.) See Gikandi, "Reason, Modernity, and the African Crisis," 143.

24. Zack-Williams, "Africa and the Project of Modernity," 34. Paul Farmer discusses perceptions of "cultural pathologies" with respect to epidemic disease in *Infections and Inequalities: The Modern Plagues.*

Zack-Williams also writes, "The task of constructing the other (African) belongs to Euro-American essentialists, who through the modernization paradigm, invented African culture by rendering a caricatured image of African value structures as traditional and dysfunctional to economic development and social change" (ibid., 21). In addition, "One important feature of discussions on modernity is the conspicuous absence of any serious reference to Africa, or how this product of the Enlightenment has shaped the African continent. The only exception to this rule is on discourse of the African Diaspora. This dearth of analysis on Africa and modernity is partly a product of the assumption that as a construct of the Enlightenment, modernity is a European project, *sui generis,* and as such Africa was and remains outside of its confines" (ibid., 20; emphasis in original).

See the end of Charles Taylor's *Modern Social Imaginaries* (196) for a brief discussion of multiple modernitites. In winter 2000, the journal *Daedalus* published a special issue on "Multiple Modernities," attempting to "challenge many of the conventional notions of how the world has changed over time, in this century predominantly, but in earlier periods as well" (Graubard, "Preface," v). The issue provides both overarching accounts of modernity theory and the arguments for multiple modernities, as well as articles focusing on specific modernities (communist, Islamic, etc.).

25. Zack-Williams, "Africa and the Project of Modernity," 34–35. See also Gikandi, "Reason, Modernity, and the African Crisis."

26. Taylor, *Modern Social Imaginaries,* 122–23, 69.

27. On this count, Rita Felski is anomalous; see *Doing Time,* 61–62.

28. Wittrock, "Modernity," 49, 55. See also the discussion on 55–56.

29. Zack-Williams and Uduku, "African Diaspora–African Development Concerns," 12–16.

30. Much of the devastation of modernity is environmental. See Bradley Lewis's discussion of this issue in "The New Global Health Movement," 466–67. See ibid., 462–73, for a discussion of the side effects of globalizing biomedicine. For Ulrich Beck, side effects are risks produced by modern systems, institutions, and technologies, the negative productions of modernity (*Risk Society,* 19). See also Zack-Williams and Uduku, "African Diaspora–African Development Concerns," 4–6.

31. Briggs, "Communicability," 284, 279; Illich, *Medical Nemesis,* 206.

32. Lewis, "The New Global Health Movement," 461.

33. Ibid., 463. Lewis suggests that medicine in the global north has, in fact, created numerous health problems that it now threatens to export to the global south: "social inequality and health disparity, social isolation and depression, consumer addiction and alienation, environmental degradation, global warming, and the increased risk factors of high fat/high sodium diets, obesity, smoking, and decreased exercise, to name a few" (ibid., 473–74). See Starfield, "Is U.S. Health Really the Best in the World?" for a discussion of iatrogenesis as a leading cause of death in the United States.

34. Ulrich Beck writes, "In this way the medical view of things *objectivizes* itself and expands ever more deeply and broadly into all aspects of life and areas of human existence" (*Risk Society*, 211; emphasis in original). Bradley Lewis writes, "The explosion in biotechnology will require consumers to support it, and medical industries, particularly the pharmaceuticals, are not content to simply let customers come to them. They actively promote a desire for their products using the latest public relations technologies" ("The New Global Health Movement," 471).

Public health practices, even ones like vaccination that are heralded as life-saving by the majority of the world's people, constitute significant medical interventions and, through the routinization of injection, may have contributed to the spread of certain blood-borne diseases like HIV/AIDS. John Illife makes this connection in *The African AIDS Epidemic*, where he writes, citing theories by Preston Marx and others, that "SIV [simian immunodeficiency virus] had been converted into HIV by a rapid passaging through African Populations during the 1950s, owing to the introduction of supposedly disposable (but often in practice re-used) syringes to inject penicillin and other new medications. Between 1952 and 1960 annual world output of syringes increased from 8 million to something approaching 1000 million" (7). This is not the theory that HIV was caused by the polio immunization campaign in the Congo region (1957–60), which allegedly used a vaccine bred on SIV-infected chimpanzee kidneys, but one which argues that the widespread use of syringes and injectable medicine introduced new interventionist medical practices precisely at a time when they could become vectors for an emerging infection. Helen Epstein, in *The Invisible Cure*, agrees, noting that reusing syringes, a common practice in Africa and the global south, can actually produce more virulent mutations of blood-borne viral illnesses (45–47).

In another section of *The African AIDS Epidemic*, Iliffe comments that other medical advances contributed to the spread of HIV/AIDS: "The leading historian of HIV/AIDS, Mirko Grimek, suggested that the epidemic was, paradoxically, in part a consequence of medical advance: that until medicine had reduced the prevalence of other infectious diseases such as tuberculosis and smallpox, death rates were too high to allow HIV to establish itself in numbers of people to reach epidemic proportions. There is no obvious way to test this intriguing suggestion, which perhaps exaggerates the extent of medical advance in sub-Saharan Africa. . . . Nevertheless it is both true and disturbing that the epidemic followed immediately on the period of greatest medical improvement in the continent's history" (61).

35. Briggs, "Modernity, Cultural Reasoning, and the Institutionalization of Social Inequality," 681; Lewis, "The New Global Health Movement," 473–74; Illich, *Medical Nemesis,* 220.

36. Lewis, "The New Global Health Movement," 470–72.

37. Briggs, "Modernity, Cultural Reasoning, and the Institutionalization of Social Inequality," 681. See Iliffe, *The African AIDS Epidemic,* 59, 61.

38. Iliffe, *The African AIDS Epidemic,* 64; Briggs, "Modernity, Cultural Reasoning, and the Institutionalization of Social Inequality," 685.

39. Briggs, "Communicability, Racial Discourse, and Disease," 275. See Farmer, *Infections and Inequalities,* for a discussion of structural violence, inequality, and epidemic infectious disease among the poor.

40. See Treichler, *How to Have Theory in an Epidemic,* 99–126, and Cindy Patton, *Inventing AIDS,* 77–97, for ideological constructions of Africa. I borrow "outbreak narrative" from Priscilla Wald's book *Contagious,* where she discusses how accounts of emerging infections portray their primitive sites of emergence (44).

CHAPTER 4

1. For example, Powell and Leiss, *Mad Cows and Mother's Milk.*

2. For example, Skolbekken, "The Risk Epidemic in Medical Journals."

3. Douglas and Wildavsky, *Risk and Culture,* 8.

4. Ibid., 10.

5. Ibid., 161. In addition, they write, "the vast increase in education and growth of service industries, both of which made hierarchy less essential after the Second World War, broadened the base of support for sectarian appeals. The civil rights movement and the revolt against the Vietnam War provided models for imitation. And in the short run, the availability of sectarian political entrepreneurs and the existence of effective technology to mobilize a mail-order membership facilitated the success of public interest groups. That is why America has become a border country," meaning that its politics are motivated by sectarian organizations and values (ibid., 173). My analysis in *Viral Mothers* does not depend on Douglas and Wildavsky's version of sectarianism, which is nevertheless crucial to their particular interpretation of American fears of environmental contamination in the 1970s. But in linking these fears to changes in core institutions of American culture, they are demonstrating a significant aspect of their argument—connections between risk perceptions and the institutional structures sustaining culture.

6. After 2001, terrorism has also been a significant focus of risk discourses.

7. Burger, "Health as a Surrogate," 133–34.

8. Helzlsouer and Gordis, "Risks to Health," 194.

9. Alcabes, "Epidemiologists Need to Shatter," B12, B11.

10. Skolbekken, "The Risk Epidemic in Medical Journals," 298.

11. Lupton, *Risk.*

12. Gary Downey has revised Douglas and Wildavsky's ideas in the following way: "Cultural identities of individuals and groups [are] constituted by relationships es-

tablished in a combination of ideological and institutionalized meaning systems" (Downey, "Risk in Culture," 409 n1).

13. Douglas and Wildavsky, *Risk and Culture*, 8.

14. Lupton, *Risk*, 86, 87, 91.

15. See Douglas and Wildavsky, *Risk and Culture*, 80, and Douglas, *Risk and Blame*, 4.

16. Douglas and Wildavsky, *Risk and Culture*, 73.

17. Lupton writes, concerning Anthony Giddens's ideas about risk society, "Risk society is thus characterized by the contradiction that the privileged have greater access to knowledge, but not enough, so that they become anxious without being able to reconcile or act upon their anxiety" (*Risk*, 69).

18. This is not to say that women are equal in the labor market or that men help out more at home. Some feminists do articulate these reasons for feeding with infant formula, although in coded terms. When feminist activists like Ellen Galinsky of the Work and Family Institute talk about maternal guilt, they are really talking about the terms of women's participation in waged labor in the United States. But the actual discussion concerning the general social acceptance of the risk of formula feeding as a consequence of modernity simply does not occur. Instead, there is equivocation concerning the scientific evidence about those risks. This situation indicates the social ambivalence about the consequences of modernity, thus demonstrating the main tenets of risk society theorists.

19. Gary Downey addresses the issue of knowledge claims based in science in "Risk in Culture," especially 391–92.

20. Douglas and Wildavsky, *Risk and Culture*, 72, 7.

21. Gary Downey's main critique of *Risk and Culture* is that Douglas and Wildavsky did not treat science itself as a cosmological system as they did other belief systems. My own presentation of the value of *Risk and Culture* to the study of American perceptions of breastfeeding risks depends upon his insight.

22. Beck, *Risk Society*, 25. See also 27.

23. Ibid., 55; emphasis in original. See also 53.

24. See ibid., 72.

25. Ibid., 58, 59, 58; emphasis in original.

CHAPTER 5

1. "Infant Likely Got West Nile in Breast Milk."

2. "CDC: Mom's Milk Gave Baby West Nile."

3. "West Nile Virus (WNV) Infection and Breastfeeding: Information for Clinicians," Division of Vector-Borne Infections Diseases. See also "Possible West Nile Virus Transmission to an Infant through Breast-Feeding—Michigan 2002." For other newspaper articles on the same day, see "West Nile-Tainted Breast Milk Likely Infected Baby, CDC Says," "West Nile's Spread to Baby Is Linked to Breast Feeding," and "Newborn Has West Nile Virus."

4. The 2002 National Immunization Survey indicated that just over 71 percent of

new mothers breastfed their babies, with approximately 35 percent still breastfeeding (at least some of the time) at six months (Li et al., "Breastfeeding Rates").

5. Bartlett, "West Nile Virus."

6. Ibid.

7. Ibid. The CDC notes, "About one in 150 people infected with WNV will develop severe illness" (Centers for Disease Control, "WNV Fact Sheet"). Lawrence and Lawrence note, "It is estimated that 150 to 300 asymptomatic cases of West Nile infection occur for every 20 febrile illnesses and for every one case of meningoencephalitis associated with West Nile virus. . . . The case-fatality rate for 2003 in the United States was approximately 2.5, but has been reported as high as 4% to 18% in hospitalized patients. The case-fatality rate for persons over 70 years of age is considered to be higher, 15% to 29% among hospitalized patients in outbreaks in Romania and Israel" (*Breastfeeding*, 678).

8. In June 2008 I was told by a park ranger at the Oregon Caves National Monument that areas of California had sprayed mosquitoes with pesticides that ended up killing local bat populations. Some species of bat can eat 600 mosquitoes per hour, suggesting that promoting bat health is a better aid to eradicating or at least controlling WNV than using pesticides that kill mosquitoes. See McAvoy, "Bats Eat Mosquitoes as Well as Numerous Garden Pests."

9. This may be a function of health news in general. Stephen Klaidman writes, "Journalists' predisposition for controversy leads to the polarization of issues" ("How Well the Media Report Health Risk," 124). One letter to the *Boston Globe* in early September 2002 did complain about unnecessarily assiduous reporting on West Nile virus, stating, "The appearance of this virus in the United States does not constitute a public health emergency or even a matter of much importance" (Laws).

10. Ruth Lawrence writes, "A high degree of antiviral activity against Japanese B encephalitis virus [part of the family that includes WNV] has been found in human milk" (*Breastfeeding*, 171). Lawrence and Lawrence write, "Nonspecific substances in human milk are active against arbovirus and murine leukemia virus" (*Breastfeeding*, 201–3). WNV is an arbovirus.

11. The "natural" way to get West Nile virus is from a bite by an infected mosquito. Mothers who are bitten by mosquitoes are often in the same place as their nursing infants. The longer version of the article on the CNN Web site states, "West Nile is rare in infants because they spend little time outdoors and the virus is usually spread by mosquito bites," providing the following evidence: "Only four children younger than 12 months have been diagnosed with West Nile since it appeared in the United States in 1999" ("CDC: Mom's Milk Gave Baby West Nile"). Other sources note the oddity of few infections in children (see Bartlett, "West Nile Virus"; Lawrence and Lawrence, *Breastfeeding*, 678).

12. A series of articles published on September 28, 2002, do a better job discussing questions concerning transmissibility of viruses through breast milk, although even these do an inadequate job of distinguishing between blood-borne and droplet infections and the action of breastfeeding immunity. See Grady, "Traces of West Nile Virus Found in Mother's Breast Milk"; Brown, "West Nile Virus Is Discovered in Breast Milk of Michigan Woman"; and Maugh, "Evidence of West Nile Virus Found in Breast Milk."

13. See Weiss, "Organ Recipients Had Virus"; Altman, "Transplants Seem Source"; Brown, "4th Organ Recipient"; Grady, "Doctors Confirm West Nile"; and Brown, "Virus's Link to Transfusions Intensifies."

14. A subsequent article identified a possible WNV infection in a newborn, indicating that the infection occurred during gestation. The article's conclusions are speculative, however. See Weiss, "Baby Had West Nile Virus."

15. Grady, "For Two Transplant Patients, a Dire Complication." The original CNN.com article on October 4, 2002, states the following: "The government discovered last month that the virus apparently can be spread through blood transfusions, as well as organ transplants. The CDC reported 15 people this year have been diagnosed with West Nile virus within a month after receiving blood transfusions" ("CDC: Mom's Milk Gave Baby West Nile"). See also "Public Health Dispatch: West Nile Virus Infection in Organ Donor and Transplant Recipients"; "Public Health Dispatch: Investigation of Blood Transfusion Recipients with West Nile Virus Infections"; and "Update: Investigations of West Nile Virus Infections in Recipients of Organ Transplantation and Blood Transfusion."

A *New England Journal of Medicine* article published in 2004 indicates that "the risk of neuroinvasive disease increases with age *and appears to be substantially higher among organ-transplant recipients than in the general population*" (Petersen and Hayes, "Westward Ho?" 2258; emphasis added). Petersen and Hayes also state, "Nearly all infections result from mosquito bites; however, transmission through transplanted organs and transfused blood, transplacental transmission, and occupational transmission by means of percutaneous exposure have occurred, and there has probably been transmission through breast milk" (2258–59).

16. Petersen and Hayes write, "Herd immunity in humans will have minimal effect on the incidence of disease, because even in areas of the United States that have had epidemics of West Nile virus, studies have shown that less than 5 percent of the population has been exposed to the virus and developed protective antibody" (2259). This leads them to believe that "the risk of West Nile virus disease is likely to vary considerably over time and place" (ibid.). All of which is to say that while "the risk of neuroinvasive disease due to West Nile virus is relatively low" (ibid.), the illness will usually seem new in any given area, a situation that lends itself to overestimation of risk because the disease is unfamiliar. West Nile virus thus constitutes an "epidemic" with high variability and unpredictability.

17. Wight, "Breastfeeding in High Risk Populations," 1.

18. "Possible West Nile Virus Transmission to an Infant through Breast-Feeding—Michigan, 2002."

19. Wight, "Breastfeeding in High Risk Populations," 4.

20. Maugh, "Evidence of West Nile Virus Found in Breast Milk." It is possible the mother was advised to stop breastfeeding for the sake of her own health. Yet any reader would see that breastfeeding women are advised to speak with their doctors about West Nile fears, but that the one woman in the news who did have the illness was herself advised to stop breastfeeding.

21. Centers for Disease Control, "Breastfeeding: Infectious Diseases and Specific Conditions Affecting Human Milk: West Nile Virus."

22. Lynn Payer, *Medicine and Culture,* 143–46.

23. Douglas and Wildavsky, *Risk and Culture,* 120.

24. Ibid., 80, 84.

25. Hausman, *Mother's Milk,* 222.

26. Davis-Floyd, "The Technocratic Body," 1137. The preceding discussion in this paragraph appears in Hausman, "Risky Business," 34–35.

CHAPTER 6

1. The Ad Council oversees public service campaigns like the National Breast-feeding Awareness Campaign. The actual ads and public service announcements (PSAs) were produced by a North Carolina advertising agency, McKinney+Silver. The Office of Women's Health, which is part of the Department of Health and Human Services, was the governmental agency involved in the project, and it worked intimately with the United States Breastfeeding Committee, "an umbrella consortia of health care organizations interested in breastfeeding" (Granju, "The Milky Way").

2. Breastfeeding advocates were tiring of emphasizing the health benefits of breastfeeding, as if breastfeeding were something extra or special to offer a child, rather than an ordinary maternal behavior. The tagline of the Ad Council campaign, "Babies were born to be breastfed," represents an attempt to make breastfeeding seem the normal mode of infant feeding, not the optimal. In the view of the NBAC's designers, too many mothers perceive the optimal as beyond their reach, and formula feeding as the "good enough" normal method. Jacqueline Wolf quotes lactation specialist Diane Wiessinger: "Our own experience tells us that optimal is not necessary. Normal is fine, and implied in this language is the absolute normalcy—and thus safety and adequacy—of artificial feeding" (Wolf, "What Feminists Can Do for Breastfeeding," 411).

3. For accounts of the controversy and reasons for the delay in the campaign launch, see Jacqueline Wolf, "What Feminists Can Do for Breastfeeding"; Petersen, "Breastfeeding Ads Delayed"; and Granju, "The Milky Way." For conflicting feminist interpretations of the campaign itself, see Kukla, "Ethics and Ideology in Breastfeeding Advocacy Campaigns"; Hausman, "Things (Not) to Do with Breasts in Public"; Joan Wolf, "Is Breast Really Best?"; and Jacqueline Wolf, "What Feminists Can Do for Breast-feeding." For specific information about the changes in the campaign when it was finally launched, see Jacqueline Wolf, "What Feminists Can Do for Breastfeeding," 413.

4. National Center for Health Statistics, *Healthy People 2000,* 206.

5. Quoted in Granju, "The Milky Way." Joan Wolf also charges that scientists supporting breastfeeding are not objective.

6. Quoted in Peterson, "Breastfeeding Ads Delayed."

7. See Susan Sontag on guilt's relation to illness (*Illness as Metaphor/AIDS and Its Metaphors,* 21–22). In Sontag's schema guilt is related to the causal mystery of certain illnesses; inculcating guilt in individuals who can be thought to cause illness in themselves or others is possible when the scientific evidence about material causality is equivocal.

8. Granju, "The Milky Way."

9. Jacqueline Wolf, "What Feminists Can Do for Breastfeeding," 409, 414, 401, 403.

10. Kukla, "Ethics and Ideology," 174; see also 160.

11. Ibid., 176.

12. Joan Wolf, "Is Breast Really Best?" 607, 608, 596.

13. Hausman, *Mother's Milk*, 195.

14. Since 2005 there has been an active group of feminist academics, breastfeeding activists, lactation consultants, and other practitioners who have met yearly in North Carolina for a series of breastfeeding symposia. I am a member of that group, which demonstrates that the seemingly louder feminist critique of breastfeeding promotion is not the only feminist voice in the debate. See Smith et al., *Breastfeeding and Feminism*, forthcoming.

15. Joan Wolf, "Rejoinder to Judy M. Hopkinson," 651.

16. Kim Gandy, president of the National Organization for Women, commented in an open letter to the secretary of Health and Human Services Mike Leavitt, "Equating a woman's decision not to breastfeed with log-rolling or mechanical bull riding while pregnant insults the millions of women who are physically unable to breastfeed, are advised not to breastfeed due to illness medical treatment [*sic*], or are unable to breastfeed for six months because of inadequate workplace accommodations."

Karen Zivi uses the term *maternal ideology* to refer to this kind of persuasive discourse. She defines maternal ideology as "the distinction of 'good' mothers from 'bad,' a distinction that encourages and rewards certain behaviors while condemning, limiting, and even criminalizing others. Maternal ideology is, in other words, used to judge women, to determine if they are engaging in acceptable mothering practices, and to decide whether the regulation of their lives and the circumscription of their rights is warranted" ("Contesting Motherhood," 349).

17. Joan Wolf, "Is Breast Really Best?" 615.

18. See ibid., 623, for an apt summation of the reasons why the NBAC was wrong in its approach.

19. Jacqueline Wolf, "What Feminists Can Do for Breastfeeding," 401.

20. Heinig writes, "All risk-based campaigns must be tempered by follow-up care from providers who are respectful of each woman's circumstances and decisions" ("The Burden of Proof," 376). Hopkinson notes that she "was, however, not entirely comfortable with the use of a fear-based campaign for two reasons. First, breast-feeding is undermined by internalized stress. . . . Second, the campaign placed the burden of change on individual women rather than on the medical and cultural practices and societal structures that undermine their breast-feeding intentions and success" ("Response to 'Is Breast Really Best?'" 645). But she adds that when "compelling evidence of efficacy was stripped from the breast-feeding campaign by removing the quantification statements regarding the degree of risk attributable to not breast-feeding," the NBAC became a fear-based campaign without important evidentiary support, thus generating "anger and resistance" that are detrimental to the uptake of beneficial health-related behaviors (646).

21. Joan Wolf, "Is Breast Really Best?" 596. See also 608, where she writes that "belief in its [breastfeeding's] superiority is so widespread that any bias, real or imagined,

might result in both publication of fewer negative studies and an association that appeared to be more consistent than it truly is."

22. Kukla writes, "We know that babies in developed countries routinely thrive on infant formula" ("Ethics and Ideology," 174). Linda Blum also talks about babies "thriving" on infant formulas (*At the Breast*, 49). I find the use of the word *thrive* interesting, as it is precisely the kind of usage that breastfeeding advocates would object to. They might use the words *survive* or *grow adequately* to describe infant development when babies are fed formula. Given their belief in the increased likelihood of acute and chronic illness, they would be reluctant to use *thrive*, which implies not just expected growth and survival but above-average health and development. *Merriam-Webster's Collegiate Dictionary*, 11th ed., offers three definitions of *thrive*, including "(1) to grow vigorously: flourish; (2) to gain in wealth or possessions: prosper; (3) to progress toward or realize a goal despite or because of circumstances." Breastfeeding advocates might concede that babies thrive based on the third definition, but this is clearly not the one meant by Kukla and Blum.

23. Joan Wolf, "Is Breast Really Best?" 605.

24. Rebecca Kukla similarly focuses on breast milk in *Mass Hysteria*, at one point arguing that getting human milk into babies by whatever means is the most important aspect of breastfeeding (163).

25. Joan Wolf, "Is Breast Really Best?" 612, 614.

26. See Penny Van Esterik, *Risks, Rights, and Regulation*, for a discussion of the evidence of the effects of chemical contaminants in breast milk.

27. See Duden, *Disembodying Women*, for an extended meditation on this issue.

28. Both Judy Hopkinson and Jane Heinig, in different ways, suggest that public health programs that do not address structural impediments present problems to the individuals targeted by the programs.

29. For some examples, see Gandy, "Open Letter."

30. Kukla, "Ethics and Ideology," 173–74 (emphasis in original).

31. This is not to say that infant formula manufacturers, leading pediatricians, and women's rights organizations worry about mothers in the same way. The fact that they all articulate the rhetoric of maternal guilt—emphasizing the unacceptability of maternal guilt—suggests how powerful a cultural consensus it commands.

32. Suzanne Haynes, senior scientist at the Office of Women's Health and one of the chief architects of the NBAC, told me that the campaign did change normative attitudes about breastfeeding in the United States (Suzanne Haynes, personal communication, March 13, 2007). However, it is not clear to me (through observation) that much has changed either discursively or socially as a result of people's changed minds.

33. See Hausman, "Things (Not) to Do with Breasts in Public."

CHAPTER 7

1. Rabin, "Breast-Feed Or Else," F1, 6.

2. See Hausman, *Mother's Milk*, 56–61, for a discussion of insufficient milk syndrome.

3. Toni Calasanti forwarded this e-mail correspondence to me. It is important to note that Joan Wolf made significant contributions to this discussion, using arguments from "Is Breast Really Best?" to promote her points, which is why the discussion seems to echo many of her ideas discussed in the previous chapter. There were a few voices in opposition to this dominant argument.

4. Jacqueline Wolf, "What Feminists Can Do for Breastfeeding," 410–13.

5. An editorial in the *New York Times* suggests that it is wrong to "hound[] those who decide they do not want to" breastfeed, even though "all things being equal, mothers should breast-feed their babies." The editorial continues: "The equation might change if it became clear that breast-feeding could protect babies from serious illnesses later in life" (Editorial, "About Breast-Feeding . . .").

6. Rabin, "Breast-Feed Or Else," F1.

7. Jacqueline Wolf, "What Feminists Can Do for Breastfeeding," 409 (emphasis added).

8. This is one of the risks of formula feeding removed from the initial version of the NBAC. See Jacqueline Wolf, "What Feminists Can Do for Breastfeeding," 401–2, for a discussion of research concerning breastfeeding and diabetes. See also 413 for an account of the risk information dropped from the campaign. See Bartick and Reinhold, "The Burden of Suboptimal Breastfeeding," for the most recent discussion of morbidity and mortality risks of not breastfeeding in the United States.

9. Lupton, "Risk as Moral Danger," 433, 432–33, 433.

10. There are small numbers of people who do make these arguments, with respect to obesity and to cosleeping, but apparently without much public support or attention.

11. Douglas and Wildavsky, *Risk and Culture,* 193.

12. Ibid., 84.

13. Maternal and Child Health Bureau, "Women's Health USA 2005."

14. See Hausman, *Mother's Milk* and "The Feminist Politics of Breastfeeding," Rima Apple, *Mothers and Medicine,* and Jacqueline Wolf, *Don't Kill Your Baby,* for discussions of these other issues.

15. See Budig and England, "The Wage Penalty for Motherhood," for an in-depth description of the maternal wage penalty and factors causing it.

16. Calnen, "Paid Maternity Leave and Its Impact on Breastfeeding in the United States," 35, 36. Jacqueline Wolf, in "What Feminists Can Do for Breastfeeding," suggests that duration in breastfeeding is what really matters and that this point is ignored even in the most commonly used statistics about breastfeeding in the United States, the Ross Mothers Survey, which mainly tracks breastfeeding initiation. Other feminist scholars, notably Rebecca Kukla in "Ethics and Ideology," refute data suggesting that breastfeeding duration beyond four to six months makes a difference to health outcomes.

17. Joan Williams, "Are Your Parental Leave Policies Legal?" One of my anonymous readers suggested that the advent of MomsRising.org has challenged the equality paradigm. I am not yet convinced of MomsRising.org's power or demographic reach.

18. "Mother's Day: More than Candy and Flowers."

19. Maternal and Child Health Bureau, "Women's Health USA 2005."

20. Budig and England do note that married and divorced women seem to suffer a more severe motherhood penalty than never-married women, suggesting, "Husbands could, in principle, provide money that allows married mothers to focus more on their children than single women can; or they could simply be a second person to share child-care responsibilities, allowing married mothers to focus more on their jobs than single mothers. The higher child penalty for married mothers suggests that the first scenario is more common" ("The Wage Penalty for Motherhood," 218).

21. For a more extended discussion of this issue, see Hausman, *Mother's Milk,* 189–232.

22. See Hausman, *Mother's Milk,* 33–68.

23. Noveck, "Strong Reaction."

24. See Kantor, "On the Job."

CHAPTER 8

1. Buell, *Writing for an Endangered World,* 31 (emphasis added), 32, 34, 45, 53.

2. Ibid., 38.

3. At one point it was the forty-fourth biggest seller on Amazon.com (Rebecca Kukla, *Mass Hysteria,* 120). Denise Copelton remarks that *What to Expect* was "the most popular book by far [in my study] . . . , read by fifty-one women in my sample [out of a total of 55] and the only pregnancy advice book to appear on the *New York Times* best seller list" ("Reading Pregnancy Advice," 4).

4. I do not address drug abuse or illegal drug use by pregnant or breastfeeding women in this chapter; that topic has had ample coverage in feminist scholarly literature (see, for example, Michie and Cahn, *Confinements,* and Roberts, *Killing the Black Body*). What concerns me here are attempts to regulate culturally normal behaviors when women are pregnant or breastfeeding. There are obvious connections between the two kinds of experiences, but I will not be elaborating on them in this analysis.

5. Buell, *Writing for an Endangered World,* 30.

6. Copelton, "Reading Pregnancy Advice," 17.

7. This is not to suggest that local, nonexpert forms of knowledge and advice are better than the guidance of strange professionals in books. See Tapias, "'Always Ready and Always Clean'?" for an interesting discussion of local concepts of bad breast milk in Bolivia. According to Tapias, neighbors and relatives often advise mothers to stop breastfeeding if their babies have certain digestive troubles, based on the perception that the mother's unexpressed anger or sadness causes the milk to go bad.

8. See Duden, *Disembodying Women,* for an extended discussion of this issue.

9. Foucault would call this kind of information a "subjugated knowledge." See *The History of Sexuality.*

10. Copelton, "Reading Pregnancy Advice," 1.

11. Sullivan, "A Mother's Final Look at Life"; Sullivan, "In Sierra Leone, Every Pregnancy Is a 'Chance of Dying.'"

12. Sullivan, "A Mother's Final Look at Life."

13. Eisenberg et al., *What to Expect,* 2nd ed., 59.

14. Ibid., 69, 70.

15. Koren, *The Complete Guide,* 141.

16. Eisenberg et al., *What to Expect,* 3rd ed., 82.

17. See Michie and Cahn, *Confinements,* 69–92; Hausman, *Mother's Milk,* 104–14; and Kukla, *Mass Hysteria,* 105–43.

18. Eisenberg et al., *What to Expect,* 3rd ed., 88 (emphasis in original). See Michie and Cahn, *Confinements,* 29. Rebecca Kukla represents the doublespeak in this way: "On the one hand, then, responsibility for keeping their uteruses pure and well-ordered is placed on pregnant women's shoulders, while on the other hand, they are subject to exhaustive, demanding, and precise scripts of self-regulation and provided with elaborate, prefabricated regimens of bodily control that are designed to elicit frightened and diligent compliance from otherwise untrustworthy bodies" (*Mass Hysteria,* 130).

19. Eisenberg et al., *What to Expect,* 3rd ed., 142, 146, 151.

20. In an informative article in the *New York Times Sunday Magazine,* Florence Williams writes that she breastfeeds in part because she "want[s] to give [her daughter] the best possible start in an uncertain world." Continuing, she comments, "I take this responsibility seriously, as most of us do; for her sake, I don't drink much alcohol or caffeine. I avoid spicy foods, strawberries and cruciferous vegetables, which are believed to cause gas in babies. I take my vitamins to ensure that I have enough calcium and iron. I don't smoke. I'm aware of concerns about pesticides and heavy metals, and I try to take precautions. Since I have been pregnant with or nursing two children for almost four years, I have been buying mostly organic food. Several years ago we installed a three-stage reverse-osmosis filter on our tap water and ice maker. I live in a leafy, scenic town in the Rocky Mountains far from brown clouds and belching diesel freeways" (Williams, "First Person," 22). What is so interesting about this passage is the utter normality of her claims for being a responsible mother, that all of these expensive and highly codified behaviors are represented as the normal consequences of being a responsible, breastfeeding mother, rather than the responses of a particular kind of mother with resources and social power. See also Deborah Lupton's comments in "Risk and the Ontology of Pregnant Embodiment," 67.

21. British Nutrition Foundation, "Maternal and Infant Nutrition."

22. Eisenberg et al., *What to Expect,* 3rd ed., 57. Later in the text, the authors state that the abuse of alcohol is a reason not to breastfeed, although "an occasional drink is okay." They add in a footnote that "when a mother has had alcohol, her baby gets less milk and generally sleeps less well. To minimize these problems, avoid breastfeeding for at least two hours after having an alcoholic drink" (ibid., 313 n8).

23. Koren, *Complete Guide,* 204–6.

24. Kukla, *Mass Hysteria,* 129–30.

25. Golden, *Message in a Bottle,* 53, 55. Golden does demonstrate that there was some resistance to the abstinence advice and shows in addition that it was a decision that developed over a number of years. Nevertheless, within a decade of the identification of fetal alcohol syndrome as a recognized medical condition, American

women were advised to abstain from all alcohol during their pregnancies, and in less than another decade there were warning labels on all bottles of alcohol sold in the United States. Recently, two articles in the *New York Times* demonstrate continued ambivalence about pregnant women's alcohol use. See Rabin, "That Prenatal Visit," and Moskin, "The Weighty Responsibility."

26. Koren, *Complete Guide*, 200.

27. See Kukla, *Mass Hysteria*, 136.

28. There is another set of concerns about genetic defects and the problems of "geriatric mothers" giving birth to disabled children, which correspond to another set of concerns that are outside of the scope of this book to address. See Lupton, "Risk and the Ontology of Pregnant Embodiment," 68.

29. Douglas, *Purity and Danger*, 95–96. In this definitive, or at least seminal, anthropology of pollutions, Douglas writes, "Both we and the Bushmen [as representatives of so-called primitive peoples] justify our pollution avoidances by fear of danger. They believe that if a man sits on the female side his male virility will be weakened. We fear pathogenicity transmitted through micro-organisms. Often our justification of our own avoidances through hygiene is sheer fantasy. The difference between us is not that our behaviour is grounded on science and theirs on symbolism. The real difference is that we do not bring forward from one context to the next the same set of ever more powerful symbols; our experience is fragmented. Our rituals create a lot of little sub-worlds, unrelated. Their rituals create one single, symbolically consistent universe" (69).

30. Buell, *Writing for an Endangered World*, 30.

31. Tsing, "Monster Stories," 297.

32. Keane, "The Toxic Womb," 265.

33. Ibid., 273.

34. Of course, pregnant women are not the only ones in U.S. society expected to regulate themselves into culturally anomalous behaviors. As medical studies continue to speculate about linkages between diet and disease, and studies interrogate the relation between environmental contamination and illness, public health advice concerning disease prevention increasingly advocates individual behaviors that contravene community norms and traditions.

CHAPTER 9

1. See *Towards Healthy Environments for Children: Frequently Asked Questions about Breastfeeding in a Contaminated Environment*, a fact sheet prepared by Penny Van Esterik with international breastfeeding advocacy organizations and environmental activist groups, as an example of an effort to ameliorate tensions between these groups.

2. Buell, *Writing for an Endangered World*, 37.

3. Steingraber, *Living Downstream*, 96, 143, 168, 238.

4. This is very different from the FAQ sheet *Towards Healthy Environments for Children*, which asks "How does the production of infant formula contribute to a pol-

luted environment?" and answers by identifying the environmental effects of infant formula "manufacture, distribution, and use" (Van Esterik, 3); Steingraber, *Living Downstream*, 238.

5. Steingraber, *Having Faith*, 253, 279; Van Esterik, *Risks, Rights, and Regulations*, esp. 31–54.

6. Giles, "Reimagining Breastfeeding."

7. See Van Esterik, *Risks, Rights, and Regulations*.

8. Steingraber, *Having Faith*, 280.

9. That many cultures enforce taboos on sexual activity while nursing suggests the strong sexual flavor of breastfeeding, even as such taboos can be interpreted within a health framework to enhance the survivability of infants.

10. Williams, "First Person," 21.

11. Schafer, "Biomonitoring: A Tool."

12. La Leche League, "Breastfeeding Remains Best Choice"; International Lactation Consultant Association, "Position on Breastfeeding," 1.

13. Milly, "Mother's Milk," 209.

14. Lunder and Sharp, *Mothers' Milk*, 17, 21, 22–24 (emphases added).

15. Emerging concerns about bisphenol A in various food containers, including baby bottles, have presented an important object lesson on this very point. Public comment has been focused on getting the compound out of the bottles' plastic, rather than on promoting breastfeeding as a way of doing away with the bottles altogether. Liquid formulas are supposed to be sterile, but powdered ones are not. This may not be widely known. Powdered formulas have caused bacterial infections in infants. See Forsythe, "*Enterobacter sakazakii* and Other Bacteria in Powdered Infant Milk Formula." Mary Rose Tully clarified these points for me and brought this source to my attention.

16. Deacon, "Toxins in Breastmilk."

17. La Leche League, "Breastfeeding Remains Best Choice"; Lunder and Sharp, *Mothers' Milk*, 45.

18. La Leche League, "Breastfeeding Remains Best Choice."

19. Van Esterik, *Risks, Rights, and Regulation*, 73. Lawrence Buell would diagnose this problem as an effect of "the totalizing rhetoric with which [toxic discourse] sets forth claims of environmental poisoning" (*Writing in an Endangered World*, 47). The cover of the EWG's *Mothers' Milk* report sports an older baby (at least six months old, because she is sitting up) staring out at the reader with a quizzical look on her face, as if to suggest that she is asking the reader "What am I going to do now?" or "What are you going to do to fix this problem of the fire retardants in my body?" which, presumably, got there through her "mother's milk" since the title is also on the cover.

20. Newman, "Toxins and Infant Feeding," 2.

21. Lawrence Buell agrees that "the paranoia of antitoxic advocacy seems a recourse made needful by the very culture of expertise" and is sustained by the inability to know definitively what the consequences of environmental contaminants are: "The culture that sustains the procedural rigor resulting in repeated findings of indeterminacy stands accused of evading the obligation to *do* something beyond critical inter-

rogation of the problem. An absolutist counterdiscourse seems from this standpoint a necessary outlet for the anxiety formal risk analysis would contain" (*Writing in an Endangered World*, 50).

22. See Davis-Floyd, "The Technocratic Body"; and Hausman, "Risky Business," for a lengthier discussion of these issues.

CHAPTER 10

1. See Glaser and Palmer, *In the Absence of Angels*.

2. Wright and Schanler, "The Resurgence of Breastfeeding," 424S.

3. Ibid., 423S. Current breastfeeding rates in other industrialized nations are variable, with Scandinavian countries enjoying high rates of initiation and duration, while others struggle with rates lower than the United States (France and Ireland, for example).

4. Many in the medical community continue to view the evidence base of breastfeeding medicine skeptically; this is a constant concern in breastfeeding advocacy circles. However, in the 1980s, with the global breastfeeding movement just beginning to have some success with international law and governing bodies, breastfeeding medicine was far less developed than it is today.

5. For an excellent short history of the Nestlé campaign, the development of the International Code of Marketing of Breastmilk Substitutes, and the issues posed to global breastfeeding promotion by HIV/AIDS, see Lerner, "Striking a Balance as AIDS Enters the Formula Fray."

6. "Chronology of the Breastfeeding Movement," *The Breastfeeding Movement*, 29. For information about the global breastfeeding movement from the early 1900s to the present, see Amin, "A Brief History of the Breastfeeding Movement."

7. Wright and Schanler, "The Resurgence of Breastfeeding," 423S. Wright and Schanler date the Innocenti declaration at 1991, not 1990.

8. According to breastfeeding advocate and researcher Ted Greiner, although the WHO invitations had not gone out to any breastfeeding experts, two such experts were able to influence the recommendation that came out of the meeting ("Perspective and Role," 25).

9. UNAIDS/WHO/UNICEF, "Policy Statement on HIV and Infant Feeding, 1997," 213.

10. UNFPA/UNICEF/WHO/UNAIDS Inter-Agency Team, *New Data*. See also De Paoli, "*To Breastfeed or Not to Breastfeed*," 17–19, for a good discussion of the development of the WHO/UNFPA guidelines.

11. Coutsoudis, Pillay, Spooner, et al., "Influence of Infant-Feeding Patterns"; and Coutsoudis, Pillay, Kuhn, et al., "Method of Feeding."

12. UNAIDS, *2006 Global Facts and Figures*.

13. UNICEF, "More HIV-Positive Children and Pregnant Women Getting AIDS Treatment."

14. Paul Farmer would suggest that instead of lack of resources to meet existing need, there is a lack of political will to provide necessary resources.

15. Ferris and Kline, "Epidemiology of Pediatric HIV Infection."

16. Kuhn et al., "Preventing Mother-to-Child HIV Transmission," 11.

17. Kuhn et al. write, "Nevirapine can cut HIV transmission from mother to child *in utero* and at parturition by half, from around 20% to around 10%. . . . A further 10% of infants are likely to be infected [through breastfeeding] during the first year of life, and another 5% during the second year" ("Preventing Mother-to-Child HIV Transmission," 10–11). The recent *HIV and Infant Feeding: Update* (based on the 2006 Interagency Task Team meeting on Prevention of HIV Infection in Pregnant Women, Mothers, and Their Infants held in Geneva) states that "the general range of HIV transmission through breastfeeding of any kind without any interventions is 5–20%. However, many health workers, even those with relevant training, over-estimate the risk of transmission. Figures lower than this range have been reported: Exclusive breastfeeding from about six weeks to six months was found to carry a risk of about 4% in South Africa" (World Health Organization, *HIV and Infant Feeding: Update,* 2).

18. Coovadia et al., "Mother-to-Child Transmission of HIV-1 Infection during Exclusive Breastfeeding," 1114. Kuhn et al. define customary breastfeeding as a practice in which "lactation is prolonged and supplemented with water and/or other liquids and solids from an early age" ("Preventing Mother-to-Child HIV Transmission," 11).

19. Coutsoudis, Pillay, Spooner et al., "Influence of Infant-Feeding Patterns." This study has since been confirmed through follow-up, although numerous other researchers continue to struggle over ways to provide safe replacement feeding in the context of maternal HIV infection. See Coutsoudis, "Infant Feeding Dilemmas," and Coutsoudis and King, "Breastfeeding Is Still a Life-Saving Formula." See also Coovadia et al., "Mother-to-Child Transmission of HIV-1 Infection during Exclusive Breastfeeding," for a 2007 study suggesting that exclusive breastfeeding can be supported with appropriate counseling.

20. World Health Organization, *WHO HIV and Infant Feeding Technical Consultation.*

21. "Informed choice" first appeared in UNAIDS/WHO/UNICEF, "Policy Statement on HIV and Infant Feeding, 1997." A technical consultation in 2000, organized by the UNFPA/UNICEF/WHO/UNAIDS Inter-Agency team on MTCT, clarified the "informed choice" policies with regard to maternal nursing in the context of HIV. Without using the language of informed choice, the technical consultation recommends, "When replacement feeding is acceptable, feasible, affordable, sustainable, and safe, avoidance of all breastfeeding by HIV-infected mothers is recommended" (UNFPA/UNICEF/WHO/UNAIDS, *New Data,* 12). The consensus statement of the 2006 technical consultation, however, begins its recommendation in the following manner: "The most appropriate infant feeding option for an HIV-infected mother should continue to depend on her individual circumstances, including her health status and the local situation, but should take greater consideration of the health services available and the counseling and support she is likely to receive. Exclusive breastfeeding is recommended for HIV-infected women for the first 6 months of life unless replacement feeding is acceptable, feasible, affordable, sustainable and safe for them and their infants before this time" (World Health Organization, *WHO HIV and Infant*

Feeding Technical Consultation, 4). The "consensus statement" is not, technically, a set of recommendations, but formal recommendations coming out of these meetings do not seem to have been published. An update was published in 2007 by the World Health Organization (*HIV and Infant Feeding: Update*).

22. See Moland and Blystad, "Counting on Mother's Love," for an excellent discussion of the difficulty of supporting informed choice in specific contexts.

23. Kuhn et al., "Preventing Mother-to-Child HIV Transmission," 13. Tanya Doherty, in "Appropriateness," a presentation at the International AIDS Conference, August 2006, discussed infrastructure criteria for assessing the feasibility of replacement feeding.

24. Some HIV-positive mothers in the United States who decided to breastfeed their babies have had their children removed from their custody.

25. Centers for Disease Control, "What Women Can Do."

26. Coutsoudis, Goga, Rollins, and Coovadia, "Free Formula Milk," 154.

27. See Chen and Rogan, "Breastfeeding and the Risk of Postneonatal Death in the United States," and Bartick and Reinhold, "The Burden of Suboptimal Breastfeeding," for discussions of enhanced infant mortality and morbidity due to not breastfeeding in the United States.

28. Kuhn et al., "Preventing Mother-to-Child Transmission," 11, 12.

29. Rollins, "HIV Transmission and Mortality."

30. Coovadia et al. note that a recent study in Côte d'Ivoire suggested no difference in mortality rates of breastfed or formula-fed infants born to HIV-positive mothers ("Mother-to-Child Transmission of HIV-1 Infection during Exclusive Breastfeeding," 1107).

31. Centers for Disease Control, "What Women Can Do." This may be because the appropriate agency, Women, Infants, and Children (WIC), is embedded in the U.S. Department of Agriculture (USDA) and its Food and Nutrition Service.

32. For example, White, *Breastfeeding and HIV/AIDS,* 69–70.

33. Ibid., 66–69; Kuhn et al., "Preventing Mother-to-Child Transmission," 11.

34. Coutsoudis, Goga, Rollins, and Coovadia indicate that mixed feeding is a common result of the free provision of formula ("Free Formula Milk," 157). Public health officials are also concerned that the free provision of infant formula will function as a tacit endorsement of replacement feeding for all infants, thereby endangering infant health far more seriously than universal breastfeeding, even in the context of high seroprevalence. Cup feeding is not perceived to threaten indigenous breastfeeding practices in the same way that bottle feeding does.

35. Linkages, *Infant Feeding Options,* 3 (emphasis added). Most HIV-positive mothers around the globe do not know their status, either because of lack of testing facilities, fear of the possibility of being positive, or lack of knowledge about HIV.

36. Stigma continues to be a significant factor in the fight against HIV/AIDS worldwide. In the *2006 Report on the Global Epidemic: Executive Summary,* UNAIDS states, "Ending the AIDS pandemic will depend largely on changing the social norms, attitudes and behaviours that contribute to its expansion. Action against AIDS-related stigma and discrimination must be supported by top leadership and at every level of society, and must address women's empowerment, homophobia, attitudes to-

ward sex workers and injecting drug users, and social norms that affect sexual behaviour—including those that contribute to the low status and powerlessness of women and girls" (19). Note that issues concerning stigma and motherhood are not addressed in this statement, which is pretty comprehensive otherwise. See also Chase, *Stigma, HIV/AIDS, and Prevention of Mother-to-Child Transmission: A Pilot Study in Zambia, India, Ukraine, and Burkina Faso.*

37. Nevertheless, increased sanitation is believed to have increased susceptibility to polio in the nineteenth and early twentieth centuries. Currently, researchers are focusing on excessive sanitary environments as one cause of increased rates of asthma and allergy.

38. The complexity of biological factors affecting perinatal HIV infection mirrors the complicated social context within which mothers and their health-care practitioners make decisions about infant feeding. Perinatal HIV infection occurs while a fetus is in utero through placental exchange, during the birth process (most common), or during breastfeeding. Infants born to HIV-positive mothers are likely to have maternal antibodies to HIV in their blood systems for a number of months, making a positive diagnosis of HIV in the newborn difficult. Transmission at any point is affected by several factors, most notably the mother's viral load during pregnancy and while breastfeeding, as well as the state of the infant's gut while nursing is ongoing and whether the mother is on ARVs.

39. Kuhn et al. comment, "A general decline in breastfeeding, resulting from present policies unmitigated, may well be a lasting heritage of the HIV epidemic" ("Preventing Mother-to-Child Transmission," 14).

40. Rosenberg, "When a Pill," 42.

41. Nevirapine is a nonnucleoside reverse transcriptase inhibitor (NNRTI). This class of drugs "inhibit[s] the synthesis of viral DNA by binding to reverse transcriptase to inhibit the enzyme's activity" (Nattrass, *Mortal Combat,* 22). In use as a prophylaxis against mother-to-child transmission, the mother gets a shot of nevirapine or takes a pill during labor and the baby is given nevirapine drops 48–72 hours following birth.

42. Tsing, "Monster Stories," 283.

43. Moland and Blystad, "Counting on Mother's Love," 473.

44. Rosenberg, "When a Pill," 43.

45. There are debates about nevirapine. Reports in 2004 suggested that the one dose of nevirapine recommended during labor, while decreasing the risk of perinatal transmission of HIV, might cause the development of drug resistance in the mothers. At the International AIDS Conference in 2006, researchers were calling for pregnant women to get regular courses of antiretrovirals rather than only receive the one dose of nevirapine to protect their unborn children, even though further research on nevirapine did not seem to bear out the initial fears expressed in 2004. See Altman, "Infant Drugs." In January 2005, the U.S. Food and Drug Administration issued a Public Health Advisory about nevirapine when used for extended periods of time in the context of a triple cocktail. Nevirapine can lead to liver toxicity. See U.S. Food and Drug Administration, "FDA Public Health Advisory."

46. Rosenberg, "When a Pill," 45, 43.

47. Ibid., 59.

48. Samuel R. Friedman, "Prevention Controversy."

49. The quintessential text with regard to this issue is Randy Shilts's *And the Band Played On*. Of particular interest to my study is his discussion of Dr. Arye Rubenstein's attempts in the early 1980s to get officials at the Centers for Disease Control (CDC), as well as editors at the *New England Journal of Medicine*, to acknowledge that the sick babies he was treating at the Albert Einstein College of Medicine in New York had what was then called "GRID" (Gay-Related Immune Deficiency) (124, 171–72).

50. Paula Treichler points out, "Western medical science is conceived as a transhistorical, transcultural model of reality; when cultural differences among human communities are taken into account, they tend to be enlisted in the service of this reality, but their status remains utilitarian" (*How to Have Theory*, 119). Biomedicine presents itself as a universal response to all human physical suffering; thus, the only role for culture is to impede biomedical advances (i.e., ignorance) or as an adjunct to biomedical truths (i.e., neutral but unnecessary).

51. Blystad and Moland, "Technologies of Hope?" 106, 115, 116, 115.

CHAPTER 11

1. Hoofnagle et al., "What Is Denialism."

2. Numerous Web sites provide counterarguments to AIDS deniers' claims. *The Body: The Complete HIV/AIDS Resource* provides a comprehensive fact sheet produced by the National Institutes of Allergy and Infectious Disease (NIAID) ("The Evidence That HIV Causes AIDS"). Tara C. Smith and Steven P. Novella provide an excellent argumentative rebuttal of AIDS denialism from a scientific perspective in "HIV Denial in the Internet Era."

3. This is not to suggest that all AIDS researchers do their work out of selfless concern for AIDS victims. A former colleague of mine, a virologist, has the following line as part of her e-mail signature: "Ambition will cure AIDS before compassion does."

4. Treichler, *How to Have Theory*, 175 (emphasis in original).

5. According to Bryce et al., "undernutrition is an underlying cause of 53% of all deaths in children aged younger than 5 years" ("WHO Estimates," 1150).

6. Cohen does not address AIDS denialism at all. Certain portions of *States of Denial* address individuals' denial of their HIV status, generally in a psychological sense. He looks more intently at Holocaust denial, but generally in terms of those present in Germany and German-dominated states during World War II, and thus not the Holocaust denialism that has flourished as a refutation of the historical record since the war.

7. See Cohen, *States of Denial*, 59, concerning "accounts" and their "public acceptability," as another way of thinking about this issue.

8. James, "AIDS Denialists."

9. Ibid.

10. Epstein, *Impure Science*.

11. Most scholars do not differentiate between the term *highly active antiretroviral treatments* (HAART) and the term *antiretrovirals* (ARVs). Because ARVs are almost always used in combination, in order to avoid resistance, the terms are basically interchangeable, and the latter is usually used.

12. Patton, *Inventing AIDS*, 61.

13. Ibid., 62.

14. Ibid., 63.

15. Treichler, *How to Have Theory*, 159 (emphasis in original). This phrase is not in quotation marks in the original text, which I take to mean that while she refers to Latour and Woolgar's 1979 study *Laboratory Life*, the phrasing of this idea is her own.

16. Ibid., 170.

17. Ibid., 173, 168, 157.

18. Epstein, *Impure Science*, 170–71.

19. Ibid., 168.

20. Peter Duesberg is perhaps the most famous scientist who is also an AIDS denialist. His perspectives on HIV/AIDS may be explored on his Web site, *Duesberg on AIDS*. He is the author of *Inventing the AIDS Virus*.

21. Epstein, *Impure Science*, 168 (emphasis added).

22. Some sources claim that Duesberg is a retrovirologist; others claim that he is not. Still others agree he is a retrovirologist but that he is not familiar with this particular kind of retrovirus.

23. Epstein, *Impure Science*, 168. *Black-boxed* is a term from Latour discussed in Treichler, *How to Have Theory*, 159. See Nattrass, *Mortal Combat*, 21–22, for an easily understood figure describing the action of antiretroviral drugs, as well as a chart describing and distinguishing the various classes of drugs.

24. This argument is a subgroup of John S. James's no. 3, "AIDS drugs are poisons, pushed by doctors corrupted by the pharmaceutical industry—so don't take any of them . . ." ("AIDS Denialists").

25. Booth, *The Rhetoric of Rhetoric*, 11.

26. Farber, "Out of Control," 37.

27. Gallo et al., "Errors in Celia Farber's March 2006 Article." I have removed the citation reference numbers in the quotations I am using from this online article.

28. Farber, "Out of Control," 37.

29. These challenges come directly out of Bauer's book *The Origin, Persistence and Failings of HIV/AIDS Theory*. I am analyzing Bauer's work, rather than more well-known denialist texts like Peter Duesberg's *Inventing the AIDS Virus*, because Bauer writes from a science studies perspective and tries to fit his account into that tradition. In addition, as a very recent addition to the denialist library, Bauer's book represents the continuation of denialist arguments into the current period.

30. Bauer, "Truth Stranger than Fiction," 9.

31. Smith and Novella, "HIV Denial."

32. Treichler, *How to Have Theory*, 160. Steven Epstein comments, "As Treichler has asserted, Gallo's group may have strengthened the credibility of their claim simply by publishing so many papers about AIDS and referencing their 1984 paper at

every turn. But in referencing it, they were no more or less likely to make either qualified or unqualified etiological claims than other scientific researchers who cited it during the same years. They promoted their product—but they did not, in any crude or blatant sense, oversell it in terms of its causal implications" (*Impure Science,* 84).

33. See Haraway, "Situated Knowledges."

34. These are the main recommendations for fighting denialism made by Smith and Novella in "HIV Denial."

35. Smith and Novella, in "HIV Denial," do suggest that "lingering denial [may be] the fault of scientists and the media for originally proclaiming AIDS a universal 'death sentence.'" They go on to comment that "even though this idea may no longer appear in the scientific literature, it remains a public perception of the disease" and suggest that a better "balance" between risk information and optimism about treatment needs to be communicated by scientists (1315). This kind of commentary again suggests their faith in information to forestall denial.

CHAPTER 12

1. Crowe is a member of the Advisory Council to AnotherLook and president of the Alberta Reappraising AIDS Society. See http://aras.ab.ca/.

2. Crowe, "Infectious HIV in Breastmilk."

3. AnotherLook, "About Us" and "AnotherLook at Breastfeeding and HIV/ AIDS."

4. *Situated knowledge* is a term that comes from Donna Haraway's chapter "Situated Knowledges: The Science Question in Feminism and the Privilege of Partial Perspective." For Haraway, the concept "situated knowledge" is used to construe scientific thinking as situated rather than transcendent: "Feminist objectivity is about limited location and situated knowledge, not about transcendence and splitting of subject and object. In this way we might become answerable for what we learn how to see" (190). It seems to me that the concept can be transposed to contexts in which it is not the production of scientific knowledge that is in question but its function in social circumstances.

5. Youde, *AIDS, South Africa, and the Politics of Knowledge,* 8.

6. Schoub, *AIDS and HIV in Perspective,* 24.

7. Youde, *AIDS, South Africa, and the Politics of Knowledge,* 6.

8. "HIV and AIDS in South Africa."

9. Koenig, "Global Health: South Africa Bolsters HIV/AIDS Plan," 1378.

10. "South Africa 'Ends' AIDS Denialism."

11. "South Africa's New Health Minister." However, Jacob Zuma, who replaced Mbeki as ANC president in December 2007, has acknowledged having unprotected sex with a woman he knew to be HIV-positive; he claimed the sex to be consensual, although charges of rape were filed against him in 2005. Zuma was acquitted of the rape charges, but his attitude about HIV and AIDS remains unclear, as he is reported to have said that taking a shower after sex was sufficient to protect him against infection. See "Jacob Zuma Cleared of Rape."

12. Nicoli Nattrass notes that the South African government pursued standard AIDS prevention policies based on the idea that HIV causes AIDS at the same time that it was refusing to provide antiretrovirals to HIV-positive patients at public clinics and hospitals. She argues that the denialists did not see the prevention programs as harmful, just "misguided." However, they were against the provision of ARVs on the theory that these caused AIDS. The bifurcation of the South African response—cohering to mainstream medicine in some respects and repudiating it in others—made addressing its denialism particularly difficult. See Nattrass, *Mortal Combat*, 78.

13. Mbali, "AIDS Discourses," 104–5, 106, 107.

14. Wang, "AIDS Denialism," 15–16, 11.

15. Butler, "South Africa's HIV/AIDS Policy," 605, 612.

16. Robins, " 'Long Live Zackie, Long Live,' " 653, 660, 662.

17. Sitze, "Denialism," 771, 773, 780.

18. Ibid., 782. At this writing (2009), Sitze's essay is five years old, and more sub-Saharan African people have access to ARVs. However, the broader claim still stands.

19. Ibid., 788; see also 790. Near the end of his essay Sitze suggests that the transition to democracy did not really change the kind of sovereign power exerted by the state during the apartheid era and which, he is inclined to argue, is the core of denialism as a kind of power exerted by states in general.

20. Craddock, "Beyond Epidemiology," 5.

21. Nattrass, "AIDS and the Scientific Governance of Medicine," 165.

22. Nattrass, *Mortal Combat*, 83, 89–90. Nattrass also questions the minister of health's alliance with Mbeki in this regard.

23. Nattrass, "AIDS and the Scientific Governance of Medicine," 176.

24. Mbali, "AIDS Discourses and the South African State," 116 (emphasis added), 117.

25. Yoube focuses on Mkebi's use of "African Renaissance" discourse in his attempt to "promote a new post-apartheid identity inspired by the ideals of the African Renaissance," which he defines in part as "a positive, self-sufficient country with the scientific capabilities to propel it into the pantheon of the world's best scientific research. Members of the government have appropriated images of liberation and resistance" to support this vision and "to justify their AIDS policies" (Yoube, *AIDS, South Africa, and the Politics of Knowledge*, 77–78).

26. Ibid., 109. Yoube notes, "In its efforts to promote its African Renaissance-inspired identity, some have noted a curious irony. While promoting African solutions to African problems, the South African government has turned to Western dissident scientists while ignoring the local scientific community which largely supports the orthodox position" (119).

27. Ibid., 116, 114.

28. Ibid., 100; Nattrass, *The Moral Economy of AIDS in South Africa*, 49–50.

29. Foucault begins a discussion of discourse in "The Discourse on Language" with the following words: "I am supposing that in every society the production of discourse is at once controlled, selected, organised and redistributed according to a certain number of procedures, whose role is to avert its powers and its dangers, to cope with chance events, to evade its ponderous, awesome materiality" (216).

30. Yoube, *AIDS, South Africa, and the Politics of Knowledge*, 108–9.

31. Meier, "In War Against AIDS," A16.

32. AnotherLook, "About Us."

33. AnotherLook, "Another Look at Breastfeeding and HIV/AIDS."

34. AnotherLook, "Call to Action."

35. Ibid.

36. There is a persistent strain of advocacy discourse and breastfeeding research itself that addresses how lack of precision in defining breastfeeding (any breastfeeding, exclusive breastfeeding, full breastfeeding, partial breastfeeding, some breastfeeding, as examples) leads to significant research deficits. Ted Greiner comments on this issue in "The Perspective and Role of the Breastfeeding Supportive NGOs," a talk he gave at the 2002 WABA-UNICEF Colloquium on HIV and Infant Feeding: "Until the 1990s, research relating health outcomes in general to feeding patterns rarely had exclusively breast-fed groups, but compared partially breastfed infants to non-breastfed infants—and found few health differences measurable using relatively small sample sizes except in the early months in very low-income populations. This was not cited as what it was—a lack of good data—it was widely cited as evidence that there were no longer any differences between formula and breast milk" ("Perspective and Role," 26).

However, the analogy between changing definitions of AIDS and known problems in defining breastfeeding is improper, given that imprecision in the definition of breastfeeding means that research findings consistently downplay the positive health impacts of breastfeeding (because few studies actually realize the importance of making sure that the "breastfeeding group" includes only mothers exclusively breastfeeding, or can in fact make sure that those claiming to be exclusively breastfeeding really are). The imprecision with respect to the conditions that lead to a diagnosis of AIDS, however, has to do with evolving biomedical understanding of the disease and the particular nature of HIV infection itself. A disease that attacks the immune system means that individuals who die from it actually die from other causes. HIV infection left unchecked causes opportunistic infections to proliferate and otherwise manageable incursions on the human immune system to become deadly. It is in the nature of AIDS not to involve a fixed definition, although HIV infection can be accurately determined by existing testing protocols. As an example, it is now commonplace to point out that early definitions of AIDS in the United States, identifying the cluster of opportunistic infections that signaled an AIDS diagnosis, focused on those illnesses suffered by HIV-positive men. Women presented with different symptoms and disease progressions. Adding new symptoms and illnesses to the list of AIDS-related illnesses was about acknowledging that the initial understanding of AIDS itself was too narrow and partial. As pointed out in Robert Gallo et al.'s response to Celia Farber's *Harper's* article, "It is true that as more was learned about AIDS, the definition of the disease changed. There is nothing unusual in this; AIDS was only discovered in 1981. It is a testimony to scientific methodology that it only took a few years to discover its cause. An accurate diagnosis of AIDS, throughout the world, does require an HIV-positive test. While there are facilities in Africa which do not even have HIV tests (one of the cheapest components of the medical response to HIV), our knowledge of HIV in Africa is based on studies that have used HIV tests. (Incidentally, facilities that cannot offer HIV testing do not offer ARVs either.)" ("Errors in Celia Farber's March 2006 article").

37. Kent and Crowe, "Infant Feeding and HIV."

38. This presentation is also available as a position paper, "Infectious HIV in Breastmilk: True or False?" on the AnotherLook position papers Web page.

39. Crowe, "Infectious HIV in Breastmillk: Fact or Fantasy?" The first bulleted point in Crowe's list is the URL of an AIDS denialist Web site mentioned in the previous chapter (and reportedly visited by Thabo Mbeki in his initial attempts to understand the relation of HIV to AIDS). See *VirusMyth: A Rethinking AID$ Website.* The second is Crowe's own organization, the Alberta Reappraising AIDS Society, which is a Canadian organization whose aims are to "challenge the dogma that HIV causes AIDS," "question whether AIDS is a true disease or just an arbitrary collection of symptoms," "challenge the accuracy of HIV tests," etc. See Alberta Reappraising AIDS Society, http://aras.ab.ca/. As discussed previously, Peter Duesberg is perhaps the most famous U.S. AIDS dissident scientist. See Duesberg, *Duesberg on AIDS.* Christine Maggiore is a prominent American AIDS denialist author whose three-year-old daughter reportedly died of AIDS-related pneumonia in 2005. Maggiore herself died in December 2008. See *Alive and Well AIDS Alternatives,* www.aliveandwell.org. The "Perth Group" does not believe that HIV itself exists. See Yoube, *AIDS, South Africa, and the Politics of Knowledge,* 106–7, for a discussion of the Perth group.

40. Morrison, "Mothers and Babies and HIV."

41. In his keynote address to the WABA-UNICEF Colloquium on HIV and infant feeding in 2002, Stephen Lewis (then special representative to the UN Secretary General on HIV/AIDS in Africa) pointed out that the American Academy of Pediatrics' breastfeeding guide has the Abbott Laboratories' logo on the cover. Abbott Labs is the larger company of which Ross, maker of the infant formula Similac, is a part. See Lewis, "Keynote," 15.

42. Greiner, "HIV—Will It Be the Death of Breastfeeding?"

43. When I visited Uganda in 2007, I found that The AIDS Service Organization (TASO) based in Kampala supported replacement feeding for HIV-positive mothers. The manager of TASO looked at me with an odd expression on his face when I asked him how HIV-positive mothers feed their babies and whether the organization had a recommended policy for mothers with regard to infant feeding, as if wondering why I would even ask such a question. Kampala is an urban area and thus piped water is more generally available, and TASO may help the mothers with formula provision. But a few days later, while talking to an AIDS worker from the Sese islands in Lake Victoria, an extremely poor community with very high seroprevalence, I found that almost all the HIV-positive women there breastfed their babies. Indeed, the worker I spoke with looked at me with an odd expression on his face when I asked about infant feeding practices in the islands. These responses to my questions about infant feeding and maternal HIV infection suggest the very local contexts of "appropriate" infant feeding practices (and the economic resources that contribute to defining certain practices as denialist or pragmatic).

44. Schoepf, "AIDS, History, and Struggles," 17.

CHAPTER 13

1. Santora, "U.S. Is Close," A1; A26. Newborn HIV antibody testing does not necessarily identify infants with positive HIV status, as infants will carry maternal antibodies in their blood for a number of months. However, newborn HIV antibody testing does indicate maternal HIV status and thus can lead to appropriate use of ARVs for the mother and infant in order to avoid infection in the infant and treat the mother. DNA PCR (polymerase chain reaction) testing of newborns has made the identification of HIV infection of infants more accurate and dependable, although it is not available in all parts of the world due to expense. There continues to be a delay after birth before PCR testing is presumed accurate in detecting HIV infection in newborns.

2. Ibid., A1.

3. Paula Treichler, writing in the late 1990s, points out that "by the end of 1987 . . . WHO's surveillance reports and seroprevalence data were sufficient to suggest three broad global patterns of AIDS. . . . According to this scheme (subsequently revised . . .) *Pattern I* is considered typical of industrialized countries with large numbers of reported cases (the 'First World,' roughly, including the United States, Canada, Western Europe, Australia, and New Zealand); it is characterized by the initial appearance of HIV infection in the late 1970s and rapid spread primarily among gay and bisexual men, intravenous drug users in urban coastal centers, and recipients of blood products. . . . Infection in the overall population is estimated to be less than 1 percent. In *Pattern II* countries (typically in sub-Saharan central Africa, the Caribbean, and Latin America), HIV infection may have appeared in the late 1970s but was not widely identified as AIDS related until 1983; heterosexual transmission is the norm, with males and females often equally infected and perinatal transmission therefore common; transmission via gay sexual contact or intravenous drug use is asserted to be low or absent. A *Pattern III* profile is attributed to the Second World countries of the then Soviet bloc as well as to much of North Africa, the Middle East, Asia, and the Pacific. . . . HIV is judged to have appeared in the early to mid-1980s, and only a small number of cases have been identified, primarily in people who have traveled to and engaged in some form of high-risk involvement with infected persons in Pattern I or II areas" (*How to Have Theory*, 111).

4. Etzioni, Letter, A27. Amitai Etzioni is also the author of an article, "HIV Testing of Infants: Privacy and Public Health," and a book, *The Limits of Privacy,* that deal with these issues in greater detail. At the time he was working on these issues, the late 1990s and 2000, newborn HIV testing was largely conducted as antibody testing, so it was largely a test of maternal HIV status. See Zivi, "Contesting Motherhood in the Age of AIDS," for a critical history of public debates on newborn HIV testing in the United States.

5. Yarney, "The Milk of Human Kindness." See also the numerous letters indicating support for Yarney's critique, in the online edition of *British Medical Journal,* www.bmj.com.

6. Freedman and Stecklow, "Bottled Up," A18.

7. Ibid., A1.

8. King, "In Zambia."

9. Rabin, "Breast-Feed Or Else."

10. Sullivan, "A Mother's Final Look at Life: In Impoverished Sierra Leone, Childbirth Carries Deadly Odds" and "In Sierra Leone, Every Pregnancy Is a 'Chance of Dying.'"

CHAPTER 14

1. The AFASS criteria ask counselors and mothers to ascertain if replacement feeding is *affordable, feasible, acceptable, sustainable,* and *safe.*

2. Farmer et al., "Structural Violence and Clinical Medicine," 1688, 1688–89. In the 2004 Partners In Health annual report, prevention strategies for MTCT are as follows: "All pregnant women are tested for HIV . . . and treated with antiretroviral therapy [if they tested positive]. Monthly education sessions for pregnant women and new mothers are a popular forum for sharing information about safe pregnancy, HIV prevention, and child care. Infant formula and all the necessary supplies for safe formula-feeding (including access to clean water) are provided to all HIV-positive mothers to prevent postpartum transmission of HIV via breast milk." These practices result in a "local vertical transmission rate of under 2 percent" (Partners In Health, *Partners In Health 2004 Annual Report,* 12). PIH also tests babies to confirm serostatus within one to four months of their birth (ibid.).

3. Coutsoudis et al., "HIV, Infant Feeding, and More Perils for Poor People," 212; Farmer et al., "Structural Violence and Clinical Medicine," 1689.

4. Partners In Health, *PIH Guide,* 33; Coutsoudis et al., "HIV, Infant Feeding, and More Perils for Poor People," 210–13.

5. Farmer et al., "Structural Violence and Clinical Medicine," 1687.

6. In this sense, the AFASS criterion of (cultural) acceptability is not pertinent: "Without exception, pregnant women found to be infected with HIV expressed interest in ART to prevent MTCT, and all requested assistance not only with procuring infant formula, but also with the means to boil water and to store the formula safely" (Farmer et al., "Structural Violence and Clinical Medicine," 1689). ART refers to antiretroviral treatment, and means the same thing as ARV.

7. My thanks to Max Stephenson for this last point. The *Partners In Health 2004 Annual Report* indicates that all pregnant women in the Zamni Lasanti project were tested for HIV (12).

8. Moland and Blystad, "Counting on Mother's Love," 448–49, 473.

9. See Coutsoudis et al., "HIV, Infant Feeding, and More Perils for Poor People," 210–11.

10. De Paoli, *"To Breastfeed or Not to Breastfeed": Infant Feeding Dilemmas Facing Women with HIV in the Kilimanjaro Region, Tanzania.*

11. Guay and Ruff, "HIV and Infant Feeding," 2463; Morrison and Greiner, "Infant Feeding Choices for HIV-Positive Mothers," 27; Buskens, "How to Counsel Infant Feeding Practices," 167, 165–66; De Paoli, *"To Breastfeed or Not to Breastfeed,"* 58, 60.

Paul Farmer, in *Infections and Inequalities,* points out that sociomedical studies have the paradoxical effect of "shift[ing] the blame onto the sick-poor by exaggerating their agency" (255). This is one claim breastfeeding advocates consistently make about "informed choice" as a policy guideline in infant feeding decisions.

12. Guay and Ruff, "HIV and Infant Feeding"; Kuhn, Stein, and Susser, "Preventing Mother-to-Child HIV Transmission in the New Millennium"; Buskens, "How to Counsel Infant Feeding Practices"; Brahmbhatt and Gray, "Child Mortality Associated with Reasons for Non-Breastfeeding and Weaning"; Coutsoudis et al., "Free Formula Milk for Infants"; Weinberg, "The Dilemma of Postnatal Mother-to-Child Transmission of HIV."

13. Nielsen, "A Tale of Two Worlds."

14. Farmer, *Infections and Inequalities,* throughout; Farmer et al., "Structural Violence and Clinical Medicine," 1689.

15. De Paoli, *"To Breastfeed or Not to Breastfeed,"* 63–64. See also Blystad and Morand, "Technologies of Hope?" and Morand and Blystad, "Counting on Mother's Love," for extended discussions of the constraints on mothers to follow particular infant feeding protocols, especially concerning the specific interventions that can make mothers change their minds or deviate from instructions.

16. Ibid., 65, 66, 69.

17. Enfamil, Mead Johnson Nutritionals, "Choosing to Breastfeed"; ibid., "Feeding Your Baby."

18. See Solinger, "Poisonous Choice" and *Beggars and Choosers.*

19. Ladd-Taylor and Umansky, "Introduction," 22.

20. Nicoli Nattrass, in *Mortal Combat,* discusses the South African health minister's "confusing discourse of choice" that overemphasized the side effects of ARVs and led to "treatment anarchy" in the country, even after denialism was officially discarded as the state position on HIV/AIDS (145).

21. See Farmer, *Infections and Inequalities,* throughout, for extensive discussion of these issues. Farmer would focus on structural inequities, analyzing "local knowledges" through structural violence, rather than as a force acting apart from economic inequality.

22. See Hausman, *Mother's Milk,* 141–50, for a discussion of how African mothers are used to represent traditional, evolutionary breastfeeding for breastfeeding advocate scholars.

Works Cited

Alcabes, Philip. "Epidemiologists Need to Shatter the Myth of a Risk-Free Life." *Chronicle of Higher Education* (May 23, 2003): B11–12.

Alive and Well AIDS Alternatives. 2007. www.aliveandwell.org/ (accessed February 23, 2009).

Altman, Lawrence. "Infant Drugs for HIV Put Mothers at Risk." *New York Times,* February 10, 2004, A22.

Altman, Lawrence. "Transplants Seem Source of West Nile Virus Cases." *New York Times,* September 4, 2002, A12.

American Academy of Pediatrics. "Special Challenges to Breastfeeding." American Academy of Pediatrics. www.aap.org/pubed/ZZZHCCBXQ7C.htm (accessed May 1, 2005).

Amin, Sarah. "A Brief History of the Breastfeeding Movement." In *The Breastfeeding Movement: A Sourcebook,* compiled by Lakshmi Menon with Anwar Fazal, Sarah Amin, and Susan Siew, 1–21. Penang, Malaysia: World Alliance for Breastfeeding Action, 2003.

AnotherLook. "About Us." www.anotherlook.org/about.php (accessed December 24, 2006).

AnotherLook. "AnotherLook at Breastfeeding and HIV/AIDS." www.anotherlook .org/index.php (accessed December 27, 2006).

AnotherLook. "Call to Action." www.anotherlook.org/call.php (accessed December 27, 2006).

Appadurai, Arjun. *Modernity at Large: Cultural Dimensions of Globalization.* Minneapolis: University of Minnesota Press, 1996.

Apple, Rima D. *Mothers and Medicine: A Social History of Infant Feeding, 1890–1950.* Wisconsin Publications in the History of Science and Medicine, no. 7. Madison: University of Wisconsin Press, 1987.

Apple, Rima D. *Perfect Motherhood: Science and Childrearing in America.* New Brunswick: Rutgers University Press, 2006.

Barthes, Roland. *Mythologies.* Translated by Annette Lavers. New York: Hill and Wang, 1972.

Bartick, Melissa, and Arnold Reinhold. "The Burden of Suboptimal Breastfeeding in the United States: A Pediatric Cost Analysis." *Pediatrics.* 5 April 2010. (10.1542/ peds.2009-1616). http://pediatricsaapublications.org/cyi/reprint/peds2009-1616 .vl (accessed April 16, 2010).

Bartlett, John G. "West Nile Virus." *Medscape Today,* 2003. www.medscape.com/ viewarticle/461720 (accessed July 17, 2006).

Bauer, Henry. *The Origin, Persistence and Failings of HIV/AIDS Theory.* Jefferson, NC: McFarland, 2007.

Bauer, Henry. "Truth Stranger than Fiction: HIV Is Not the Cause of AIDS." Seminar, Edward Via School of Osteopathic Medicine, Blacksburg, VA. September 12, 2007. http://failingsofhivaidstheory.homestead.com/MedSeminar.pdf (accessed October 23, 2008).

Beck, Ulrich. *Risk Society: Towards a New Modernity.* Translated by Mark Ritter. London: Sage, 1992.

Beck-Gernsheim, Elisabeth. "Life as a Planning Project." In *Risk, Environment, and Modernity: Towards a New Ecology,* edited by Scott Lash, Bronislaw Szerszynski, and Brian Wynne, 139–53. London: Sage, 1996.

Blum, Linda. *At the Breast: Ideologies of Breastfeeding and Motherhood in the Contemporary United States.* Boston: Beacon Press, 1999.

Blystad, Astrid, and Karen Marie Moland. "Technologies of Hope? Motherhood, HIV, and Infant Feeding in Eastern Africa." *Anthropology and Medicine* 16, no. 2 (August 2009): 105–18.

Booth, Wayne C. *The Rhetoric of Rhetoric: The Quest for Effective Communication.* Blackwell Manifestoes. Malden, MA: Blackwell, 2004.

Boswell-Penc, Maia. *Tainted Milk: Breastmilk, Feminisms, and the Politics of Environmental Degradation.* Albany: State University of New York Press, 2006.

Brahmbhatt, Heena, and Ronald H. Gray. "Child Mortality Associated with Reasons for Non-Breastfeeding and Weaning: Is Breastfeeding Best for HIV-Positive Mothers?" *AIDS* 17 (2003): 879–85.

"Breast-Feeding by Mother with H.I.V. an Issue in Custody Case." *New York Times,* April 18, 1999, A17.

Brenna, J. Thomas. "Infant Formulas Containing DHA and ARA." *Cornell Cooperative Extension Food and Nutrition, Ask the Nutrition Expert,* January 2003. www.cce.cor nell.edu/food/expfiles/topics/brenna/brennaoverview.html (accessed November 13, 2004).

Briggs, Charles L. "Communicability, Racial Discourse, and Disease." *Annual Review of Anthropology* 34 (2005): 269–91.

Briggs, Charles L. "Modernity, Cultural Reasoning, and the Institutionalization of Social Inequality: Racializing Death in a Venezuelan Cholera Epidemic." *Comparative Studies in Society and History* 43, no. 4 (October 2001): 665–700.

British Nutrition Foundation. "Maternal and Infant Nutrition." 2004. www.nutri tion.org.uk (accessed October 21, 2006).

Brown, David. "4th Organ Recipient Has West Nile Virus, CDC Officials Say." *Washington Post,* September 6, 2002, A3.

Brown, David. "Virus's Link to Transfusions Intensifies." *Washington Post,* September 13, 2002, A3.

Brown, David. "West Nile Virus Is Discovered in Breast Milk of Michigan Woman." *Washington Post,* September 28, 2002, A11.

Bryce, Jennifer, Cynthia Boschi-Pinto, Kenji Shibuya, Robert E. Black, and the WHO Child Health Epidemiology Reference Group. "WHO Estimates of the Causes of Death in Children." *Lancet* 365 (March 26, 2005): 1147–52.

Budig, Michelle J., and Paula England. "The Wage Penalty for Motherhood." *American Sociological Review* 66 (April 2001): 204–25.

Buell, Lawrence. *Writing for an Endangered World: Literature, Culture, and the Environment in the U.S. and Beyond.* Cambridge: Harvard University Press, 2001.

Burger, Edward J., Jr. "Health as a Surrogate for the Environment." *Daedalus* 119, no. 4 (Fall 1990): 133–54.

Buskens, Ineke. "How to Counsel Infant Feeding Practices in Southern Africa in a Time of HIV/AIDS?" *Medimond International Proceedings,* E710L8237 (2004): 163–68.

Butler, Anthony. "South Africa's HIV/AIDS Policy, 1994–2004: How Can It Be Explained?" *African Affairs* 104, no. 417 (2005): 591–614.

Calnen, Gerald. "Paid Maternity Leave and Its Impact on Breastfeeding in the United States: An Historic, Economic, Political, and Social Perspective." *Breastfeeding Medicine* 2, no. 1 (November 2007): 34–44.

Cauvin, Henri E. "South African Court Orders Medicine for H.I.V. Infected Mothers." *New York Times,* December 15, 2001, A9.

CBS News. "South Africa's AIDS Stance Criticized." August 19, 2006. www.cbsnews .com/stories/2006/08/19/health/main1913718.shtml (accessed December 22, 2006).

"CDC: Mom's Milk Gave Baby West Nile." *CNN.com,* October 3, 2002. cnn.health.com (accessed October 4, 2002).

Celia Farber: Index. VirusMyth.com. www.virusmyth.net/aids/index/cfarber.htm (accessed January 4, 2007).

Centers for Disease Control. "Breastfeeding: Infectious Diseases and Specific Conditions Affecting Human Milk: West Nile Virus." Department of Health and Human Services, United States Government, September 28, 2005. www.cdc.gov/breast feeding/disease/west_nile_virus.htm (accessed July 17, 2006).

Centers for Disease Control. "HIV/AIDS and Women." Department of Health and Human Services, United States Government, June 28, 2007. www.cdc.gov/hiv/top ics/women/index.htm (accessed November 6, 2008).

Centers for Disease Control. "What Women Can Do." Department of Health and Human Services, United States Government, February 21, 2007. www.cdc.gov/ hiv/topics/perinatal/protection.htm (accessed February 17, 2009).

Centers for Disease Control. "WNV Fact Sheet." Department of Health and Human Services, United States Government, September 27, 2005. www.cdc.gov/westnile (accessed July 17, 2006).

Chase, Elaine, with Peter Aggleton, Virginia Bond, Shubhada Maitra, Alexander Golubov, and Idrissa Ouedraogo. *Stigma, HIV/AIDS, and Prevention of Mother-to-Child Transmission: A Pilot Study in Zambia, India, Ukraine, and Burkina Faso.* London: UNICEF and the Panos Institute, 2001.

Chen, Aimin, and Walter J. Rogan. "Breastfeeding and the Risk of Postneonatal Death in the United States." *Pediatrics* 113, no. 5 (2004): 435–39.

"Chronology of the Breastfeeding Movement." In *The Breastfeeding Movement: A Sourcebook,* compiled by Lakshmi Menon, with Anwar Fazal, Sarah Amin, and Susan Siew, 22–32. Penang, Malaysia: World Alliance for Breastfeeding Action, 2003.

Cohen, Stanley. *States of Denial: Knowing about Atrocities and Suffering.* Malden, MA: Polity, 2001.

Conrad, Peter. *The Medicalization of Society: On the Transformation of Human Conditions into Treatable Disorders.* Baltimore: Johns Hopkins University Press, 2007.

Coovadia, Hoosen M., Nigel C. Rollins, Ruth M. Bland, Kirsty Little, Anna Coutsoudis, Michael L. Bennish, and Marie-Louise Newell. "Mother-to-Child Transmission of HIV-1 Infection during Exclusive Breastfeeding in the First 6 Months of Life: An Intervention Cohort Study." *Lancet* 369 (March 31, 2007): 1107–16.

Copelton, Denise. "Reading Pregnancy Advice: An Exploration of How and Why Women Consult Popular Pregnancy Advice Books." Paper presented at the annual meeting of the American Sociological Association, San Francisco, August 14, 2004. www.allacademic.com/meta/p110750_index.html (accessed October 13, 2008).

Coutsoudis, Anna. "Infant Feeding Dilemmas Created by HIV: South African Experiences." *Journal of Nutrition* 135, no. 4 (April 2005): 956–59.

Coutsoudis, Anna, Hoosen M. Coovadia, and Catherine M. Wilfert. "HIV, Infant Feeding, and More Perils for Poor People: New WHO Guidelines Encourage Review of Formula Milk Policies." *Bulletin of the World Health Organization* 86, no. 3 (March 2008): 210–14.

Coutsoudis, Anna, A. E. Goga, N. Rollins, and Hoosen M. Coovadia. "Free Formula Milk for Infants of HIV-Infected Women: Blessing or Curse?" *Health Policy and Planning* 17, no. 2 (2002): 154–60.

Coutsoudis, Anna, and Judith King. "Breastfeeding Is Still a Life-Saving Formula." *ChildrenFIRST* 42 (April–May 2002). www.childrenfirst.org/za (accessed February 16, 2005).

Coutsoudis, Anna, Kubendran Pillay, Louise Kuhn, Wei-Yann Tsai, and Hoosen M. Coovadia. "Method of Feeding and Transmission of HIV-1 from Mothers to Children by 15 Months of Age: Prospective Cohort Study from Durban, South Africa." *AIDS* 15 (February 16, 2001), 379–87.

Coutsoudis, Anna, Kubendran Pillay, Elizabeth Spooner, Louise Kuhn, and Hoosen M. Coovadia. "Influence of Infant-Feeding Patterns on Early Mother-to-Child Transmission of HIV-1 in Durban, South Africa: A Prospective Cohort Study." *Lancet* 354, no. 9177 (1999): 471–76.

Craddock, Susan. "Beyond Epidemiology: Locating AIDS in Africa." In *HIV and AIDS in Africa: Beyond Epidemiology,* edited by Ezekiel Kalipeni, Susan Craddock, Joseph R. Oppong, and Jayati Gosh, 1–10. Malden, MA: Blackwell, 2004.

Creyghton, Marie-Louise. "Breast-feeding and *Baraka* in Northern Tunisia." In *The*

Anthropology of Breast-Feeding: Natural Law or Social Construct, edited by Vanessa Maher, 37–58. Oxford: Berg Publishers, 1992.

Crowe, David. "Infectious HIV in Breastmilk: Fact or Fantasy?" Presentation to La Leche League International Conference, Chicago, July 2005. Session 205: Perspectives on HIV, AIDS, and Breastfeeding Research. www.anotherlook.org/presenta tions/LLLI-200107-factorfantasy.pdf (accessed January 4, 2007).

Crowe, David, George Kent, Pamela Morrison, and Ted Greiner. "Commentary: Revisiting the Risk of HIV Infection from Breastfeeding." www.anotherlook.org/papers/g/english.pdf (accessed January 4, 2007).

Davis-Floyd, Robbie. "The Technocratic Body: American Childbirth as Cultural Expression." *Social Science and Medicine* 38 (1994): 1125–40.

Deacon, Caroline. "Toxins in Breastmilk (referenced)." *BabyCentre,* March 2006. www.babycentre.co.uk/miscellaneous/referencedarticles/toxinsinbreastmilk/ (accessed September 12, 2006).

De Paoli, Marina Manuela. *"To Breastfeed or Not to Breastfeed": Infant Feeding Dilemmas Facing Women with HIV in the Kilimanjaro Region, Tanzania.* Dissertation, Department of Nutrition, Faculty of Medicine, University of Oslo. Oslo, Norway: Unipub AS, 2004.

Department of Health and Human Services, National Women's Health Information Center. "New Breastfeeding Rates Published." *Women's Health.Gov,* January 2005. www.4woman.gov/news/pr/2005.breastfeeding.htm (accessed September 5, 2006).

De Wagt, Arjan, and David Clark. "UNICEF's Support to Free Infant Formula for Infants of HIV-Infected Mothers in Africa: A Review of UNICEF Experience." LINKAGES Art and Science of Breastfeeding Presentation Series, Washington, DC, April 14, 2004. http://www.waba.org.my/whatwedo/hiv/usefulresearch.htm (accessed June 30, 2008).

Doherty, Tanya. "Appropriateness of Infant Feeding Decisions by HIV-Positive Women: Implications for Infant Outcomes." HIV and Infant Feeding Satellite Session no. 113. International AIDS Conference, Toronto, Canada, August 15, 2006. www.path.org/news/an060813_AIDSconf_infant_feeding.php (accessed September 5, 2006).

Douglas, Mary. *Purity and Danger: An Analysis of the Concepts of Pollution and Taboo.* New York: Routledge and Kegan Paul, 1966.

Douglas, Mary. *Risk and Blame: Essays in Cultural Theory.* London: Routledge, 1992.

Douglas, Mary, and Aaron Wildavsky. *Risk and Culture.* Berkeley: University of California Press, 1982.

Downey, Gary L. "Risk in Culture: The American Conflict Over Nuclear Power." *Cultural Anthropology* 1, no. 4 (November 1986): 388–412.

Dreyfus, Herbert L., and Paul Rabinow. "What Is Maturity? Habermas and Foucault on 'What Is Enlightenment?'" In *Foucault: A Critical Reader,* edited by David Couzens Hoy, 109–21. Oxford: Basil Blackwell, 1986.

Dubos, René, and Jean Dubos. *The White Plague: Tuberculosis, Man, and Society.* Boston: Little, Brown, 1952.

Duden, Barbara. *Disembodying Women: Perspectives on Pregnancy and the Unborn.* Translated by Lee Hoinacki. Cambridge: Harvard University Press, 1993.

Duesberg, Peter. *Duesberg on AIDS*, 2003. www.duesberg.com (accessed February 23, 2009).

Duesberg, Peter. *Inventing the AIDS Virus.* Washington, DC: Regnery, 1996.

The Durban Declaration. *The Body: The Complete HIV/AIDS Resource. Body Positive* magazine, October 2000. www.thebody.com/bp/oct00/durban.html (accessed December 21, 2006).

Editorial. "About Breast-Feeding . . ." *New York Times,* July 2, 2006, Week in Review, 9.

Eisenberg, Arlene, Heidi E. Murkoff, and Sandee E. Hathaway. *What to Expect When You're Expecting.* 2nd ed., New York: Workman, 1991; 3rd ed., 2002.

Enfamil, Mead Johnson Nutritionals. "Choosing to Breastfeed." 1998. www.enfamil.com (accessed September 17, 2007).

Enfamil, Mead Johnson Nutritionals. "Feeding Your Baby." 1998. www.enfamil.com (accessed September 17, 2007).

Epstein, Helen. *The Invisible Cure: Africa, the West, and the Fight Against AIDS.* New York: Farrar, Straus and Giroux, 2007.

Epstein, Steven. *Impure Science: AIDS, Activism, and the Politics of Knowledge.* Berkeley: University of California Press, 1996.

Escobar, Arturo. *Encountering Development: The Making and Unmaking of the Third World.* Princeton: Princeton University Press, 1994.

Etzioni, Amitai. "HIV Testing of Infants: Privacy and Public Health." *Health Affairs* 17, no. 4 (1998): 170–83.

Etzioni, Amitai. Letter to the Editor. *New York Times,* July 20, 2000, A27.

Etzioni, Amitai. *The Limits of Privacy.* New York: Basic Books, 1999.

Farber, Celia. "HIV and Breastfeeding. The Fears. The Misconceptions. The Facts." *Mothering* (September–October 1998). www.virusmyth.net/aids/data/cfbreast .htm (accessed February 6, 2002).

Farber, Celia. "Out of Control: AIDS and the Corruption of Medical Science." *Harper's Magazine* 312, no. 1870 (March 2006): 37–52.

Farber, Celia. "Sins of Omission: The AZT Scandal." *Spin* 5, no. 8 (November 1989): 40–44, 115–17. www.virusmyth.net/aids/data/cfsins.htm (accessed January 4, 2007).

Farmer, Paul. *Infections and Inequalities: The Modern Plagues.* Berkeley: University of California Press, 1999.

Farmer, Paul E., Bruce Nizeye, Sara Stulac, and Salmaan Keshavjee. "Structural Violence and Clinical Medicine." *Public Library of Science: Medicine* 3, no. 10 (October 2006): e449, 1686–91. www.plosmedicine.org (accessed January 23, 2009).

Feder, Ellen K. *Family Bonds: Genealogies of Race and Gender.* New York: Oxford University Press, 2007.

Feldberg, Georgina D. *Disease and Class: Tuberculosis and the Shaping of Modern North American Society.* New Brunswick: Rutgers University Press, 1995.

Felski, Rita. *Doing Time: Feminist Theory and Postmodern Culture.* New York: New York University Press, 2000.

Ferris, Meg Gwynne, and Mark W. Kline. "Epidemiology of Pediatric HIV Infection." *UpToDate* 10, no. 2 (2002). www.uptodateonline.com (accessed July 28, 2002).

Fildes, Valerie. *Breasts, Bottles, and Babies: A History of Infant Feeding.* Edinburgh: Edinburgh University Press, 1986.

Forsythe, Stephen J. "*Enterobacter sakazakii* and Other Bacteria in Powdered Infant Milk Formula." *Maternal and Child Nutrition* 1 (2005): 44–50.

Foucault, Michel. "The Discourse on Language." In *The Archaeology of Knowledge and The Discourse on Language,* translated by A. M. Sheridan Smith, 215–37. New York: Pantheon, 1972.

Foucault, Michel. *The History of Sexuality.* Vol. 1, *An Introduction.* Translated by Robert Hurley. New York: Random House/Vintage, 1980.

Foucault, Michel. "The Politics of Health in the Eighteenth Century." In *Power/Knowledge: Selected Interviews and Other Writings, 1972–1977,* edited by Colin Gordon, 166–82. New York: Pantheon, 1980.

Freedman, Alix M., and Steve Stecklow. "Bottled Up: As Unicef Battles Baby-Formula Makers, African Infants Sicken." *Wall Street Journal,* December 5, 2000, A1, 18.

Friedman, Samuel R., chair. "Prevention Controversy: Controversy and Common Ground." International AIDS Conference, August 15, 2006, Toronto, Canada.

Gallo, Robert, Nathan Geffen, Gregg Gonsalves, Richard Jeffereys, Daniel R. Kuritzke, Bruce Mirken, John P. Moore, and Jeffrey T. Saffrit. "Errors in Celia Farber's March 2006 article in Harper's Magazine." March 25, 2006. www.tac.org.za/Documents/ErrorsInFarberArticle.pdf (accessed January 4, 2007). Also available at "Responses to Harper's Magazine's *Out of Control.* 2006–2009." www.aidstruth.org/ new/denialism/harpers-farber (accessed February 23, 2009).

Gandy, Kim. Open Letter to the Department of Health and Human Services Secretary Mike Leavitt. *The National Organization for Women.* www.now.org/issues/mothers/060718breastfeeding.html (accessed August 8, 2006).

Giddens, Anthony. *The Consequences of Modernity.* Stanford: Stanford University Press, 1990.

Giddens, Anthony. *Modernity and Self-Identity.* Stanford: Stanford University Press, 1991.

Gikandi, Simon. "Reason, Modernity, and the African Crisis." In *African Modernities: Entangled Meanings in Current Debate,* edited by Jan-Georg Deutsch, Peter Probst, and Heike Schmidt, 135–57. Portsmouth, NH: Heinemann, 2002.

Giles, Fiona. "Reimagining Breastfeeding: Return to the Lactating Subject." Paper presented at the Society for Literature and Science Conference, Pasadena, CA, October 2002.

Glaser, Elizabeth, and Laura Palmer. *In the Absence of Angels: A Hollywood Family's Courageous Story.* New York: G. P. Putnam's Sons, 1991.

Golden, Janet. *Message in a Bottle: The Making of Fetal Alcohol Syndrome.* Cambridge: Harvard University Press, 2005.

Golden, Janet. *A Social History of Wet Nursing in America: From Breast to Bottle.* Cambridge History of Medicine. Cambridge: Cambridge University Press, 1996.

Gottlieb, Alma. *The Afterlife Is Where We Come From: The Culture of Infancy in West Africa.* Chicago: University of Chicago Press, 2004.

Grady, Denise. "Doctors Confirm West Nile in a 4th Transplant Patient." *New York Times,* September 6, 2002, A16.

Grady, Denise. "For Two Transplant Patients, a Dire Complication: West Nile." *New York Times,* May 16, 2006. www.nytimes.com/2006/05/16/health/16viru.html (accessed May 16, 2006).

Grady, Denise. "Traces of West Nile Virus Found in Mother's Breast Milk." *New York Times,* September 28, 2002, A12.

Granju, Katie Allison. "The Milky Way of Doing Business." *Hip Mama,* December 19, 2003. www.hipmama.com/node/view/588 (accessed March 8, 2004).

Graubard, Stephen R. "Preface to the Issue 'Multiple Modernities.'" *Daedalus* 129, no. 1 (Winter 2000): v–xii.

Gray, Ethan A. "What the Nurse Should Know about Tuberculosis." *Public Health Nurse* 12, no. 7 (July 1920): 556–58.

Greiner, Ted. "HIV—Will It Be the Death of Breastfeeding? Examining the Infant Feeding Component of the Prevention of Mother-to-Child Transmission." *Ted Greiner's Breastfeeding Website: Breastfeeding Papers.* www.welcome.to/breastfeeding / (accessed December 26, 2006). Now available at http://global-breastfeeding.org/2002/03/04/hiv-will-it-be-the-death-of-breastfeeding/ (accessed April 18, 2010).

Greiner, Ted. "The Perspective and Role of the Breastfeeding Supportive NGOs." In *HIV and Infant Feeding: A Report of a WABA-UNICEF Colloquium,* edited by Ted Greiner, 25–28. Penang, Malaysia: World Alliance for Breastfeeding Action, 2003.

Guay, Laura A., and Andrea J. Ruff. "HIV and Infant Feeding—An Ongoing Challenge." *Journal of the American Medical Association* 286, no. 19 (November 21, 2001): 2462–64.

Gunderloy, Mike. "Breastfeeding, HIV, and Disease Transmission." *Attachment Parenting.* www.larkfarm.com/AP/breastfeeding_hiv.htm (accessed May 1, 2005).

Hacking, Ian. *The Taming of Chance.* Cambridge: Cambridge University Press, 1990.

Haraway, Donna. "Situated Knowledges: The Science Question in Feminism and the Privilege of Partial Perspective." In *Simians, Cyborgs, and Women,* 183–201. New York: Routledge, 1991.

Hausman, Bernice L. "The Feminist Politics of Breastfeeding." *Australian Feminist Studies* 19, no. 45 (November 2004): 273–85.

Hausman, Bernice L. *Mother's Milk: Breastfeeding Controversies in American Culture.* New York: Routledge, 2003.

Hausman, Bernice L. "Risky Business: Framing Childbirth in Hospital Settings." *Journal of Medical Humanities* 26, no. 1 (Spring 2005): 23–38.

Hausman, Bernice L. "Things (Not) to Do with Breasts in Public: Maternal Embodiment and the Biocultural Politics of Infant Feeding." *New Literary History* 38, no. 3 (Summer 2007): 479–504.

Heinig, M. Jane. "The Burden of Proof: A Commentary on 'Is Breast Really Best? Risk and Total Motherhood in the National Breastfeeding Awareness Campaign.'" *Journal of Human Lactation* 23, no. 4 (2007): 374–76.

Helzlsouer, Kathy J., and Leon Gordis. "Risks to Health in the United States." *Daedalus* 119, no. 4 (Fall 1990): 193–206.

"HIV and AIDS in South Africa." November 2, 2006. www.avert.org/aidsouthafrica .htm (accessed December 21, 2006).

Hoofnagle, Mark, Chris Hoofnagle, and PalMD. "What Is Denialism." *denialism blog.* 2005–8. scienceblogs.com/denialism/about.php (accessed November 13, 2008).

Hopkinson, Judy M. "Response to 'Is Breast Really Best? Risk and Total Motherhood in the National Breastfeeding Awareness Campaign.'" *Journal of Health Politics, Policy, and Law* 32, no. 4 (August 2007): 637–48.

Hoy, David Couzens. "Introduction." In *Foucault: A Critical Reader,* edited by David Couzens Hoy, 1–25. Oxford: Basil Blackwell, 1986.

Iliffe, John. *The African AIDS Epidemic: A History.* Athens: Ohio University Press; Oxford: James Curry; Cape Town: Double Storey, 2006.

Illich, Ivan. *Medical Nemesis: The Expropriation of Health.* New York: Random House/Pantheon, 1976.

Inda, Jonathan Xavier. "Analytics of the Modern: An Introduction." In *Anthropologies of Modernity: Foucault, Governmentality, and Life Politics,* edited by Jonathan Xavier Inda, 1–2. Malden, MA: Blackwell, 2005.

"Infant Likely Got West Nile in Breast Milk." *Roanoke Times,* October 4, 2002, A9.

International Lactation Consultant Association. "Position on Breastfeeding, Breast Milk, and Environmental Contaminants." October 2001. www.ilca.org/pubs/Envi ronContPP.pdf (accessed November 14, 2006).

"Jacob Zuma Cleared of Rape." *Guardian.co.uk.* May 8, 2006. www.guardian.co.uk/ world/2006/may/08/aids.southafrica (accessed January 2, 2009).

Jaggar, Alison M. "Is Globalization Good for Women?" *Comparative Literature* 53, no. 4 (Autumn 2001): 298–314.

James, John S. "AIDS Denialists: How to Respond." *AIDS Treatment News* no. 342 (May 5, 2000). *The Body: The Complete HIV/AIDS Resource.* www.thebody.com/ atn/342/denialists.html (accessed December 21, 2006).

Kantor, Jodi. "On the Job, Nursing Mothers Are Finding a 2-Class System." *New York Times,* September 1, 2006, A1, 14.

Keane, Helen. "The Toxic Womb: Fetal Alcohol Syndrome, Alcoholism, and the Female Body." *Australian Feminist Studies* 11, no. 24 (1996): 263–76.

Kelly, Michael, ed. *Critique and Power: Recasting the Foucault/Habermas Debate.* Cambridge: MIT Press, 1994.

Kent, George, and David Crowe. "Infant Feeding and HIV: The Importance of Language in Shaping Policy." 2001. www.anotherlook.org/papers/f/index.php (accessed January 4, 2006).

King, Karisa. "In Zambia, a Formula to Fight AIDS." *San Antonio Express-News,* December 18, 2006. www.mysanantonio.com/news/metro/stories/MYSA121706.01A .ZambiaAIDS.304c9dc.html (accessed December 29, 2006).

Klaidman, Stephen. "How Well the Media Report Health Risk." *Daedalus* 119, no. 4 (Fall 1990): 119–32.

Knöbl, Wolfgang. "Modernization Theory, Modernization, and African Modernities." In *African Modernities: Entangled Meanings in Current Debate,* edited by Jan-

Georg Deutsch, Peter Probst, and Heike Schmidt, 158–78. Portsmouth, NH: Heinemann, 2002.

Koenig, Robert. "Global Health: South Africa Bolsters HIV/AIDS Plan, but Obstacles Remain." *Science* 314, no. 5804 (December 2006): 1378–79. www.sciencemag.org/cgi/content/full/314/5804/1378 (accessed December 21, 2006).

Koren, Gideon. *The Complete Guide to Everyday Risks in Pregnancy and Breastfeeding.* Toronto: Robert Rose, 2004.

Kuhn, Louise, Zena Stein, and Mervyn Susser. "Preventing Mother-to-Child HIV Transmission in the New Millennium: The Challenge of Breast Feeding." *Pediatric and Perinatal Epidemiology* 18 (2004): 10–16.

Kukla, Rebecca. "Ethics and Ideology in Breastfeeding Advocacy Campaigns." *Hypatia* 21, no. 1 (Winter 2006): 157–80.

Kukla, Rebecca. *Mass Hysteria: Medicine, Culture, and Mothers' Bodies.* Lanham, MD: Rowman and Littlefield, 2005.

Ladd-Taylor, Molly, and Lauri Umansky. "Introduction." In *"Bad" Mothers: The Politics of Blame in Twentieth-Century America,* edited by Molly Ladd-Taylor and Lauri Umansky, 1–28. New York: New York University Press, 1998.

La Leche League International. "Breastfeeding Remains Best Choice in a Polluted World." *Media Releases,* August 2003. www.lalecheleague.org/Release/contaminants.html (accessed September 12, 2006).

La Leche League International. *The Womanly Art of Breastfeeding.* 6th ed. Schaumburg, IL: La Leche League International, 1997.

La Motte, Ellen N. *The Tuberculosis Nurse.* 1915. Reprint, The History of American Nursing, edited by Susan Reverby. New York: Garland Publishing, 1985.

Law, Jules. "The Politics of Breastfeeding: Assessing Risk, Dividing Labor." *Signs* 25 (Winter 2000): 407–50.

Lawrence, Ruth A. *Breastfeeding: A Guide for the Medical Profession.* 4th ed. St. Louis: Mosby, 1994.

Lawrence, Ruth A. "Major Difficulties in Promoting Breastfeeding: U.S. Perspectives." In *Programmes to Promote Breastfeeding,* edited by Derrick B. Jelliffe and E. F. Patrice Jelliffe, 267–71. Oxford: Oxford University Press, 1988.

Lawrence, Ruth A., and Robert M. Lawrence. *Breastfeeding: A Guide for the Medical Profession.* 6th ed. Philadelphia: Elsevier Mosby, 2005.

Laws, M. Barton. Letter to the Editor. *Boston Globe,* September 5, 2002, 3rd ed., A14 (available on LexisNexis Academic).

Lears, T. J. Jackson. *No Place of Grace: Antimodernism and the Transformation of American Culture, 1880–1920.* New York: Pantheon, 1981.

Lerner, Sharon. "Striking a Balance as AIDS Enters the Formula Fray." *Ms. Magazine* (March–April 1998): 14–21.

Lewis, Bradley. "High Theory/Mass Markets: *Newsweek* Magazine and the Circuits of Medical Culture." *Perspectives in Biology and Medicine* 50, no. 3 (Summer 2007): 363–78.

Lewis, Bradley. "The New Global Health Movement: Rx for the World?" *New Literary History* 38, no. 3 (Summer 2007): 459–77.

Lewis, Stephen. "Keynote Address." In *HIV and Infant Feeding: A Report of a WABA-UNICEF Colloquium*, edited by Ted Greiner, 12–17. Penang, Malaysia: World Alliance for Breastfeeding Action, 2003.

Li, Ruowei, Natalie Darling, Emmanuel Maurice, Lawrence Barker, and Laurence M. Grummer-Strawn. "Breastfeeding Rates in the United States by Characteristics of the Child, Mother, or Family: The 2002 National Immunization Survey." *Pediatrics* 115, no. 1 (January 2005): e31–e37.

Linkages. *Infant Feeding Options in the Context of HIV*. Washington, DC: Academy for Educational Development, April 2004. www.linkagesproject.org (accessed October 15, 2004).

Lunder, Sonya, and Renee Sharp. *Mothers' Milk: Record Levels of Toxic Fire Retardants Found in American Mothers' Breast Milk*. Washington, DC: Environmental Working Group, 2006. www.ewg.org/reports/mothersmilk (accessed November 14, 2006).

Lupton, Deborah. *Risk*. Key Ideas Series, edited by Peter Hamilton. London: Routledge, 1999.

Lupton, Deborah. "Risk and the Ontology of Pregnant Embodiment." In *Risk and Sociocultural Theory: New Directions and Perspectives*, edited by Deborah Lupton, 59–85. Cambridge: Cambridge University Press, 1999.

Lupton, Deborah. "Risk as Moral Danger: The Social and Political Functions of Risk Discourse in Public Health." *International Journal of Health Services* 23, no. 3 (1993): 425–35.

Maher, Vanessa. "Breast-Feeding in Cross-Cultural Perspective: Paradoxes and Proposals." In *The Anthropology of Breast-Feeding: Natural Law or Social Construct*, edited by Vanessa Maher, 1–36. Oxford: Berg Publishers, 1992.

Martin, Emily. *Bipolar Expeditions: Mania and Depression in American Culture*. Princeton: Princeton University Press, 2007.

Martin, Emily. *Flexible Bodies: Tracking Immunity in American Culture—From the Days of Polio to the Age of AIDS*. Boston: Beacon, 1994.

Martin, Emily. "The Pharmaceutical Person." *BioSocieties* 1, no. 3 (2006): 273–87.

Maternal and Child Health Bureau. "Child Health USA 2002." U.S. Department of Health and Human Services, Health Resources and Services Administration. mchb.hrsa.gov/chusa02/main_pages/page_18.htm (accessed July 27, 2006).

Maternal and Child Health Bureau. "Women's Health USA 2005—Breastfeeding." U.S. Department of Health and Human Services Administration. mchb.hrsa.gov/whusa_05/pages/0428breastfeed.htm (accessed August 11, 2006).

Maugh, Thomas H., II. "Evidence of West Nile Virus Found in Breast Milk." *Los Angeles Times*, September 28, 2002, A14.

Mbali, Mandisa. "AIDS Discourses and the South African State: Government Denialism and Post-Apartheid AIDS Policy-Making." *Transformation* 54 (2004): 104–22.

McAvoy, Gene. "Bats Eat Mosquitoes as Well as Numerous Garden Pests." Hendry County Horticultural News, Hendry County Extension Service, University of Florida. No date. hendry.ifas.ufl.edu/HCHortNews_Bats.htm (accessed August 18, 2008).

Meier, Barry. "In War Against AIDS, Battle Over Baby Formula Reignites." *New York Times,* June 8, 1997, A1, 16.

Menon, Lakshmi, compiler. *The Breastfeeding Movement: A Sourcebook.* Compiled with Answar Fazal, Sarah Amin, and Susan Siew. Penang, Malaysia: World Alliance for Breastfeeding Action, 2003.

Meyer, Dagmar Estermann, and Dora Lúcia de Oliveira. "Breastfeeding Policies and the Production of Motherhood: A Historical-Cultural Approach." *Nursing Inquiry* 10, no. 1 (2003): 11–18.

Michie, Helena, and Naomi Cahn. *Confinements: Fertility and Infertility in Contemporary Culture.* New Brunswick: Rutgers University Press, 1997.

Millard, Ann V. "The Place of the Clock in Pediatric Advice: Rationales, Cultural Themes, and Impediments to Breastfeeding." *Social Science and Medicine* 31, no. 2 (1990): 211–21.

Milly, Pascal, with assistance from William Leiss. "Mother's Milk: Communicating the Risks of PCBs in Canada and the Far North." In *Mad Cows and Mother's Milk: The Perils of Poor Risk Communication,* edited by Douglas Powell and William Leiss, 183–209. Montreal: McGill-Queen's University Press, 1997.

Moland, Karen Marie, and Astrid Blystad. "Counting on Mother's Love: The Global Politics of Prevention of Mother-to-Child Transmission of HIV in Eastern Africa." In *Anthropology and Public Health: Bridging Differences in Culture and Society,* 2nd ed., edited by Robert A. Hahn and Marcia C. Inhorn, 447–79. New York: Oxford University Press, 2009.

Morrison, Pamela. "Mothers and Babies and HIV: What Is the Risk of Breastfeeding?" March 2002. www.anotherlook.org/papers/e/index.php (accessed January 4, 2007).

Morrison, Pamela, and Ted Greiner. "Infant Feeding Choices for HIV-Positive Mothers." *Breastfeeding Abstracts* 19, no. 4 (May 2000): 27–28.

Moskin, Julia. "The Weighty Responsibility of Drinking for Two." *New York Times,* November 29, 2006. www.nytimes.com (accessed November 29, 2006).

"Mother's Day: More than Candy and Flowers, Working Parents Need Time-Off." *Clearinghouse on International Developments in Child, Youth, and Family Policies.* Issue Brief (Spring 2002). www.childpolicyintl.org/issuebrief/issuebrief5.htm (accessed July 29, 2006).

National Center for Health Statistics. *Healthy People 2000 Final Review.* Hyattesville, MD: Public Health Service, 2001.

National Institutes of Allergy and Infectious Disease. "The Evidence that HIV Causes AIDS." *The Body: The Complete HIV/AIDS Resource.* February 27, 2003. www.thebody.com/content/whatis/art6541.html (accessed November 9, 2008).

National Institutes of Health. *State-of-the-Science Conference Statement: Cesarean Delivery on Maternal Request,* March 27–29, 2006. http://consensus.nih.gov/2006/CesareanStatement_Final053106.pdf (accessed November 2, 2006).

National Institutes of Health, National Institute of Child Development and Human Development. *Breastfeeding.* January 31, 2007. http://www.nichd.nih.gov/health/topics/Breastfeeding.cfm (accessed September 30, 2007).

Nattrass, Nicoli. "AIDS and the Scientific Governance of Medicine in Post-Apartheid South Africa." *African Affairs* 107, no. 427 (2008): 157–76.

Nattrass, Nicoli. *The Moral Economy of AIDS in South Africa.* Cambridge: Cambridge University Press, 2004.

Nattrass, Nicoli. *Mortal Combat: AIDS Denialism and the Struggle for Antiretrovirals in South Africa.* Scottsville, South Africa: University of KwaZulu-Natal Press, 2007.

"Newborn Has West Nile Virus." *Washington Post,* October 4, 2002, A21.

Newman, Jack. "Toxins and Infant Feeding." Handout no. 28, January 2005. www.bflrc.com/newman/handouts/0501-HO28-Toxins_and_Infant_Feeding .htm (accessed November 14, 2006).

Nielsen, Karin. "A Tale of Two Worlds: Stopping Global Mother-to-Child HIV Transmission." 8th Conference on Retroviruses and Opportunistic Infections (February 5, 2001). *Medscape.* www.medscape.com/medscape/cno/2001/RETRO (accessed December 23, 2001).

Noveck, Jocelyn. "Strong Reaction to Public Feeding Revealed." *Roanoke Times,* July 28, 2006, A8.

Ott, Katherine. *Fevered Lives: Tuberculosis in American Culture since 1870.* Cambridge: Harvard University Press, 1996.

Partners In Health. *Partners In Health 2004 Annual Report.* Boston: Partners In Health, 2005.

Partners In Health. *PIH Guide to Community-Based Treatment of HIV in Resource-Poor Settings.* 2nd ed. Boston: Partners In Health, 2006. www.pih.org/issues/ hivaids.html (accessed January 23, 2009).

Patton, Cindy. *Globalizing AIDS.* Minneapolis: University of Minnesota Press, 2002.

Patton, Cindy. *Inventing AIDS.* New York: Routledge, 1990.

Payer, Lynn. *Medicine and Culture: Varieties of Treatment in the United States, England, West Germany, and France.* 2nd ed. New York: Henry Holt, 1996.

Petersen, Lyle R., and Edward B. Hayes. "Westward Ho?—The Spread of West Nile Virus." *New England Journal of Medicine* 351, no. 22 (November 25, 2004): 2257–59.

Petersen, Melody. "Breastfeeding Ads Delayed by a Dispute Over Content." *New York Times,* December 4, 2003. www.nytimes.com (accessed March 8, 2004).

"Possible West Nile Virus Transmission to an Infant through Breast-Feeding—Michigan 2002." *Morbidity and Mortality Weekly Report* 51, no. 39 (October 4, 2002): 877–88. www.cdc.gov/mmwr/preview/mmwrhtml/mm5139a1.htm (accessed July 17, 2006).

Powell, Douglas, and William Leiss, eds. *Mad Cows and Mother's Milk: The Perils of Poor Risk Communication.* Montreal: McGill-Queen's University Press, 1997.

"Public Health Dispatch: Investigation of Blood Transfusion Recipients with West Nile Virus Infections." *Morbidity and Mortality Weekly Report* 51, no. 36 (September 13, 2002): 823. www.cdc.gov/mmwr/preview/mmwrhtml/mm5136a5.htm (accessed July 17, 2006).

"Public Health Dispatch: West Nile Virus Infection in Organ Donor and Transplant Recipients—Georgia and Florida, 2002." *Morbidity and Mortality Weekly Report*

51, no. 35 (September 6, 2002): 790. www.cdc.gov/mmwr/preview/mmwrhtml/mm5135a5.htm (accessed July 17, 2006).

Rabin, Roni. "Breast-Feed Or Else." *New York Times,* June 13, 2006, F1, 6.

Rabin, Roni. "That Prenatal Visit May Be Months Too Late." *New York Times,* November 28, 2006. www.nytimes.com (accessed November 30, 2006).

Roberts, Dorothy. *Killing the Black Body: Race, Reproduction, and the Meaning of Liberty.* New York: Pantheon, 1997.

Robins, Steven. " 'Long Live Zackie, Long Live': AIDS Activism, Science, and Citizenship after Apartheid." *Journal of Southern African Studies* 30, no. 3 (September 2004): 651–72.

Roche, Mary Margaret. "Reducing Infant Mortality." *Public Health Nurse* 12, no. 7 (July 1920): 604–6.

Rollins, Nigel. "HIV Transmission and Mortality Associated with Exclusive Breastfeeding: Implications for Counseling HIV-Infected Women." HIV and Infant Feeding Satellite Session no. 113. International AIDS Conference, Toronto, Canada (August 15, 2006). www.path.org/files/Nigel_Rollins.pdf (accessed September 5, 2006).

Rosenberg, Tina. "When a Pill Is Not Enough." *New York Times Magazine,* August 6, 2006, 42–45, 52, 58–59.

Ross Products Division of Abbott Laboratories. "2006 Breastfeeding Trends." Cleveland: Ross Products Division of Abbott Laboratories, 2006.

Rothman, Sheila M. *Living in the Shadow of Death: Tuberculosis and the Social Experience of Illness in American History.* New York: Basic Books, 1994.

Santora, Marc. "U.S. Is Close to Eliminating AIDS in Infants, Officials Say." *New York Times,* January 30, 2005, A1, 26.

Schaefer, George. *Tuberculosis in Obstetrics and Gynecology.* Boston: Little, Brown, 1956.

Schafer, Kristin S. "Biomonitoring: A Tool Whose Time Has Come." *Pesticide Action Network North America.* From *Global Pesticide Campaigner* 14, no. 1 (April 2004). www.panna.org/resources/gpc/gpc_200404.14.1.02.dv.html (accessed September 12, 2006).

Scheper-Hughes, Nancy. *Death without Weeping: The Violence of Everyday Life in Brazil.* Berkeley: University of California Press, 1992.

Schoepf, Brooke Grundfest. "AIDS, History, and Struggles over Meaning." In *HIV and AIDS in Africa: Beyond Epidemiology,* edited by Ezekiel Kalipeni, Susan Craddock, Joseph R. Oppong, and Jayati Gosh, 15–28. Malden, MA: Blackwell, 2004.

Schoub, Barry D. *AIDS and HIV in Perspective: A Guide to Understanding the Virus and Its Consequences.* New York: Cambridge University Press, 1999.

Shilts, Randy. *And the Band Played On: Politics, People, and the AIDS Epidemic.* New York: St. Martin's, 1987.

Sitze, Adam. "Denialism." *South Atlantic Quarterly* 193, no. 4 (Fall 2004): 769–811.

Skolbekken, John-Arne. "The Risk Epidemic in Medical Journals." *Social Science and Medicine* 40, no. 3 (1995): 291–305.

Smith, Paige Hall, Bernice L. Hausman, and Miriam Labbok, eds. *Breastfeeding and Feminism: Informing Public Health Approaches.* Forthcoming.

Smith, Tara C., and Steven P. Novella. "HIV Denial in the Internet Era." *Public Library of Science: Medicine* 4, no. 8 (August 2007): e256. www.plosmedicine.org.

Solinger, R. *Beggars and Choosers: How the Politics of Choice Shapes Abortion, Adoption, and Welfare in the United States.* New York: Hill and Wang, 2001.

Solinger, R. "Poisonous Choice." In *"Bad" Mothers: The Politics of Blame in Twentieth-Century America,* edited by Molly Ladd-Taylor and Lauri Umansky, 381–402. New York: New York University Press, 1998.

Sontag, Susan. *Illness as Metaphor/AIDS and Its Metaphors.* New York: Doubleday/Anchor, 1989.

"South Africa 'Ends' AIDS Denialism." *Global Network of People Living with HIV/AIDS.* November 8, 2006. www.gnpplus.net/cms/article.php/20061110155 858521 (accessed December 22, 2006).

"South Africa's New Health Minister Reverses Policy on HIV/AIDS." *Los Angeles Times,* October 14, 2008. www.latimes.com/news/nationworld/world/la-fg-aids14-2008oct14,0,7510285.story (accessed October 20, 2008).

Starfield, Barbara. "Is U.S. Health Really the Best in the World?" *Journal of the American Medical Association* 284, no. 4 (2001): 483–85.

Stehlin, Isadora B. "Infant Formula: Second Best But Good Enough." *FDA Consumer Magazine,* June 1996. www.fda.gov/fdac/features/596_baby.html (accessed November 21, 2004).

Steingraber, Sandra. *Having Faith: An Ecologist's Journey to Motherhood.* Cambridge, MA: Perseus Publishing, 2001.

Steingraber, Sandra. *Living Downstream: An Ecologist Looks at Cancer and the Environment.* Reading, MA: Addison-Wesley, 1997.

Sullivan, Kevin. "A Mother's Final Look at Life: In Impoverished Sierra Leone, Childbirth Carries Deadly Odds." *Washington Post,* October 12, 2008, A1, A16–17.

Sullivan, Kevin. "In Sierra Leone, Every Pregnancy Is a 'Chance of Dying.'" *Washington Post,* October 12, 2008. www.washingtonpost.com/wp-dyn/content/article/2008/10/12/AR2008101201886.html (accessed February 20, 2006).

Szalavitz, Maia. "10 Ways We Get the Odds Wrong." *Psychology Today* 41, no. 1 (January–February 2008): 96–102.

Tapias, Maria. "'Always Ready and Always Clean'?: Competing Discourses of Breast-Feeding, Infant Illness, and the Politics of Mother-Blame in Bolivia." *Body and Society* 12, no. 2 (2006): 83–108.

Taylor, Charles. *Modern Social Imaginaries.* Durham: Duke University Press, 2004.

Treichler, Paula. *How to Have Theory in an Epidemic: Cultural Chronicles of AIDS.* Durham: Duke University Press, 1999.

Tsing, Anna Lowenhaupt. "Monster Stories: Women Charged with Perinatal Endangerment." In *Uncertain Terms: Negotiating Gender in American Culture,* edited by Faye Ginsburg and Anna Lowenhaupt Tsing, 282–99. Boston: Beacon Press, 1990.

Turner, Brian. *Regulating Bodies: Essays in Medical Sociology.* London: Routledge, 1992.

UNAIDS. *2006 Global Facts and Figures.* Geneva: UNAIDS Press Office, 2006.

UNAIDS. *2006 Report on the Global AIDS Epidemic: Executive Summary.* A UNAIDS 10th Anniversary Special Edition. Geneva: UNAIDS, 2006.

UNAIDS. *2008 Report on the Global HIV/AIDS Epidemic: Executive Summary.* Geneva: UNAIDS, 2008.

UNAIDS. "A Global Overview of the AIDS Epidemic." 2004. www.unaids.org/bangkok2004/GAR2004.html/GAR2004_00_en.htm (accessed October 15, 2004).

UNAIDS/WHO/UNICEF. "UNAIDS/WHO/UNICEF Policy Statement on HIV and Infant Feeding, 1997." In *The Breastfeeding Movement: A Sourcebook,* compiled by Lakshmi Menon with Anwar Fazal, Sarah Amin, and Susan Siew, 212–13. Penang, Malaysia: World Alliance for Breastfeeding Action, 2003.

UNFPA/UNICEF/WHO/UNAIDS Inter-Agency Team. *New Data on the Prevention of Mother-to-Child Transmission of HIV and Their Policy Implications: Technical Consultation.* 2001. www.who.int/reproductive-health/new_data_prevention_mtct_hiv/index.html (accessed January 3, 2007).

UNICEF. "More HIV-Positive Children and Pregnant Women Getting AIDS Treatment, New Report Says." Joint Press Release with UNAIDS and WHO. *UNICEF Press Centre.* April 3, 2008. www.unicef.org/media/media_43458.html (accessed October 16, 2008).

"Update: Investigations of West Nile Virus Infections in Recipients of Organ Transplantation and Blood Transfusion." *Morbidity and Mortality Weekly Report* 51, no. 37 (September 20, 2002): 833–36. www.cdc.gov/mmwr/preview/mmwrhtml/mm5137a5.htm (accessed July 17, 2006).

U.S. Congress Committee on Oversight and Government Reform. *HIV/AIDS TODAY Factsheets.* 2008. http://oversight.house.gov/features/hivaids/ (accessed October 16, 2008).

U.S. Food and Drug Administration. "FDA Public Health Advisory for Nevirapine (Viramune)." January 19, 2005. www.fda.gov/cder/drug/advisory/nevirapine.htm (accessed January 4, 2006).

Van Esterik, Penny. *Beyond the Breast-Bottle Controversy.* New Brunswick: Rutgers University Press, 1989.

Van Esterik, Penny. *Risks, Rights, and Regulation: Communicating about Risk and Infant Feeding.* Penang, Malaysia: World Alliance for Breastfeeding Action, 2002. Also published online at www.waba.org.my/whatwedo/environment/penny.htm (accessed April 18, 2010).

Van Esterik, Penny. *Towards Healthy Environments for Children: Frequently Asked Questions (FAQ) about Breastfeeding in a Contaminated Environment.* Fact Sheet. Penang, Malaysia: World Alliance for Breastfeeding Action, 2003.

Verghese, Abraham, Steve L. Berk, and F. Sarubbi. "Urbs in Rure: Human Immunodeficiency Virus Infection in Rural Tennessee." *Journal of Infectious Disease* 160, no. 6 (December 1989): 1051–55.

VirusMyth: A Rethinking AID$ Website. July 7, 2003. www.virusmyth.net/aids/ (accessed December 24, 2006).

Wald, Priscilla. *Contagious: Cultures, Carriers, and the Outbreak Narrative.* Durham: Duke University Press, 2008.

Wang, Joy. "AIDS Denialism and 'The Humanisation of the African.'" *Race and Class* 49, no. 3 (2007): 1–18.

Weinberg, Geoffrey A. "The Dilemma of Postnatal Mother-to-Child Transmission of HIV: To Breastfeed or Not?" *Birth* 27, no. 3 (September 2000): 199–205.

Weiss, Rick. "Baby Had West Nile Virus." *Washington Post,* December 20, 2002, A2.

Weiss, Rick. "Organ Recipients Had Virus." *Washington Post,* September 4, 2002, A1.

"West Nile-Tainted Breast Milk Likely Infected Baby, CDC Says." *Los Angeles Times,* October 4, 2002, A29.

"West Nile's Spread to Baby is Linked to Breast Feeding." *Wall Street Journal,* October 4, 2002, B4.

"West Nile Virus (WNV) Infection and Breastfeeding: Information for Clinicians." Division of Vector-Borne Infections Diseases, Centers for Disease Control. July 16, 2003. www.cdc.gov/ncidod/dvbid/westnile/clinican_breastfeeding.htm (accessed March 8, 2004).

White, Edith. *Breastfeeding and HIV/AIDS: The Research, the Politics, the Women's Responses.* Jefferson, NC: McFarland, 1999.

Wight, Nancy E. "Breastfeeding in High Risk Populations: The Mom with Hepatitis." *Breastfeeding Update* (San Diego County Breastfeeding Coalition) 1, no. 4 (December 2001): 1, 4. www.breastfeeding.org/newsletter/v1i4 (accessed March 8, 2004).

Wildavsky, Aaron, and Karl Dake. "Theories of Risk Perception." *Daedalus* 119, no. 4 (Fall 1990): 41–60.

Williams, Cicely. "Milk and Murder." Speech, Singapore Rotary Club (1939). Reprinted in *The Breastfeeding Movement: A Sourcebook,* compiled by Lakshmi Menon with Anwar Fazal, Sarah Amin, and Susan Siew, 34–36. Penang, Malaysia: World Alliance for Breastfeeding Action, 2003.

Williams, Florence. "First Person: Toxic Breast Milk?" *New York Times Magazine,* January 9, 2005, 21–24.

Williams, Joan. "Are Your Parental Leave Policies Legal?" *Chronicle of Higher Education* 51, no. 23 (November 2, 2005): C1. http://chronicle.com/weekly/v51/i23/23c0o101.htm (accessed July 27, 2006).

Williams, Raymond. *The Long Revolution.* 1961. Reprint, Peterborough, Ontario: Broadview Press, 2001.

Wittrock, Björn. "Modernity: One, None, or Many? European Origins and Modernity as a Global Condition." *Daedalus* 129, no. 1 (Winter 2000): 31–60.

Wolf, Jacqueline H. *Don't Kill Your Baby: Public Health and the Decline of Breastfeeding in the Nineteenth and Twentieth Centuries.* Columbus: Ohio State University Press, 2001.

Wolf, Jacqueline H. "Low Breastfeeding Rates and Public Health in the United States." *American Journal of Public Health* 93, no. 12 (December 2003): 2000–2010.

Wolf, Jacqueline H. "What Feminists Can Do for Breastfeeding and What Breastfeeding Can Do for Feminists." *Signs* 31, no. 2 (Winter 2006): 397–424.

Wolf, Joan B. "Is Breast Really Best? Risk and Total Motherhood in the National

Breastfeeding Awareness Campaign." *Journal of Health Politics, Policy, and Law* 32, no. 4 (August 2007): 595–636.

Wolf, Joan B. "Rejoinder to Judy M. Hopkinson." *Journal of Health Politics, Policy, and Law* 32, no. 4 (August 2007): 649–54.

World Health Organization. *HIV and Infant Feeding: Update.* Geneva: WHO, 2007. www.who.int/child_adolescent_health/documents/9789241595964/en/index.html (accessed October 16, 2008).

World Health Organization. *WHO HIV and Infant Feeding Technical Consultation: Consensus Statement.* 2006. www.who.int/child_adolescent_health/documents/if_consensus/en/index.html (accessed June 30, 2008).

Wright, Anne L., and Richard J. Schanler. "The Resurgence of Breastfeeding at the End of the Second Millennium." *Journal of Nutrition* 131 (2001): 421S–425S.

Yarney, Gavin. "The Milk of Human Kindness." *British Medical Journal* 322 (January 6, 2001): 57. www.bmj.com (accessed September 20, 2002).

Youde, Jeremy R. *AIDS, South Africa, and the Politics of Knowledge.* Hampshire, UK: Ashgate Press, 2007.

Zack-Williams, Alfred B. "Africa and the Project of Modernity: Some Reflections." In *Africa Beyond the Post-Colonial: Political and Socio-Cultural Identities,* edited by Ola Uduku and Alfred B. Zack-Williams, 20–38. Hampshire, UK: Ashgate, 2004.

Zack-Williams, Alfred B., and Ola Uduku. "African Diaspora–African Development Concern: An Introduction." In *Africa Beyond the Post-Colonial: Political and Socio-Cultural Identities,* edited by Ola Uduku and Alfred B. Zack-Williams, 1–19. Hampshire, UK: Ashgate, 2004.

Zivi, Karen. "Contesting Motherhood in the Age of AIDS: Maternal Ideology in the Debate of Mandatory HIV Testing." *Feminist Studies* 31, no. 2 (Summer 2005): 347–74.

Index